Clinical Applications of Pathophysiology

Assessment, Diagnostic Reasoning, and Management

Clinical Applications of Pathophysiology

Assessment, Diagnostic Reasoning, and Management

Valentina L. Brashers, MD
Associate Professor of Nursing
Clinical Assistant Professor of Medicine
University of Virginia
Charlottesville, Virginia

Second Edition

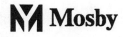

An Affiliate of Elsevier

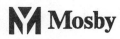

Mosby

An Affiliate of Elsevier

Vice President and Publishing Director: Sally Schrefer
Executive Editor: Darlene Como
Managing Editor: Brian Dennison
Project Manager: Gayle May Morris
Cover Design: Kathi Gosche
Design and Layout: Sue Anne Meeks

A NOTE TO THE READER:
Pharmacology is an ever-changing field. Standard safety precautions must be followed, but as new research and clinical experience broaden our knowledge, changes in treatment and drug therapy may become necessary or appropriate. Readers are advised to check the most current product information provided by the manufacturer of each drug to be administered to verify the recommended dose, the method and duration of administration, and contraindications. It is the responsibility of the licensed health care provider, relying on experience and knowledge of the patient, to determine dosages and the best treatment for each individual patient. Neither the publisher nor the editor assumes any liability for any injury and/or damage to persons or property arising from this publication.

Printed in the United States of America

Mosby, Inc.
An Affiliate of Elsevier
11830 Westline Industrial Drive
St. Louis, Missouri 63146

International Standard BookNumber 0-323-01623-5

04 05 / 9 8 7 6 5

Contributors

Leslie Buchanan, MSN, RN, ENP
Clinician 4; Emergency Nurse Practitioner
Department of Emergency Medicine
University of Virginia Health System
Charlottesville, Virginia

Suzanne M. Burns, MSN, RN, RRT, ACNP-CS, CCRN, FAAN
Clinician 5; Associate Professor of Nursing
University of Virginia Health Sciences Center
Charlottesville, Virginia

Eugene C. Corbett, Jr., MD, FACP
Anne L. and Bernard B. Brodie Teaching
Associate Professor of Internal Medicine
Assistant Professor of Nursing
Department of Medicine
University of Virginia
Charlottesville, Virginia

Mikel Gray, PhD, CUNP, CCCN, FAAN
Professor of Nursing
University of Virginia School of Nursing
Nurse Practitioner
Department of Urology
University of Virginia
Charlottesville, Virginia

Kathleen R. Haden, MSN, RN, CS, ANP, OCN
Adult Nurse Practitioner
Adjunct Faculty
University of Virginia School of Nursing
Charlottesville, Virginia

Richard P. Keeling, MD
CEO, Rethinkinc
Executive Consultant, Richard P. Keeling and Associates
Editor, *Journal of the American College of Health*
New York, New York

Gail L. Kongable, MSN, FNP, CNRN
Associate Professor
Departments of Neurology and Neurosurgery
University of Virginia Health System
Charlottesville, Virginia

Patrice Y. Neese, MSN, RN, CS, ANP
Nurse Practitioner
Breast and Melanoma Teams
Department of Surgery/Oncology
University of Virginia
Charlottesville, Virginia

Lucy R. Paskus, BA, BSN, RN
Clinical Coordinator
Pediatric Intensive Care Unit
The Children's Hospital
Denver, Colorado

Kathryn B. Reid, MSN, RN, CCRN, FNP
Instructor of Nursing
University of Virginia School of Nursing
Charlottesville, Virginia

Juanita Reigle, MSN, RN, ACNP-CS
Clinician 5; Associate Professor of Nursing
Heart Center
University of Virginia Health System
Charlottesville, Virginia

Reviewers

Charlé C.F. Avery, MSN, RN, CS, ANP
Advanced Practice Nurse
Baylor Senior Health Center - Hillside
Dallas, Texas

Janie B. Butts, DSN, RN
Instructor
University of Southern Mississippi
College of Nursing
Hattiesburg, Mississippi

Sue E. Huether, PhD, RN
Professor
University of Utah College of Nursing
Salt Lake City, Utah

Kathryn L. McCance, PhD, RN
Professor
University of Utah College of Nursing
Salt Lake City, Utah

Kristynia M. Robinson, PhD, RN, FNPc
Associate Professor
Department of Nursing
Idaho State University
Pocatello, Idaho

Lorraine M. Wilson, PhD, RN
Professor of Nursing
Pathophysiology Instructor
Director, MSN Program - Adult Health
Eastern Michigan University
Ypsilanti, Michigan

Preface

Welcome to the second edition of *Clinical Applications of Pathophysiology: Assessment, Diagnostic Reasoning, and Management.* As with the first edition, the purpose of this book is to provide a summary of the pathophysiology of selected common diseases or illnesses and the application of that information to clinical assessment, diagnosis, and management. Case studies are provided to reinforce the skills learned in each chapter, and an up-to-date list of suggested readings is included. This second edition is filled with new figures and tables. Two new chapters have been added that present immunologic diseases, and the case studies have all been significantly updated. The Suggested Solutions and Rationales to the case study questions are no longer contained within this volume; instructors who adopt the book for course use may obtain the Solutions from their Mosby sales representative or by calling Faculty Support at 1-800-222-9570.

This text is designed to be used by the health care clinician, student, and educator. By understanding the underlying pathophysiologic processes, the reader can better predict clinical manifestations, choose evaluative studies, initiate appropriate therapies, and anticipate potential complications. In addition, insights into the underlying disease process can prepare the practitioner for the use of new and innovative interventions and drugs.

This book is organized by body system, with 27 selected diagnoses that are not only common to clinical practice but represent concepts of pathophysiology, evaluation, and management that can be applied to many other illnesses. Each chapter has two distinct sections.

The first section contains a concise summary of the disease, including Definition, Epidemiology, Pathophysiology, Patient Presentation, Differential Diagnosis, Keys to Evaluation, and Keys to Management. Figures and tables illustrate important points. This information is followed by a unique "Pathophysiology → Clinical Link" diagram that emphasizes how an understanding of the pathophysiologic principles can guide patient care. A list of selected recent articles is included for each chapter.

The second section of each chapter contains a representative case study in a fill-in-the-blank format that can be used by clinicians and students to practice their skills and by educators to evaluate their students.

Acknowledgments

This book would not exist without the generous and kind support of Drs. Kathy McCance and Sue Huether of the University of Utah. They not only encouraged me to write the first edition of this book but also supported me in developing this much-improved second edition. I have used their nationally-renowned text *Pathophysiology: The Biologic Basis for Disease in Adults and Children* in my classes for years, and am honored to be a contributing author to their outstanding scholarly works. They set the standard for the teaching of pathophysiology, and I am grateful for the opportunity to learn from them both. They are the very best of mentors, role models, and friends.

This second edition would not have been possible without the hard work and support of Managing Editor Brian Dennison at Harcourt Health Sciences who has joined me in my commitment to turning out the very best and most accurate book possible. Sue Meeks did an outstanding job of finalizing the chapters and getting them ready for this exciting new second edition.

I am endlessly grateful to the expert clinical nurses who contributed many of the case studies for this book. Their expertise has guided my teaching, my writing, and my practice for many years. I would also like to thank my students for their enthusiasm for pathophysiology; they are my inspiration and my reason for coming to work each day. I would like to especially thank Lucy Paskus for her hard work and scholarly contribution to two chapters. I am convinced that her name will appear on many important publications in the future. Eugene Corbett, Jr., MD, and Richard Keeling, MD, provided their valuable expertise to this book. They have my respect and gratitude for all their contributions to my teaching and writing.

My colleagues at the University of Virginia School of Nursing have been supportive in both word and deed of my unique role in the School. It is my privilege to work with such a knowledgeable, dedicated, and caring a group of professionals. I would like to especially thank Dr. Sharon Utz, who is my mentor, my boss, and my constant support in helping me grow professionally and personally as a part of nursing education. I would also like to thank my Dean, Dr. Jeanette Lancaster, who has always given me the opportunity to express my energies and ideas in creative ways.

Finally, I would like to thank my family and friends, especially Patty, for putting up with my long hours and distracted ways for yet another edition of this book.

Contents

1

Hypertension

DEFINITION

- Hypertension (HTN) is defined as sustained abnormal elevation of the arterial blood pressure.

- The Sixth Report of the Joint National Committee on Detection, Evaluation, and Treatment of High Blood Pressure (JNC VI) defines high blood pressure in adults as follows:

Category	Systolic (mmHg)	Diastolic (mmHg)
Optimal	<120	<80
Normal	<130	<85
High normal	130 – 139	85 – 89
Hypertension		
Stage 1 (mild)	140 – 159	90 – 99
Stage 2 (moderate)	160 – 179	100 – 109
Stage 3 (severe)	≥180	≥110

- The category "High normal" indicates the group at risk for developing HTN for which there is an opportunity to prevent progression with lifestyle modification.

- The 1999 World Health Organization definition is essentially the same but includes a separate category for isolated systolic hypertension (systolic ≥140 mmHg and diastolic <90 mmHg).

- 95% is primary (essential) HTN; 5% is secondary HTN.

- There are many contributing processes to primary HTN (see below).

- Secondary HTN can be caused by renal parenchymal disease, renal vascular disease, adrenocortical disease (Cushings or hyperaldosteronism), pheochromocytoma, hyperthyroidism, hyperparathyroidism, and some drugs.

EPIDEMIOLOGY

- It is estimated that 50 million U.S. adults have hypertension.

- HTN is a risk factor for coronary artery disease, congestive heart failure, stroke, and renal failure.

- African Americans tend to develop more severe HTN at an earlier age and have nearly twice the risk of stroke and myocardial infarction (MI) as whites.

- The elderly population tends to have more isolated systolic HTN, which has been clearly associated with an increased risk for MI and stroke.

- Patient awareness and adequacy of management remain surprisingly low.

- Risk factors in all populations include age, obesity, sedentary lifestyle, family history, smoking, alcohol, high sodium intake (especially in African America, the elderly, and diabetics), and low potassium or magnesium intake (especially in African Americans).

PATHOPHYSIOLOGY

- Essential hypertension involves an extremely complicated interaction between genetics and the environment mediated by host of neurohormonal mediators.

- Generally caused by increased peripheral resistance and/or increased blood volume.

- The genes implicated in primary hypertension (heritability accounts for an estimated 30% to 40% of primary hypertension) include angiotensin II receptor, angiotensinogen and renin genes; endothelial nitric oxide synthetase gene; G protein receptor kinase gene; adrenergic receptor genes; calcium transport and sodium-hydrogen antiporter genes (affect salt sensitivity); and genes that are associated with insulin resistance, obesity, hyperlipidemia, and hypertension as a cluster of traits.

- Current theories of primary hypertension include:

  - Increased activity of the sympathetic nervous system (SNS).

    1) Maladaptive responses to sympathetic stimulation.

    2) Genetic changes in receptors plus sustained serum catecholamine levels.

  - Increased activity of the renin-angiotensin-aldosterone system (RAA).

    1) Directly vasoconstricts but also increases SNS activity and decreases vasodilatory prostaglandins and nitric oxide levels.

    2) Mediates arteriolar remodeling (structural changes in vessel walls).

    3) Mediates end-organ damage to heart (hypertrophy), blood vessels and kidney.

  - Defects in salt and water transport.

    1) Altered activity of brain natriuretic peptide (BNF), atrial natriuretic peptide (ANF), adrenomedullin, urodilatin, and endothelin.

    2) Related to poor dietary intake of calcium, magnesium, and potassium.

  - A complex interaction involving insulin resistance and endothelial function.

    1) Hypertension is common in diabetes, and insulin resistance is found in many hypertensive patients without clinical diabetes.

    2) Insulin resistance is associated with decreased endothelial release of nitric oxide and other vasodilators and affects renal function.

    3) Insulin resistance and high insulin levels increase SNS and RAA activity.

- These theories would explain elevations in peripheral resistance due to an increase in vasoconstrictors (SNS, RAA) or a decrease in vasodilators (ANF, adrenomedullin, urodilatin, nitric oxide) AND are felt to mediate changes in what is called the "pressure-natriuresis relationship" which states that hypertensive individuals have less renal sodium excretion for a given increase in blood pressure (Fig. 1-1).

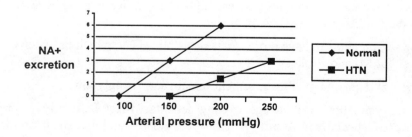

Fig. 1-1 Pressure Natriuresis Relationship

(From Crowley, A. W., & Roman, R. J. [1996]. The role of the kidney in hypertension. *Journal of the American Medical Association, 275,* 1581.)

- An understanding of this pathophysiology supports the current interventions employed in the management of HTN, such as salt restriction, weight loss, and diabetic control, SNS blockers, RAA blockers, nonspecific vasodilators, diuretics, and new experimental drugs that modulate ANF and endothelin.

PATIENT PRESENTATION

History

Family history; childhood history of increased BP; other cardiac risk factors, such as diabetes or dyslipidemia; history of stroke; smoking; alcohol abuse; high salt intake; recent changes in weight or obesity; medications; herbal remedies; or illicit drugs.

Symptoms

Usually asymptomatic in early stages; if BP rises acutely, patient may develop epistaxis, headache, blurred vision, tinnitus, dizziness, transient neurologic deficits, or angina; if more slowly progressive, the patient may present with symptoms related to end-organ damage, such as congestive heart failure, stroke, renal failure, or retinopathy.

Examination

Systolic or diastolic HTN; skin striae; retinopathy with vasoconstriction, arterial nicking, hemorrhages, or exudates; focal neurologic deficits; cardiomegaly (displaced point of maximal impulse [PMI]), heave, or gallops (S_3 or S_4); decreased peripheral pulses or bruits; abdominal bruits or masses; peripheral or pulmonary edema; if severe or sudden HTN, look for encephalopathic changes with cerebral edema and papilledema.

DIFFERENTIAL DIAGNOSIS

- First differentiate an isolated increase in blood pressure from true HTN (see Keys to Assessment below).
- Then rule out secondary HTN.
    - Renal parenchymal disease
    - Renal vascular disease
    - Cushing disease or primary hyperaldosteronism
    - Pheochromocytoma
    - Hyperthyroidism
    - Hyperparathyroidism

KEYS TO ASSESSMENT

- Goals of evaluation are to establish the true diagnosis of HTN, rule out secondary HTN, assess for end-organ damage, and evaluate for overall cardiovascular and neurovascular risk profile.
- Diagnosis requires the measurement of blood pressure on at least three separate occasions averaging two readings at least 2 minutes apart with the patient seated, the arm supported at heart level, after 5 minutes rest, with no smoking or caffeine intake in the past 30 minutes; consider beginning treatment immediately if initial measurement reveals a systolic >160 mm Hg or diastolic >105 mm Hg.
- 24-hour ambulatory blood pressure monitoring has a better correlation with end-organ damage, helps to screen out "white coat HTN" (occurs only in the clinic), and aids in the selection of antihypertensive therapy; it is recommended for patients with drug resistance, hypotensive symptoms with medications, episodic HTN, and autonomic dysfunction; may also be a better indicator of cardiovascular risk in patients with isolated systolic hypertension.

- Isolated systolic hypertension is an important risk factor for stroke and cardiovascular disease and must be recognized and managed; in the elderly the pulse pressure is an indicator of cardiovascular risk.

- Examine for abdominal masses, bruits, manifestations of Cushings (truncal obesity, striae), manifestations of pheochromocytoma (tachycardia, sweating, tremor).

- Funduscopic, vascular, cardiac, pulmonary, extremity and neurologic exam.

- **Laboratory:** urinalysis; chemistries including sodium, potassium, fasting glucose, blood urea nitrogen (BUN) and creatinine (Cr), serum calcium, and magnesium; lipid profile; and electrocardiogram (ECG).

- Microalbuminuria is an important indicator of early hypertensive renal disease.

- Consider more specific tests, such as renin, cortisol, urine catecholamines, renal ultrasound, echocardiogram, and vascular studies, if history, physical, and severity of HTN indicate possible secondary cause or significant end-organ involvement.

- A comprehensive review of lifestyle issues is key to designing a management program that is effective and suited to the individual needs of the patient (thus improving adherence).

KEYS TO MANAGEMENT

- **Prevention:** target persons with high-normal blood pressure, a family history of HTN, and one or more lifestyle contributors to age-related increases in BP, such as obesity, high sodium intake, physical inactivity, and excessive alcohol intake.

- **Decisions:** therapy for hypertensive patients are based on the following (Table 1-1).
  - The degree of blood pressure elevation.
  - The presence of target organ damage.
  - The presence of clinical cardiovascular disease or other risk factors.

Table 1-1 Risk Stratification and Treatment[*]

Blood Pressure Stages (mmHg)	Risk Group A (no risk factors; no TOD/CDD)[1]	Risk Group B (at least 1 risk factor not including diabetes; no TOD/CDD)	Risk Group C (TOD/CDD and/or diabetes with or without other risk factors)
High normal (130-139/85-89)	Lifestyle modification	Lifestyle modification	Drug therapy[2]
Stage 1 (140-159/90-99)	Lifestyle modification[3] (up to 12 months)	Lifestyle modification (up to 6 months)	Drug therapy
Stages 2 and 3 ($\geq$160/$\geq$110)	Drug therapy	Drug therapy	Drug therapy

[*]Lifestyle modification should be adjunctive therapy for all patients recommended for pharmacologic therapy.
[1]TOD/CCD indicates target-organ disease/clinical cardiovascular disease.
[2]For those with heart failure, renal insufficiency, or diabetes.
[3]For multiple risk factors, clinicians should consider drugs as initial therapy plus lifestyle modifications.

(From The Sixth Report of the Joint National Committee on Prevention, Detection, Evaluation, and Treatment of High Blood Pressure. [1997]. *Archives of Internal Medicine 157*, 2420.)

- Lifestyle modification
  - Weight reduction (single most effective method of prevention; individualize the program).
  - Exercise (regular aerobic exercise to achieve moderate physical fitness).
  - Low-salt diet (goal of <6 gm salt per day); increase potassium, calcium, and magnesium intake.

  - Decrease alcohol intake (no more than 2 beers, 10 oz of wine, or 2 oz of whiskey per day for men; half that amount for women).
  - Cessation of smoking.
- Pharmacologic (Fig. 1-2 [next page])
  - Pharmacologic therapy is indicated for patients who have failed lifestyle modification alone, have hypertension stage 2 or 3, have target organ damage, or have other significant cardiovascular risk factors.
  - JNC VI continues to recommend diuretics or β-blockers as first line agents for uncomplicated HTN.
  - Other conditions are associated with indications for certain antihypertensive choices.
  - A general principle is to fit the choice of antihypertensive to the individual patient.
  - There is a relatively new class of drugs known as angiotensin II receptor blockers; these agents have fewer side effects than the classic angiotensin converting enzyme (ACE) inhibitors and are effective in controlling blood pressure in many patients but their long-term protection against target organ damage is unknown.
  - Fixed-dose combinations of 2 agents from different classes often contain very low doses of each agent, thus minimizing adverse effects while providing good antihypertensive efficacy (e.g., low dose diuretic + ACE inhibitor).
- After 1 year of successful blood pressure control, especially if there has been significant lifestyle modification, patients with uncomplicated HTN can be considered for step-down therapy including the following:
  - Medication reductions should be made slowly with close follow-up.
  - Patient should continue to be checked regularly as HTN can return even months or years after discontinuance.
- Adequate therapy results in a significant decrease in risk for ischemic heart disease, stroke, and congestive heart failure.
- Success of therapy rests on patient education, proper drug selection, careful follow-up, and repeated review of strategies with the patient.

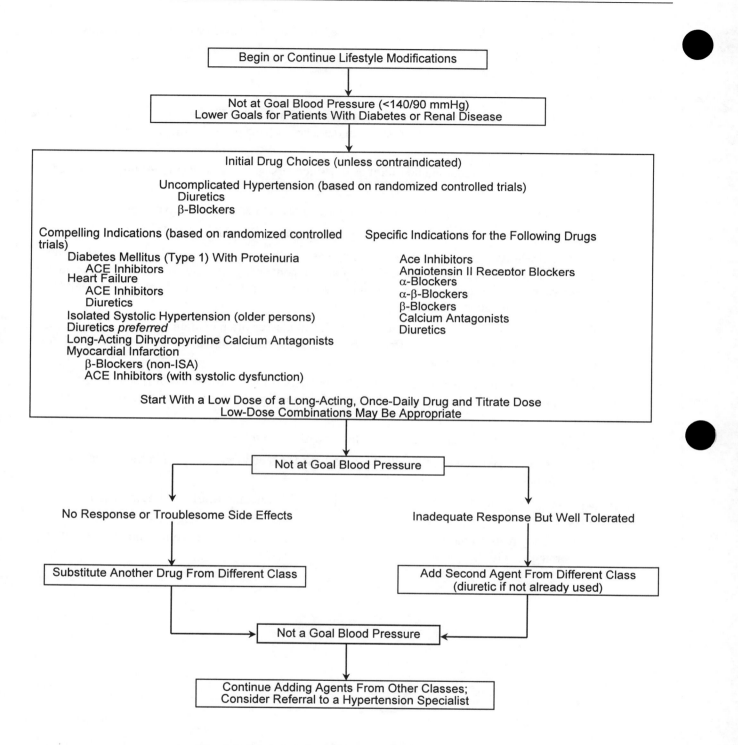

Fig. 1-2 Pharmacologic Therapy for Hypertension

(From The Sixth Report of the Joint National Committee on Prevention, Detection, Evaluation, and Treatment of High Blood Pressure. (1997). *Archives of Internal Medicine, 157*, 2430.)

Pathophysiology $\rightarrow$ Clinical Link

What is going on in the disease process that influences how the patient presents and how he or she should be managed?

What should you do now that you understand the underlying pathophysiology?

Patients whose blood pressures fall between 130 to 139 mmHg systolic and 85 to 89 mmHg diastolic are at increased risk for developing HTN.	It is critical to identify at-risk patients (family history, race, older age, smoker, high-salt diet, diabetes, dyslipidemia) and intervene with lifestyle modification.
The pathophysiology of the hemodynamic manifestations of HTN includes increased peripheral resistance and increased circulating volume.	HTN results in increased work for the heart, making cardiac complications (such as hypertrophy and ischemia) likely; the blood pressure will usually respond to vasodilators and diuresis.
Renal parenchyma disease, renal artery stenosis, and adrenal diseases result in hormonally-induced increases in peripheral resistance and circulating volume and, therefore, HTN.	The initial assessment of a patient with HTN should include evaluation for possible secondary causes, including a careful physical exam (rule out abdominal bruits or masses, striae) and laboratory tests (chemistries, urinalysis, BUN, and Cr).
One of the most important putative mediators of primary HTN is the over activity of the RAA system; angiotensin II has been implicated in the pathogenesis of other HTN-related diseases, such as congestive heart failure, MI, and diabetic renal disease.	Angiotensin-converting enzyme inhibitors (and the new angiotensin II receptor blockers) are effective in many patients with HTN and are specifically indicated in patients with congestive heart failure, MI with systolic dysfunction, and diabetes.
The proposed mechanism of primary HTN include effects on the pressure/natriuresis relationship; this relationship is also influenced by calcium, potassium and magnesium intake.	Recent studies have reconfirmed the importance of salt restriction for most patients (especially African Americans, older people, and diabetics) in uncomplicated HTN. Adequate potassium, calcium and magnesium intake is recommended.
Insulin resistance and associated endothelial dysfunction have been implicated as a cause of primary hypertension, even in the absence of diabetes, and is influenced by activity of the RAA and SNS.	Treatment of insulin resistance with hypoglycemic agents can reduce blood pressure in many patients, and treatment of hypertension with angiotensin-converting enzyme inhibitors can improve insulin sensitivity and protect against renal damage in diabetes.
HTN is usually asymptomatic and target organ damage develops slowly.	Patient education about HTN and its potential complications improves adherence to therapy.

Suggested Reading

Anonymous. (1997). Effects of weight loss and sodium reduction intervention on blood pressure and hypertension incidence in overweight people with high-normal blood pressure. The Trials of Hypertension Prevention, phase II. The trials of Hypertension Prevention Collaborative Research Group. *Archives of Internal Medicine, 157*(6), 657-667.

Anonymous. (1997). Five-year findings of the hypertension detection and follow-up program. I. Reduction in mortality of persons with high blood pressure, including mild hypertension. Hypertension Detection and Follow-up Program Cooperative Group. *Journal of the American Medical Association, 277*(2), 157-166.

Anonymous. (1997). The sixth report of the Joint National Committee on Prevention, Detection, Evaluation, and Treatment of High Blood Pressure. *Archives of Internal Medicine, 157*, 2413-2446.

Anonymous. (1999). World Health Organization-International Society of Hypertension guidelines for the management of hypertension. Guidelines subcommittee. *Journal of Hypertension, 17*(2), 151-183.

Appel, L. J., Moore, T. J., Obarzanek, E., Vollmer, W. M., Svetkey, L. P., Sacks, F. M., Bray, G. A., Vogt, T. M., Cutler, J. A., Windhauser, M. M., Lin, P. H., & Karanja, N. (1997). A clinical trial of the effects of dietary patterns on blood pressure. DASH Collaborative Research Group. *New England Journal of Medicine, 336*(16), 1117-1124.

Arauz-Pacheco, C., Lender, D., Snell, P. G., Huet, B., Ramirez, L. C., Breen, L., Mora, P., & Raskin, P. (1996). Relationship between insulin sensitivity, hyperinsulinemia, and insulin-mediated sympathetic activation in normotensive and hypertensive subjects. *American Journal of Hypertension, 9*(12 Pt 1), 1172-1178.

Bianchi, S., Bigazzi, R., & Campese, V. M. (1999). Microalbuminuria in essential hypertension: Significance, pathophysiology, and therapeutic implications. *American Journal of Kidney Disease, 34*(6), 973-995.

Brooks D. P., & Ruffolo, R. R., Jr. (1999). Pharmacological mechanism of angiotensin II receptor antagonists: Implications for the treatment of elevated systolic blood pressure. *Journal of Hypertension, 17*(2 supp), S27-S32.

Burnier, M., & Brunner, H. R. (2000). Angiotensin II receptor antagonists. *Lancet, 355*, 637-645.

Carretero, O. A., & Oparil, S. (2000). Essential hypertension. Part I: Definition and etiology. *Circulation, 101*, 329-335.

Carretero, O. A., & Oparil, S. (2000). Essential hypertension. Part II: Treatment. *Circulation, 101*, 446-453.

Cleland. S. J., Petrie. J. R., Small, M., Elliott, H. L., & Connell, J. M. (2000). Insulin action is associated with endothelial function in hypertension and type 2 diabetes. *Hypertension, 35*(1 Pt 2), 507-511.

Cowley, A. W. J. (1997). Genetic and nongenetic determinants of salt sensitivity and blood pressure. *American Journal of Clinical Nutrition, 65*(2 Suppl), 587S-593S.

Deedwania, P. C. (2000). Hypertension and diabetes: New therapeutic options. *Archives of Internal Medicine, 160*, 1585-1594.

DeWan, A. T., Arnett, D. K., Atwood, L. D., Province, M. A., Lewis, C. E., Hunt, S. C., & Eckfeldt, J. (2001). A genome scan for renal function among hypertensives: The HyperGEN study. *American Journal of Human Genetics, 68*, 136-144.

Dominiczak, A. F., Negrin, D. C., Clark, J. S., Brosnan, M. J., McBride, M. W., & Alexander, M. Y. (2000). Genes and hypertension: From gene mapping in experimental models to vascular gene transfer strategies. *Hypertension, 35*, 164-172.

Ferro, C. J., & Webb, D. J. (1997). Endothelial dysfunction and hypertension. *Drugs, 53*(Suppl 1), 30-41.

Frohlich, E. D. (1997). Current pathophysiologic considerations in essential hypertension. *Medical Clinics of North America, 81*, 1113-1129.

Fuller, J., Stevens, L. K., Chaturvedi, N., & Holloway, J. F. (2000). Antihypertensive therapy for preventing cardiovascular complications in people with diabetes mellitus. *Cochrane Database of Systematic Reviews [computer file]*, CD002188.

Gandhi, S. K., Powers, J. C., Nomeir, A. M., Fowle, K., Kitzman, D. W., Rankin, K. M., & Little, W. C. (2001). The pathogenesis of acute pulmonary edema associated with hypertension. *New England Journal of Medicine, 344*, 17-22.

Gibbons, G. H. (1998). The pathophysiology of hypertension. The importance of angiotensin II in cardiovascular remodeling. *American Journal of Hypertension, 11*, 177S-181S.

Giner, V., Poch, E., Bragulat, E., Oriola, J., Gonzalez, D., Coca, A., & De La Sierra, A. (2000). Renin-angiotensin system genetic polymorphisms and salt sensitivity in essential hypertension. *Hypertension, 35*(1 Pt 2), 512-517.

Gordon, N. F., Scott, C. B., & Levine, B. D. (1997). Comparison of single versus multiple lifestyle interventions: Are the antihypertensive effects of exercise training and diet-induced weight loss additive? *American Journal of Cardiology, 79*(6), 763-767.

Granger, J. P., & Alexander, B. T. (2000). Abnormal pressure-natriuresis in hypertension: Role of nitric oxide. *Acta Physiologica Scandinavica, 168*, 161-168.

Grimm, R. H. J., Grandits, G. A., Cutler, J. A., Stewart, A. L., McDonald, R. H., Svendsen, K., Prineas, R. J., & Liebson, P. R. (1997). Relationships of quality-of-life measures to long-term lifestyle and drug treatment in the Treatment of Mild Hypertension Study. *Archives of Internal Medicine, 157*(6), 638-648.

Gueyffier, F., Boutitie, F., Boissel, J. P., Pocock, S., Coope, J., Cutler, J., Ekbom, T., Fagard, R., Friedman, L., Perry, M., Prineas, R., & Schron, E. (1997). Effect of antihypertensive drug treatment on cardiovascular outcomes in women and men. A meta-analysis of individual patient data from randomized, controlled trials. The INDANA Investigators. *Annals of Internal Medicine, 126*(10), 761-767.

Hansson, L. (1999). The hypertension optimal treatment study and the importance of lowering blood pressure. *Journal of Hypertension, 1*(Supp 17), S9-S13.

Jamerson, K. A. (2000). Treating high-risk hypertensive patients. *American Journal of Hypertension, 13,* 68S-73S.

Julius, S. (2000). Worldwide trends and shortcomings in the treatment of hypertension. *American Journal of Hypertension, 13,* 57S-61S.

Kannel, W. B. (1999). Historical perspectives on the relative contributions of diastolic and systolic blood pressure elevation to cardiovascular risk profile. *American Heart Journal, 138*(3 Part 2), S2205-S2210.

Kaplan, N. M. (2000). Evidence in favor of moderate dietary sodium reduction. *American. Journal of Hypertension, 13,* 8-13.

Kato, J., Kitamura, K., Matsui, E., Tanaka, M., Ishizaka, Y., Kita, T., Kangawa, K., & Eto, T. (1999). Plasma adrenomedullin and natriuretic peptides in patients with essential or malignant hypertension. *Hypertension Research, 22*(1), 61-65.

Kohno, M., Yokokawa, K., Yasunari, K., Kano, H., Minami, M., Hanehira, T., & Yoshikawa, J. (1997). Changes in plasma cardiac natriuretic peptides concentrations during 1 year treatment with angiotensin-converting enzyme inhibitor in elderly hypertensive patients with left ventricular hypertrophy. *International Journal of Clinical Pharmacology & Therapeutics, 35*(1), 38-42.

Kotchen, T. A., & Kotchen, J. M. (1997). Dietary sodium and blood pressure: Interactions with other nutrients *American Journal of Clinical Nutrition, 65*(2 Suppl), 708S-711S.

Lender, D., Arauz-Pacheco, C., Breen, L., Mora-Mora, P., Ramirez, L. C., & Raskin, P. (1999). A double blind comparison of the effects of amlodipine and enalapril on insulin sensitivity in hypertensive patients. *American Journal of Hypertension. 12*(3), 298-303.

Mancia, G., Grassi, G., Giannattasio, C., & Seravalle, G. (1999). Sympathetic activation in the pathogenesis of hypertension and progression of organ damage. *Hypertension, 34*(4 Pt 2), 724-728.

Moore, T. J., Vollmer, W. M., Appel, L. J., Sacks, F. M., Svetkey, L. P., Vogt, T. M., Conlin, P. R., Simons-Morton, D. G., Carter-Edwards, L., & Harsha, D. W. (1999). Effect of dietary patterns on ambulatory blood pressure: Results from the Dietary Approaches to Stop Hypertension (DASH) Trial. DASH Collaborative Research Group. *Hypertension, 34*(3), 472-477.

Mulrow, C. D., Chiquette, E., Angel, L., Cornell, J., Summerbell, C., Anagnostelis, B., Grimm, R., Jr., & Brand, M. B. (2000). Dieting to reduce body weight for controlling hypertension in adults. *Cochrane Database of Systematic Reviews [computer file],* CD000484.

Mulrow, C., Lau, J., Cornell, J., & Brand, M. (2000). Pharmacotherapy for hypertension in the elderly. *Cochrane Database of Systematic Reviews [computer file],* CD000028.

Nowson, C. A., McMurchie, E. J., Burnard, S. L., Head, R. J., Boehm, J., Hoang, H. N., Hopper, J. L., & Wark, J. D. (1997). Genetic factors associated with altered sodium transport in human hypertension: A twin study. *Clinical and Experimental Pharmacology & Physiology, 24*(6), 424-426.

O'Brien, E., Coats, A., Owens, P., Petrie, J., Padfield, P. L., Littler, W. A., de Swiet, M., & Mee, F. (2000). Use and interpretation of ambulatory blood pressure monitoring: Recommendations of the British Hypertension Society. *British Medical Journal, 320,* 1128-1134.

O'Keefe, J. H., Wetzel, M., Moe, R. R., Bronsnahan, K., & Lavie, C. J. (2001). Should an angiotensin-converting enzyme inhibitor be standard therapy for patients with atherosclerotic disease? *Journal of the American College of Cardiology, 37,* 1-8.

Osei, K. (1999). Insulin resistance and systemic hypertension. *American Journal of Cardiology, 84*(1A), 33J-36J.

Palmieri, V., Bella, J. N., Arnett, D. K., Liu, J. E., Oberman, A., Schuck, M. Y., Kitzman, D. W., Hopkins, P. N., Morgan, D., Rao, D. C., & Devereux, R. B. (2001). Effect of type 2 diabetes mellitus on left ventricular geometry and systolic function in hypertensive subjects: Hypertension Genetic Epidemiology Network (HyperGEN) study. *Circulation [Online], 103,* 102-107.

Pickering, T. (1999). Advances in the treatment of hypertension. *Journal of the American Medical Association, 281*(2), 114-116.

Port, S., Demer, L., Jennrich, R., Walter, D., & Garfinkel, A. (2000). Systolic blood pressure and mortality. *Lancet, 355*(9199), 175-180.

Rahman, M., Douglas, J. G., & Wright, J. T. J. (1997). Pathophysiology and treatment implications of hypertension in the African-American population. *Endocrinology and Metabolism Clinics of North America, 26*(1), 125-144.

Romero, J. C., & Reckelhoff, J. F. (1999). State-of-the-art lecture. Role of angiotensin and oxidative stress in essential hypertension. *Hypertension, 34*(4 Pt 2), 943-949.

Ruitenberg, A., Skoog, I., Ott, A., Aevarsson, O., Witteman, J. C., Lernfelt, B., van Harskamp, F., Hofman, A., & Breteler, M. M. (2001). Blood pressure and risk of dementia: Results from the Rotterdam study and the Gothenburg H-70 study. *Dementia & Geriatric Cognitive Disorders, 12,* 33-39.

Schmieder, R. E., Erdmann, J., Delles, C., Jacobi, J., Fleck, E., Hilgers, K., & Regitz-Zagrosek, V. (2001). Effect of the angiotensin II type 2-receptor gene (+1675 G/A) on left ventricular structure in humans. *Journal of the American College of Cardiology, 37,* 175-182.

Schussheim, A. E., Diamond, J. A., & Phillips, R. A. (2001). Left ventricular midwall function improves with antihypertensive therapy and regression of left ventricular hypertrophy in patients with asymptomatic hypertension. *American Journal of Cardiology, 87,* 61-65.

Siragy, H. M. (2000). The role of the AT2 receptor in hypertension. *American Journal of Hypertension, 13,* 62S-67S.

Smulyan, H., & Safar, M. E. (2000). The diastolic blood pressure in systolic hypertension. *Annals of Internal Medicine, 132,* 233-237.

Stevens, V. J., Obarzanek, E., Cook, N. R., Lee, I. M., Appel, L. J., Smith, W. D., Milas, N. C., Mattfeldt-Beman, M., Belden, L., Bragg, C., Millstone, M., Raczynski, J., Brewer, A., Singh, B., Cohen, J., & Trials for the Hypertension Prevention Research Group. (2001). Long-term weight loss and changes in blood pressure: Results of the trials of hypertension prevention, phase II. *Annals of Internal Medicine, 134,* 1-11.

Verdecchia, P. (2000). Prognostic value of ambulatory blood pressure: Current evidence and clinical implications. *Hypertension, 35,* 844-851.

White, W. B., Prisant, L. M., & Wright, J. T., Jr. (2000). Management of patients with hypertension and diabetes mellitus: Advances in the evidence for intensive treatment. *American Journal of Medicine, 108,* 238-245.

Zizek, B., Poredos, P., & Videcnik, V. (2001). Endothelial dysfunction in hypertensive patients and in normotensive offspring of subjects with essential hypertension. *Heart [British Cardiac Society: Online], 85,* 215-217.

Zusman, R. M. (2000). The role of alpha 1-blockers in combination therapy for hypertension. *International Journal of Clinical Practice, 54,* 36-40.

Case Study

Hypertension

INITIAL HISTORY

- Age 47, male, African American.
- Coming in for physical exam after having his blood pressure checked at a health fair and being told it was high.
- Works as an executive for an insurance firm.
- No specific complaints.

Question 1   What questions would you like to ask this patient?

ADDITIONAL HISTORY

- No other health problems, on no medications.
- Father and older brother both have hypertension.
- History of MI and stroke at young ages in paternal grandparents.
- Denies cardiac or neurologic symptoms.

Question 2   Are there other questions you would like to ask this patient?

MORE HISTORY
- Eats significant amounts of prepackaged and snack foods.
- Nonsmoker, drinks an average of 3 to 4 beers most evenings.
- Has gained 12 pounds over the past year due to physical inactivity.
- Last cholesterol checked 3 years ago; can only remember that his total cholesterol was 252 mg/dl; has "tried" to watch his diet.

Question 3   What are his risk factors for HTN?

PHYSICAL EXAMINATION
- Mildly obese male in no distress.
- T=37 orally; P = 95 and regular; RR = 14; BP = 156/98 in both arms, sitting.

HEENT, Neck
- PERRLA, fundi with vasoconstriction but with no nicking, hemorrhages, or exudates
- Pharynx clear
- Neck supple without bruits or thyromegaly

Lungs
- Good lung expansion bilaterally
- Percussion without dullness throughout
- Breath sounds clear

Cardiac
- RRR, PMI 5th ICS at midclavicular line
- No murmurs
- Soft S_4 gallop heard at apex

Abdomen
- Mildly obese
- No abdominal bruits heard
- Soft without tenderness or organomegaly, liver 8 cm at midclavicular line
- No masses felt

Extremities
- No edema, no clubbing, no bruits
- Pulses full in all extremities

Neurological
- Alert and oriented
- Strength 5/5 throughout
- DTR 2+ and symmetrical
- Sensory intact to pin prick and light touch throughout
- Proprioception normal
- Gait steady

Question 4 What are the pertinent positives and negatives on the physical exam and what might they mean?

Question 5 What should be done now?

Question 6 How should he prepare for his next visit, and how should his blood pressure be measured when he returns?

PATIENT'S RETURN VISIT
- Patient continues to feel well, no complaints.
- BP 160/100 both arms, sitting with arm elevated to heart level.
- Rest of exam unchanged.

Question 7 What now?

PATIENT RETURNS FOR HIS THIRD VISIT
- Still no complaints.
- BP = 158/102.
- Rest of exam unchanged.

Question 8 What now? Would you order laboratory tests? If so, what?

LABORATORY
- All blood chemistries, including sodium, potassium, BUN, Cr, and calcium, are normal.
- Complete blood count normal.
- Urinalysis negative for protein or glucose, microscopy without cells or cellular casts.
- Total cholesterol and LDL elevated; HDL slightly low.
- ECG shows increased QRS voltage in the chest leads.

Question 9 What do the lab results mean?

Question 10 How should this patient be managed?

2

Dyslipidemia and Atherosclerosis

DEFINITION

- Dyslipidemia includes those changes in the lipid profile that are associated with an increased risk for atherosclerosis:

	Desirable	Borderline Risk	High Risk
Total Cholesterol (mg/dl)	<200	200 – 239	≥240
LDL Cholesterol (mg/dl)	<130	130 – 159	≥160
HDL Cholesterol (mg/dl)	≥50	35 – 49	>35
LDL/HDL ratio			>1.3
Tryglycerides (TG, mg/dl)	>250 (fasting) considered a probable risk		

- Atherosclerosis is a chronic disease characterized by thickening and hardening of the arterial wall. Lesions contain lipid deposits and become calcified, leading to vessel obstruction, platelet aggregation, and abnormal vasoconstriction.

EPIDEMIOLOGY

- Hyperlipidemia
  - Estimates of the overall incidence of dyslipidemia in the United States range from 38% to 50%.
  - Relative dyslipidemia with changes in the vascular wall are common in children in the United States.
  - 1/500 persons have an identifiable heterozygous or homozygous familial hypercholesterolemia.
  - There is a high incidence of dyslipidemia in persons with diabetes, hypertension, and in African Americans.
  - The causes of dyslipidemia include:
    1) Common (polygenic) hypercholesterolemia
    2) Familial hypercholesterolemias
    3) Diet high in saturated fats and/or cholesterol
    4) Diabetes
    5) Renal failure
    6) Drugs (thiazides, steroids)
    7) Smoking
    8) Hypothyroidism
- Atherosclerosis
  - Atherosclerotic coronary disease is the leading cause of death in the United States.
  - Atherosclerotic cerebrovascular disease is the leading cause of stroke in the United States.

- The risk factors and probable mechanisms of injury for atherosclerosis include:
  1) Dyslipidemia
     a) Increased total cholesterol or LDL cholesterol; especially small dense LDL.
     b) Decreased HDL; most important single risk factor in dyslipidemia.
     c) Increased triglycerides; especially if LDL is also high.
     d) Increased lipoprotein(a) [Lp(a)]; hereditary risk factor predictive in women.
  2) Smoking
  3) Hypertension
  4) Male gender
  5) Female after menopause (estrogen deficiency)
  6) Age >50
  7) Diabetes (insulin resistance)
  8) Increased serum fibrinogen
  9) Increased serum homocysteine
  10) High-fat diet, obesity, sedentary lifestyle
  11) Family history
  12) "Novel" risk factors that are being studied include C-reactive protein, increased serum uric acid, antiphospholipid antibodies, soluble intercellular adhesion molecule-1, antibodies to infectious agents, and serum endotoxin.

PATHOPHYSIOLOGY

- The process begins with *endothelial injury* (Fig. 2-1, p. 20).
  - Aging
    1) Decreased vessel compliance with increased shear forces.
    2) Increased vulnerability to endothelial injury.
  - Dyslipidemia
    1) Oxidized LDL promotes superoxide anion production and degrades nitric oxide.
    2) Lack of HDL results in increased LDL deposition in vessels, smooth muscle proliferation and decreased endothelial repair.
  - Hyperhomocystinemia
    1) Usually due to dietary insufficiency of cobalamin, pyridoxin, and folate.
    2) Increased toxic oxygen radicals, decreased nitric oxide, increased smooth muscle and collagen production, increased thrombosis.
  - Hypertension
    1) Increased shear forces and decreased nitric oxide synthesis.
    2) Angiotensin II (Ang II) causes vessel remodeling and upregulates the receptor for oxidized LDL on endothelial cells.
  - Smoking
    1) Increased oxidation of LDL.
    2) Decreased nitric oxide.

- Diabetes (insulin resistance)
    1) Glycation of vessels walls and decreased nitric oxide synthesis.
    2) "Insulin resistance syndrome" (diabetes, hypertension, dyslipidemia, hyperinsulinemia and obesity) suggests a complex interaction of genes and environment.
- Estrogen deficiency
    1) Increased risk of dyslipidemia including elevated Lp[a].
    2) Alterations in vessel healing and vasomotor tone.
- Autoimmune processes
    1) T lymphocytes found in endothelial lesions may contribute to injury.
    2) Some patients have measurable levels of antibodies to oxidized LDL which may also contribute to tissue injury.
- Infections
    1) *Chlamydia pneumoniae* is found in a large number of atherosclerotic lesions especially in early onset atherosclerosis (ages 15 to 34); cause and effect being debated.
    2) *Cytomegalovirus* and *Helicobacter pylori* have also been found in atherosclerotic lesions but are less prevalent than Chlamydia.
    3) Periodontal disease and endotoxemia are risk factors for atherosclerosis (mechanism unknown).

- The injured endothelial cells
    - Secrete monocyte chemoattractants and express inducible cell surface adhesion molecules to which monocytes and lymphocytes bind and *promote the recruitment of macrophages* to the area of injury.
    - Release cytokines and *stimulate inflammation.*
    - Release less nitric oxide (vasodilator).
    - Secrete growth factors *that promote smooth muscle cell migration and proliferation.*
- *LDL is oxidized* by the oxygen radicals, is phagocytosed by the macrophages, and then is carried into the vessel wall (LDL oxidation is promoted by increased serum LDL, increased lipoxygenase activity, and increased in oxygen radicals).
- Macrophages filled with oxidized LDL are called *foam cells.* Accumulations of these cells form a pathologic lesion called a *fatty streak* that induces further immunologic and inflammatory changes that result in progressive vessel damage.
- Leukocytes and macrophages release a host of inflammatory cytokines and mitogens that further stimulate smooth muscle proliferation (Ang II, growth factors) and inhibit endothelial synthesis and release of endogenous vasodilators, such as nitric oxide.
- Smooth muscle cells migrate into the area overlying the foam cells forming a cap called *a fibrous plaque.* Vascular remodeling occurs with calcification and fibrosis, apoptosis and necrosis of the lesion, perilesional vessel wall thickening, and protrusion into the vessel lumen.
- As the plaque progresses, it can *ulcerate or rupture* due to (1) mechanical shear forces; (2) macrophage-derived collagenases, elastases, and stromelysin; and (3) apoptosis of cells at the edges of the plaque cause continued necrosis of the vessel wall. The amount of collagen and elastin deposition in the cap (made by smooth muscle cells and fibroblasts) and the amount of LDL in the core determine its stability and vulnerability to rupture. In addition, T lymphocytes produce interferon gamma that decreases collagen production and weakens the plaque (autoimmunity).

- Platelets aggregate and adhere to the surface of the ruptured plaque due to decreased endothelial anticoagulants and exposure of platelet glycoprotein IIb/IIIa surface receptors, the coagulation cascade is initiated, and a thrombus forms over the lesion that may completely obstruct the lumen of the vessel; the release of thromboxane A with resultant vasoconstriction further narrows the vessel lumen.

- The overall result is an artery that is narrowed and vulnerable to *abnormal vasoconstriction and thrombosis.*

- Lifestyle and pharmacologic interventions are possible at every step in this cascade of events that may prevent or reverse the process (see Pathophysiology → Clinical Link).

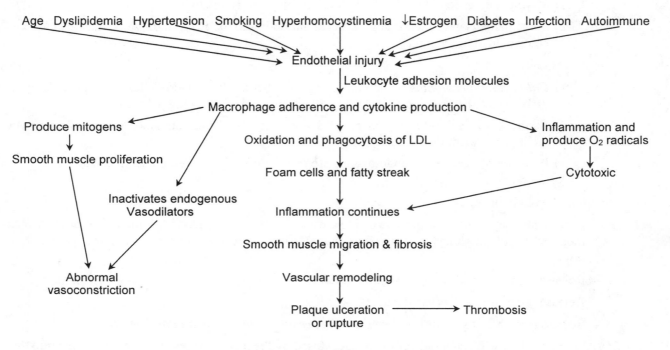

Fig. 2-1 Pathogenesis of Atherosclerosis

PATIENT PRESENTATION

- Dyslipidemia and atherosclerosis are often asymptomatic and the decision to assess a patient is based on a history of risk factors.

- If the patient does present with symptoms, the symptoms are most often the result of atherosclerotic obstruction of major vessels with ischemia of target organs such as the heart, the kidneys, the brain, or the extremities.

History

High-fat diet; weight gain; sedentary lifestyle; age; gender; race; postmenopausal; smoking; diabetes; hypertension; family history; past medical history of high blood pressure or cardiac, cerebrovascular, or peripheral vascular disease.

Symptoms

Chest pain; shortness of breath; transient or permanent neurologic deficits; intermittent claudication (pain in leg with walking, relieved with rest); hair loss and skin ulcers on extremities; worsening headaches, dizziness, or epistaxis.

Examination

Corneal arcus; xanthomas; increased blood pressure; abdominal bruits; bruits and decreased pulses in extremity arteries; obesity; evidence of congestive heart failure; focal neurologic deficits.

DIFFERENTIAL DIAGNOSIS

- Familial dyslipidemia vs common polygenic dyslipidemia vs secondary dyslipidemia (renal failure, diabetes, drug-induced, hypothyroidism).
- Hypertension; primary as a risk factor, secondary due to renal vascular disease as a target organ effect.
- Ischemic heart disease.
- Cerebrovascular disease.
- Peripheral vascular disease.

KEYS TO ASSESSMENT

- The goals are to identify modifiable risk factors and to assess for target organ effects.
- Remember, if one arterial system is diseased, it is likely that others are, too.
- Lipid profile:
    1) Current recommendations include a screening of total cholesterol in all adults over 20 years old every 5 years; the initial measurement should include an HDL.
    2) The patient should be seated for 30 minutes, after fasting for 12 hours, and have had no recent major changes in weight, exercise, smoking, or blood pressure.
    3) If the total cholesterol is <200, the patient should return for a repeat screening in 5 years.
    4) If the total cholesterol is >200, a repeat measurement should be obtained and the results should be averaged to guide subsequent care decisions.
    5) If the total cholesterol is 200 to 239 (borderline) and the patient has no coronary risk factors, he or she should be given diet guidelines and should return in 1 year.
    6) If the total cholesterol is 200 to 239 and the patient has definite coronary artery disease or coronary risk factors, or if the total cholesterol is ≥240, he or she should receive a complete lipoprotein analysis and consideration for pharmacologic therapy.
- Lp(a) is a genetically determined risk factor especially in women and diabetics; a test should be ordered if there is advanced atherosclerosis without the conventional risk factors.
- Fasting blood glucose or glycosylated hemoglobin.
- Serum electrolytes and blood urea nitrogen (BUN) and creatinine (Cr).
- Thyroid stimulating hormone (TSH).
- Liver function tests (aspartate aminotransferase [AST], alanine aminotransferase [ALT], alkaline phosphatase, lactate dehydrogenase [LDH]).
- Serum homocysteine; not yet recommended for routine screening.
- Electrocardiogram (ECG).
- Doppler ultrasound evaluation of selected arterial systems (popliteal, femoral, carotid) is done if the physical exam and history suggest involvement.
- Evaluation for evidence of coronary artery disease (see Chapter 3) or cerebrovascular disease (see Chapter 19).

KEYS TO MANAGEMENT

- Prevention
  - There is increasing evidence that atherosclerosis begins in childhood. Good diet habits and exercise with weight control should begin early in life and continue throughout life.
  - Smoking cessation and exercise are associated with increased HDL.
  - Aggressive recognition and management of risk factors such as familial dyslipidemia, obesity, hypertension and diabetes is crucial.
  - The decision to use diet therapy alone or in combination with pharmacologic therapy is based on the level of dyslipidemia and the presence or absence of other risk factors (Table 2-1).

Table 2-1 **National Cholesterol Education Program II Treatment Decisions**

	LDL level (mmol/L)	
	Diet Therapy	Drug Therapy
Without coronary disease and with <2 risk factors	≥160	≥190
Without coronary disease and with ≥2 risk factors	≥130	≥160
With coronary disease	≥100	≥130

- Diet therapy
  - A stepwise approach as recommended by National Cholesterol Education Program.

Nutrient	Step I	Step II
Total fat	≤30% of total calories	
Saturated fat	8% to 10% of total calories	≤7% of total calories
Polyunsaturated fat	≤10% of total calories	
Monounsturated fat	≤15% of total calories	
Carbohydrates	≥55% of total calories	
Protein	~15% of total calories	
Cholesterol	<300 mg/dl	<200 mg/dl
Total calories	Sufficient to achieve and maintain desirable weight	

  - Evidence suggests that a modest increase in the percentage of monounsaturated and ω-3 and ω-6 polyunsaturated fats is as important as reducing total saturated fats.
  - Increased folate intake that lowers homocysteine levels and increased antioxidant intake (especially vitamin E); both have been associated with decreased risk of atherosclerotic disease.
  - Moderate alcohol intake raises HDL, decreases platelet aggregation, and may improve insulin sensitivity.
  - Soy protein, oat fiber, fish oils, and garlic have all been found to reduce cholesterol.
- Pharmacologic intervention
  - **Lipid lowering**
    1) *HMG-CoA reductase inhibitors* (pravastatin, lovastatin, atorvastatin, etc.) lower serum total cholesterol and LDL and raise HDL with few side effects. Their long-term safety and efficacy and are well-established (cause regression of atherosclerotic lesions, reduce the risk of ischemic heart disease) and should be first-line drug therapy.
    2) *Fibric acid derivatives* (gemfibrozil) decrease cholesterol slowly but are more effective than HMG-CoA reductase inhibitors in decreasing triglycerides but have considerable gastrointestinal side effects.

3) *Nicotinic acid* reduces total cholesterol, triglycerides and LDL, and raises HDL, but is associated with flushing, gastrointestinal upset, and can impair glucose tolerance in prediabetic patients.

4) *Bile acid sequestrants* (cholestyramine and colestipol) decrease LDL slowly but increase triglycerides and have significant gastrointestinal side effects.

- **Anticoagulation:** may be indicated to prevent thrombus formation on established plaques; aspirn, dipyridamole, clopidogrel, ticlopidine, anti-platelet GPIIb/IIIa receptor antibodies (abciximab, eptifibatide, tirofiban, etc.); warfarin and heparin are options for selected patients.

- **Others**

1) Probucol and other antioxidants, such as vitamin E, have been shown to alter lipids and reduce atherosclerosis.

2) Estrogens have been shown to have a beneficial effect on lipid profiles. Retrospective observational studies suggest that hormone replacement therapy (HRT) for postmenopausal women can reduce coronary disease by up to 50%. However, recent prospective studies have found an increase in coronary events during the first year after HRT is begun, and current recommendations are to avoid using HRT as secondary prevention in women with known coronary disease. In addition, there is evidence that HRT may increase some measures of inflammation (including C-reactive protein). Early results from large studies of HRT as primary prevention for coronary disease are not yielding positive results and the role of HRT in the prevention of atherosclerosis remains controversial.

3) Angiotensin converting enzyme (ACE) inhibitors increase endogenous vasodilators, reduce smooth muscle hypertrophy, and decrease fibrosis in arterial walls and reduce the risk of coronary events in hypertension and should be considered for patients with hypertension and atherosclerotic disease.

4) *Antiinflammatories:* aspirin's effect in reducing coronary events is now believed to be in part due to its antiinflammatory effects as well as its antithrombotic effects. Other antinflammatories are being evaluated.

5) *Antibiotics:* several studies are underway to evaluate the effect of antibiotics on the prevention and treatment of atherosclerosis.

- Specific interventions for vascular systems

  - Once vessel obstruction becomes significant (by plaque rupture or superimposed thrombus formation), there may not be time to wait for diet and drugs to cause atherosclerotic regression.

  - Alternatives for reestablishing vessel patency include percutaneous transluminal angioplasty (with or without stenting), atherectomy, laser, or bypass grafting.

  - In the event of acute thrombus formation, thrombolysis may be indicated.

Pathophysiology → Clinical Link

What is going on in the disease process that influences how the patient presents and how he or she should be managed?

What should you do now that you understand the underlying pathophysiology?

There is a high incidence of dyslipidemia in the United States population, including children.	→ Patient screening should begin early in life with measurement of total cholesterol HDL initially, with further evaluation if indicated by a total cholesterol >200.
Serum plasma lipoprotein levels are determined by many factors including genetics, diet, drugs, gender, age, and other diseases such as diabetes.	→ A careful history with attention to modifiable risk factors can improve the lipoprotein profile, and patients should be evaluated for diet therapy, exercise, estrogen replacement, and lipid-lowering drugs when appropriate.
Endothelial injury begins the whole process of atherosclerosis.	→ Risk factor modification can prevent the initiation of atherosclerosis.
Macrophages and leukocytes are involved in inflammatory and immune processes that promote the atherosclerotic lesion, especially via the production of toxic oxygen radicals.	→ Antiinflammatories and antioxidants are all current or future therapies for the prevention and treatment of atherosclerosis.
Abnormal smooth muscle proliferation and inactivation of endogenous vasodilators result in vasoconstriction which is an important contributor to arterial ischemic syndromes.	→ Modulation of the role that macrophages and leukocytes play in atherogenesis not only reduces plaque formation but also prevents additional vessel obstruction due to vasoconstriction.
Oxidation of LDL is a vital step in atherogenesis and results in the formation of the fatty streak as well as promotes further inflammation and plaque generation.	→ Reduction in LDL (and possibly the intake of antioxidants) reduces atherogenesis and can result in regression of established lesions.
Once fibrosis begins in the fatty streak, the atherosclerotic process becomes less reversible and more likely to result in plaque ulceration and rupture.	→ Antiinflammatories may also help prevent maturation of the plaque, making the lesion more responsible to lipid-lowering and other risk factor reductions, as well as reduce the risk of sudden vessel occlusion.
Endothelial dysfunction due to injury and plaque formation results in superimposed thrombosis which is the major cause of complete vessel obstruction and infarction of distal tissues.	→ Antithrombotic drugs help prevent the adhesion of platelets to the injured endothelium, thus preventing thrombus formation and reducing the risk of infarction.

Suggested Reading

Adams, M. R., Kinlay, S., Blake, G. J., Orford, J. L., Ganz, P., & Selwyn, A. P. (2000) Atherogenic lipids and endothelial dysfunction: Mechanisms in the genesis of ischemic syndromes. *Annual Review of Medicine, 51*, 149-167.

Albert, C. M., Manson, J. E., Cook, N. R., Ajani, U. A., Gaziano, J. M., & Hennekens, C. H. (1999). Moderate alcohol consumption and the risk of sudden cardiac death among US male physicians. *Circulation, 100*(9), 944-950.

Andrews, N. P., Prasad, A., & Quyyumi, A. A. (2001). N-acetylcysteine improves coronary and peripheral vascular function. *Journal of the American College of Cardiology, 37,* 117-123.

Ansell, B. J., Watson, K. E., Fogelman, A. M. (1999). An evidence-based assessment of the NCEP Adult Treatment Panel II guidelines. National Cholesterol Education Program. *Journal of the American Medical Association, 282*(21), 2051-2057.

Batalla, A., Reguero, J. R., Hevia, S., Cubero, G. I., & Cortina, A. (2001). Mild hypercholesterolemia and premature heart disease. *Journal of the American College of Cardiology, 37,* 331-332.

Berenson, G. S., Srinivasan, S. R., Bao, W., Newman, W. P., Tracy, R. E., & Wattigney, W. A. (1998). Association between multiple cardiovascular risk factors and atherosclerosis in children and young adults. The Bogalusa Heart Study. *New England Journal of Medicine, 338*(23), 1650-1656.

Blumenthal, R. S. (2000). Statins: Effective antiatherosclerotic therapy. *American Heart Journal, 139*(4), 577-583.

Britten, M. B., Zeiher, A. M., & Schachinger, V. (1999). Clinical importance of coronary endothelial vasodilator dysfunction and therapeutic options. *Journal of Internal Medicine, 245*(4), 315-327.

Busse, R., & Fleming, I. (1996). Endothelial dysfunction in atherosclerosis. *Journal of Vascular Research, 33*(3), 181-194.

Danesh, J., Muir, J., Wong, Y. K., Ward, M., Gallimore, J. R., & Pepys, M. B. (1999). Risk factors for coronary heart disease and acute-phase proteins. A population-based study. *European Heart Journal, 201*(13), 954-959.

Danesh, J. (1999). Coronary heart disease, *Helicobacter pylori*, dental disease, *Chlamydia pneumoniae*, and cytomegalovirus: Meta-analyses of prospective studies. *American Heart Journal, 138*(5, Part 2), S434-S437.

Danesh, J. (1999). Smoldering arteries? Low-grade inflammation and coronary heart disease. *Journal of the American Medical Association, 82*(22), 2169-2171.

De Meyer, G. R., & Herman, A. G. (1997). Vascular endothelial dysfunction. *Progress in Cardiovascular Diseases, 39*(4), 325-342.

Dieplinger, H. (1996). Lipoprotein(a) in health and disease. *Critical Reviews in Clinical Laboratory Sciences, 33*(6), 495-543.

Dusting, G. J. (1996). Nitric oxide in coronary artery disease: Roles in atherosclerosis, myocardial reperfusion and heart failure [review, 108 refs]. *EXS, 76,* 33-55.

Epstein, S., Zhou, Y. F., Zhu, J. (1999). Potential role of cytomegalovirus in the pathogenesis of restenosis atherosclerosis. *American Heart Journal, 138*(5, Part 2), S476-S478.

Galton, D. J. (1997). Genetic determinants of atherosclerosis-related dyslipidemias and their clinical implications. *Clinica Chimica Acta, 257*(2), 181-197.

Gaziano, J.M., Gaziano, T. A., Glynn, R. J., Sesso, H. D., Ajani, U. A., Stampfer, M. J., Manson, J. E., Hennekens, C. H., & Buring, J. E. (2000). Light-to-moderate alcohol consumption and mortality in the Physicians' Health Study enrollment cohort. *Journal of the American College of Cardiology, 35*(1), 96-105.

Gielen, S., Schuler, G., & Hambrecht, R. (2001). Exercise training in coronary artery disease and coronary vasomotion. *Circulation, 103,* E1-E6.

Giles, S. H., Croft, J. B., Greenlund, K. J., Ford, E. S., & Kittner, S. J. (2000). Association between total homocysteine and the likelihood for a history of acute myocardial infarction by race and ethnicity: Results from the Third National Health and Nutrition Examination Survey. *American Heart Journal, 139,* 446-455.

Gimbrone, M. A., Jr., Topper, J. N., Nagel, T., Anderson, K. R., & Garcia-Cardena, G. (2000). Endothelial dysfunction, hemodynamic forces, and atherogenesis. *Annals of the New York Academy of Sciences, 902,* 230-239.

Gonzalez, E. R. (1998). Antiplatelet therapy in atherosclerotic cardiovascular disease. *Clinical Therapeutics, 20*(Suppl B), B18-B41.

Gotto, A. M., Jr. (1998). Triglyceride as a risk factor for coronary artery disease. *American Journal of Cardiology, 82*(9A), 22Q-25Q.

Grundy, S. M. (1999). Primary prevention of coronary heart disease: Integrating risk assessment with intervention. *Circulation, 100*(9), 988-998.

Gupta, S. (1999). *Chlamydia pneumoniae*, monocyte activation, and azithromycin in coronary heart disease. *American Heart Journal, 138*(5, Part 2), S539-S541.

Haroon, Z. A., Wannenburg, T., Gupta, M., Greenberg, C. S., Wallin, R., & Sane, D. C. (2001). Localization of tissue transglutaminase in human carotid and coronary artery atherosclerosis: Implications for plaque stability and progression. *Laboratory Investigation, 81,* 83-93.

Hamilton, C. A. (1997). Low-density lipoprotein and oxidised low-density lipoprotein: Their role in the development of atherosclerosis. *Pharmacology and Therapeutics, 74*(1), 55-72.

He, J., Vupputuri, S., Allen, K., Prerost, M. R., Hughes, J., & Whelton, P. K. (1999). Passive smoking and the risk of coronary heart disease—A meta-analysis of epidemiologic studies. *New England Journal of Medicine, 340*(12), 920-926.

He, J., & Whelton, P. K. (1999). Elevated systolic blood pressure as a risk factor for cardiovascular and renal disease. *Journal of Hypertension—Supplement, 17*(2), S7-S13.

Hoffmeister, A., Rothenbacher, D., Bazner, U., Frohlich, M., Brenner, H., Hombach, V., & Koenig, W. (2001). Role of novel markers of inflammation in patients with stable coronary heart disease. *American Journal of Cardiology, 87*(3), 262-266.

Hughes, S. (2000). Novel risk factors for coronary heart disease: Emerging connections. *Journal of Cardiovascular Nursing, 14,* 91-103.

John, S., & Schmieder, R. E. (2000). Impaired endothelial function in arterial hypertension and hypercholesterolemia: Potential mechanisms and differences. *Journal of Hypertension, 18*(4), 363-374.

Kinlay, S., Fang, J. C., & Hikita, H. (1999). Plasma alpha tocopherol and coronary endothelium-dependent vasodilator function. *Circulation,100,* 219-221.

Koenig, W., Sund, M., Frohlich, M., Fischer, H. G., Lowel, H., Doring, A., Hutchinson, W. L., & Pepys, M. B. (1999). C-reactive protein, a sensitive marker of inflammation, predicts future risk of coronary heart disease in initially healthy middle-aged men: Results from the MONICA (Monitoring Trends and Determinants in Cardiovascular Disease) Augsburg Cohort Study, 1984 to 1992. *Circulation, 99*(2), 237-242.

Kullo, I. J., Gau, G. T., & Tajik, A. J. (2000). Novel risk factors for atherosclerosis. *Mayo Clinic Proceedings, 75,* 369-380.

Kwiterovich, P. O., Jr. (1998). The antiatherogenic role of high-density lipoprotein cholesterol. *American Journal of Cardiology, 82*(9A), 13Q-21Q.

LaRosa, J. C., He, J., & Vupputuri, S. (1999). Effect of statins on risk of coronary disease: A meta-analysis of randomized controlled trials. *Journal of the American Medical Association, 282*(24), 2340-2346.

Lee, R. T., & Libby, P. (1997). The unstable atheroma. *Arteriosclerosis, Thrombosis and Vascular Biology, 17*(10), 1859-1867.

Libby, P. (2000). Changing concepts of atherogenesis. *Journal of Internal Medicine, 247*(3), 349-358.

Libby, P., & Ridker, P. (1999). Novel inflammatory markers of coronary risk: Theory versus practice. *Circulation, 100,* 1148-1150.

Malek, A. M., Alper, S. I., & Izumo, S. (1999). Hemodynamic shear stress and its role in atherosclerosis. *Journal of the American Medical Association, 282*(21), 2035-2042.

McGill, H. C. J., McMahan, C. A., Malcom, G. T., Oalmann, M. C., & Strong, J. P. (1997). Effects of serum lipoproteins and smoking on atherosclerosis in young men and women. The PDAY Research Group. Pathobiological Determinants of Atherosclerosis in Youth. *Arteriosclerosis, Thrombosis and Vascular Biology, 17*(1), 95-106.

Mehta, J. L., & Romeo, F. (2000). Inflammation, infection and atherosclerosis: Do antibacterials have a role in the therapy of coronary artery disease? *Drugs, 59,* 159-170.

Miller, M., Dolinar, C., Cromwell, W., & Otvos, J. D. (2001). Effectiveness of high doses of simvastatin as monotherapy in mixed hyperlipidemia. *American Journal of Cardiology, 87,* 232-234.

Miwa, K., Nakagawa, K., Yoshida, N., Taguchi, Y., & Inoue, H. (2000). Lipoprotein(a) is a risk factor for occurrence of acute myocardial infarction in patients with coronary vasospasm. *Journal of the American College of Cardiology, 35*(5), 1200-1205.

Muhlestein, J. B., Horne, B. D., Bair, T. L., Li, Q., Madsen, T. E., Pearson, R. R., & Anderson, J. L. (2001). Usefulness of in-hospital prescription of statin agents after angiographic diagnosis of coronary artery disease in improving continued compliance and reduced mortality. *American Journal of Cardiology, 87,* 257-261.

Nathan, L., & Chaudhuri, G. (1997). Estrogens and atherosclerosis. *Annual Review of Pharmacology and Toxicology, 37,* 477-515.

National Cholesterol Education Program (NCEP) Expert Panel. (1993). Summary of the second report of the National Cholesterol Expert Panel on detection, evaluation, and treatment of high blood cholesterol in adults (adult treatment panel II). *Journal of the American Medical Association, 269*(3), 3015-3023.

Neunteufl, T., Priglinger, U., Heher, S., Zehetgruber, M., Soregi, G., Lehr, S., Huber, K., Maurer, G., Weidinger, F., & Kostner, K. (2000). Effects of vitamin E on chronic and acute endothelial dysfunction in smokers. *Journal of the American College of Cardiology, 35*(2), 277-283.

Nicoletti, A., Caligiuri, G., & Hansson, G. K. (2000). Immunomodulation of atherosclerosis: Myth and reality. *Journal of Internal Medicine, 247,* 397-405.

Ockene, I. S., & Miller, N. H. (1997). Cigarette smoking, cardiovascular disease, and stroke: A statement for healthcare professionals from the American Heart Association. American Heart Association Task Force on Risk Reduction. *Circulation, 96,* 3243-3247.

O'Keefe, J. H., Wetzel, M., Moe, R. R., Bronsnahan, K., & Lavie, C. J. (2001). Should an angiotensin-converting enzyme inhibitor be standard therapy for patients with atherosclerotic disease? *Journal of the American College of Cardiology, 37,* 1-8.

Ornish, D., Scherwitz, L. W., Billings, J. H., et al. (1998). Intensive lifestyle changes for reversal of coronary heart disease. *Journal of the American Medical Association, 280,* 2001-2007.

Pasterkamp, G., de Kleijn, D. P., & Borst, C. (2000). Arterial remodeling in atherosclerosis, restenosis and after alteration of blood flow: Potential mechanisms and clinical implications. *Cardiovascular Research, 45,* 843-852.

Pentikainen, M. O., Oorni, K., Ala-Korpela, M., & Kovanen, P. T. (2000). Modified LDL—Trigger of atherosclerosis and inflammation in the arterial intima. *Journal of Internal Medicine, 247,* 359-370.

Raitakari, O. T., Seale, J. P., & Celermajer, D. S. (2001). Impaired vascular responses to nitroglycerin in subjects with coronary atherosclerosis. *American Journal of Cardiology, 87,* 217-219.

Rimm, E. B., Williams, P., Fosher, K., Criqui, M., Stampfer, M. J. (1999). Moderate alcohol intake and lower risk of coronary hart disease: Meta-analysis of effects on lipids and haemostatic factors. *British Medical Journal, 319*, 1523-1528.

Ross, R. (1999). Mechanisms of disease: Atherosclerosis—An inflammatory disease. *New England Journal of Medicine, 340*(2), 115-126.

Rothwell, P. M., Villagra, R., Gibson, R., Donders, R. C., & Warlow, C. P. (2000). Evidence of a chronic systemic cause of instability of atherosclerotic plaques. *Lancet, 335*, 19-24.

Saikku, P. (2000). *Chlamydia pneumoniae* in atherosclerosis. *Journal of Internal Medicine, 247*, 391-396.

Schachinger, V., Britten, M. B., Elsner, M., Walter, D. H., Scharrer, I., & Zeiher, A. M. (1999). A positive family history of premature coronary artery disease is associated with impaired endothelium-dependent coronary blood flow regulation. *Circulation, 100*(14), 1502-1508.

Selwyn, A. P., Kinlay, S., Creager, M., Libby, P., & Ganz, P. (1997). Cell dysfunction in atherosclerosis and the ischemic manifestations of coronary artery disease. *American Journal of Cardiology, 79*(5A), 17-23.

Sinisalo, J., Paronen, J., Mattila, K. J., Syrjala, M., Alfthan, G., Palosuo, T., Nieminen, M. S., & Vaarala, O. (2000). Relation of inflammation to vascular function in patients with coronary heart disease. *Atherosclerosis, 149*(2), 403-411.

Sniderman, A. D., Bergeron, J., & Frohlich, J. (2001). Apolipoprotein B versus lipoprotein lipids: Vital lessons from the AFCAPS/TexCAPS trial. *CMAJ: Canadian Medical Association Journal, 164*, 44-47.

Sparling, P. B., Snow, T. K., & Beavers, B. D. (1999). Serum cholesterol levels in college students: Opportunities for education and intervention. *Journal of American College Health, 48*(3), 123-127.

Spencer, A. P., Carson, D. S., & Crouch, M. A. (1999). Vitamin E and coronary disease. *Archives of Internal Medicine, 159*, 1313-1320.

Stary, H. C. (2000). Natural history and histological classification of atherosclerotic lesions: An update. *Arteriosclerosis, Thrombosis & Vascular Biology, 20*, 1177-1178.

Steinberg, D. (1997). Lewis A. Conner Memorial Lecture. Oxidative modification of LDL and atherogenesis. *Circulation, 95*(4), 1062-1071.

Steinberg, D., & Gotto, A. M. (1999). Preventing coronary artery disease by lowering cholesterol levels. Fifty years from bench to bedside. *Journal of the American Medical Association, 282*(21), 2043-2050.

Susic, D. (1997). Hypertension, aging, and atherosclerosis. The endothelial interface. *Medical Clinics of North America, 81*(5), 1231-1240.

Villablanca, A. C., McDonald, J. M., & Rutledge, J. C. (2000). Smoking and cardiovascular disease. *Clinics in Chest Medicine, 21*, 159-172.

Virmani, R., Kolodgie, F. D., Burke, A. P., Farb, A., & Schwartz, S. M. (2000). Lessons from sudden coronary death: A comprehensive morphological classification scheme for atherosclerotic lesions. *Arteriosclerosis, Thrombosis & Vascular Biology, 20*, 1262-1275.

Vogel, R. A. (1997). Coronary risk factors, endothelial function, and atherosclerosis: A review. *Clinical Cardiology, 20*(5), 426-432.

Wagner, J. D. (2000). Rationale for hormone replacement therapy in atherosclerosis prevention. *Journal of Reproductive Medicine, 45*, 245-258.

Welch, G. N., & Loscalzo, J. (1998). Homocysteine and atherothrombosis. *New England Journal of Medicine, 338*(15), 1042-1050.

Welch, G. N., Upchurch, G. J., & Loscalzo, J. (1997). Hyperhomocyst(e)inemia and atherothrombosis. *Annals of the New York Academy of Sciences, 811*, 48-58, discussion 58-59.

Willinek, W. A., Ludwig, M., Lennarz, M., Holler, T., & Stumpe, K. O. (2000). High-normal serum homocysteine concentrations are associated with an increased risk of early atherosclerotic carotid artery wall lesions in healthy subjects. *Journal of Hypertension, 18*(4), 425-430.

Wu, T., Trevisan, M., Genco, R. J., Falkner, K. L., Dorn, J. P., & Sempos, C. T. (2000). Examination of the relation between periodontal health status and cardiovascular risk factors: Serum total and high density lipoprotein cholesterol, C-reactive protein, and plasma fibrinogen. *American Journal of Epidemiology, 151*(3), 273-282.

Yuan, S., Liu, Y., & Zhu, L. (1999). Vascular complications of diabetes mellitus. *Clinical & Experimental Pharmacology & Physiology, 26*(12), 977-978.

Yusuf, S., Dagenais, G., Pogue, J., Bosch, J., & Sleight, P. (2000). Vitamin E supplementation and cardiovascular events in high-risk patients. The Heart Outcomes Prevention Study Investigators. *New England Journal of Medicine, 342*, 154-160.

Zaman, A. G., Helf, G., Worthley, S. G., & Badimon, J. J. (2000). The role of plaque rupture and thrombosis in coronary artery disease *Atherosclerosis, 149*(2), 251-266.

Case Study*

Dyslipidemia and Atherosclerosis

INITIAL HISTORY
- 69-year-old white male.
- Complains of excruciating left leg pain.
- Reports sudden onset 45 minutes ago while sitting on a bench at the shopping mall, unrelieved with massage/rest, pain is nonradiating.
- Reports has previously had occasional left leg aching discomfort when walking long distances.

Question 1 What other questions would you like to ask about his medical, family, and social history?

PREVIOUS MEDICAL HISTORY AND HOME MEDICATIONS
- Denies any history of chest pain or focal neurological symptoms.
- No significant previous medical history; does not think he has ever been told he has hypertension, diabetes, or dyslipidemia.
- 75 pack/year smoking history (continues to smoke).
- Uses alcohol occasionally.
- He is not on any medications and he has no allergies.

ADDITIONAL FAMILY AND SOCIAL HISTORY
- Father died of myocardial infarction at age 78, mother is alive and suffers from hypertension and cerebrovascular disease; 1 brother, age 62, 1 sister, age 58—both alive and well.
- Patient lives with wife of 45 years, is a retired civil engineer (retired 4 years ago), and enjoys gardening and travel.
- He feels healthy overall and does not seek regular medical care.

*Kathryn B. Reid contributed this case study.

INITIAL PHYSICAL FINDINGS
- Left leg is mottled and cyanotic, distal to the knee, cool to touch.
- Right leg is pink and warm.
- Doppler of the left dorsalis pedis (DP) and posterior tibialis (PT) pulses reveal decreased pulses with faint bruits heard.
- Right DP and PT pulses are palpable.

Question 2   What is your initial diagnosis?

Question 3   What are the possible causes of this patient's problem?

Question 4   What are the potential general sequelae if this problem is not resolved?

PHYSICAL EXAMINATION
- T = 36.9 PO; sitting BP = 160/90 mmHg left arm, 166/92 mmHg right arm; P = 96 beats/minute, regular rate; RR = 20 breaths/minute, unlabored.
- Slightly obese man complaining of left lower leg and calf aching/throbbing pain, "8" on a scale of 1 to 10.

HEENT, Neck, Lungs, Cardiac
- Unremarkable, fundi without lesions.
- Supple, no adenopathy or thyromegaly, no bruits.
- Bilateral and symmetrical chest expansion with clear breath sounds.
- $S_1 S_2$ clear; no rub, gallop, or murmur; regular rate.

Abdomen, Neurological
- Abdomen with +bowel sounds throughout, nontender, nondistended.
- Alert and oriented, appropriately anxious; cranial nerves X to XII intact; strength 5/5 throughout, DTRs 2+ and symmetrical, sensation intact.

Skin, Extremities
- Skin intact, warm, pink except for left leg (cool and mottled distal to knee).
- Peripheral pulses all palpable except for left DP and PT.
- Faint bruits by doppler.
- No edema.

Question 5 What are the immediate therapeutic alternatives for restoring perfusion to this man's leg and which do you feel would be most appropriate in this case?

Question 6 What studies would you initiate at this time?

LABORATORY RESULTS
- Glucose = 225; urine myoglobin = negative.
- Triglycerides = 315; cholesterol = 353; HDL = 40; LDL = 165.
- All other blood work within normal limits; 12-lead ECG is normal.
- Rectal exam normal, stool guaiac negative.

Question 7 What risk factors for atherosclerotic peripheral vascular disease do you identify for this man?

PATIENT UPDATE

- The patient is admitted to the hospital, is anticoagulated, and undergoes urokinase therapy. Resolution of his blood clot is noted on fluoroscopy, as well as improved distal pulses. Two hours later, however, his status changes as follows:
    - Left DP is absent by doppler, left PT is unchanged.
    - Left leg is increasingly mottled.
    - Left leg demonstrates increased calf size, edema, and tightness.
    - Urine is positive for myoglobin.
    - Patient reports numbness and tingling in his left leg and foot.

Question 8 Based on these new findings, what complications is this patient exhibiting and what precautions must be taken?

PATIENT UPDATE

- A left calf fasciotomy is performed with the following results:
    - Left DP pulse improves to present pulsatile flow by doppler; left PT pulse also is present by doppler.
    - Patient reports resolving numbness and tingling.
    - Mottled appearance of the left leg begins to disappear.

PATIENT COURSE

- The patient's left femoral artery clot is successfully dissolved with urokinase therapy, and normal perfusion is restored to his left leg. The fasciotomy site is sutured and closed 2 days later.
- The angiographic findings of a severe distal femoral artery stenosis is successfully opened through percutaneous transluminal angioplasty. Angiography findings are consistent with peripheral atherosclerotic vascular disease.
- The patient's diastolic blood pressure remains 88 to 98 mmHg and his blood glucose levels remain 150 to 270 during his hospital course.

Question 9 What are the priorities for medical aspects of care now that this patient's acute problem has been resolved?

Question 10 What essential information and education do you need to provide this patient prior to discharge?

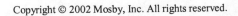

3

Ischemic Heart Disease

DEFINITION

- Ischemic heart disease (IHD) is an imbalance between the demand for myocardial perfusion and the supply of oxygenated blood by the coronary arteries.
- Results in either transient myocardial ischemia (angina) or prolonged ischemia resulting in myocyte damage (acute coronary syndromes).
- Most commonly caused by obstruction of coronary flow by atherosclerotic disease of the coronary vessels, especially when accompanied by an increase in myocardial demand (e.g., exercise) and/or thrombus formation on a ruptured atherosclerotic plaque.

EPIDEMIOLOGY

- Number 1 killer of both men and women in the United States.
- Over 1 million myocardial infarctions (MI) per year in the United States.
- Cardiovascular deaths have decreased 50% in the past 3 decades; this rate of decline is greatest in white males and lowest in black females.
- It is estimated that over 2 million Americans have silent myocardial ischemia with an increased risk of MI and sudden death.
- Risk factors are the same as those for atherosclerosis.
    - The male gender or female after menopause
    - Smoking
    - Dyslipidemia
    - Hypertension
    - Diabetes
    - Family history of ischemic heart disease, especially before age 50
    - Hyperhomocystinemia
    - Increased fibrinogen
    - Obesity
    - Sedentary lifestyle
    - "Novel" risk factors, such as C-reactive protein, infectious agents, serum endotoxin, and increased uric acid

PATHOPHYSIOLOGY

- Atherosclerotic lesions form in coronary vessels (see Chapter 2).

Transient Coronary Ischemic Syndromes

- Stable angina

- The atherosclerotic lesion partially obstructs flow. Stenoses of proximal "conduit" vessels results in autoregulation of distal "resistive" vessels to maintain flow; if stenoses exceed the resistance of the distal bed (60% to 75% occlusion), autoregulation can no longer compensate.

- Slowly increasing atherosclerotic coronary obstructions allow for collateral perfusion such that there is less risk of infarction and overall prognosis is fairly good, however, risk of MI and death increases as the number of affected vessels and the severity of the obstructions increase.

- Transient ischemia occurs when there is increased myocardial demand for coronary flow.

    - Anaerobic metabolism leads to lactate stimulation of pain receptors and inhibition of myocardial contractility resulting in transient decreases in ejection fraction with pulmonary congestion and poor peripheral perfusion of tissues.

    - Although there is no acute infarction of myocardial tissue in stable angina, repetitive ischemia results in ischemic myocardial remodeling and a risk of heart failure.

    - There is increasing evidence for ischemic preconditioning which suggests that brief episodes of repetitive ischemia can induce adaptive mechanisms in myocardial tissue that are protective during prolonged ischemic events.

- The resultant anaerobic metabolism by the myocytes release lactic acid, which causes stimulation of sympathetic afferents giving the sensation of pain in the substernal area; cross stimulation of other sympathetic afferents results in the "radiation" of pain to the neck, jaw, left shoulder, or arm.

- Silent ischemia:

    - Silent ischemia is significant transient myocardial ischemia without associated symptoms.

    - It may be due to less severe ischemia ± high pain threshold ± autonomic dysfunction.

    - It is common in elderly and diabetic patients and in a significant number of men aged 45 to 65.

    - It may indicate higher risk for myocardial infarction in patients with chronic stable angina or in asymptomatic patients with a history of recent myocardial infarction or bypass surgery.

- Prinzmetal angina:

    - It presents with chest pain attributable to transient ischemia of myocardium that occurs unpredictably and at rest; the pain frequently occurs at night during rapid-eye-movement sleep and may have a cyclic pattern of occurrence.

    - It is caused by vasospasm of one or more major coronary arteries with or without atherosclerosis.

    - It may result from hyperactivity of sympathetic nervous system, increased calcium flux in arterial smooth muscle, or impaired production or release of prostaglandin or thromboxane (imbalance of coronary vasodilators and vasoconstrictors).

Acute Coronary Syndromes

- The acute coronary syndromes result when there is sudden coronary obstruction due to thrombus formation over an atherosclerotic plaque.

- The American Heart Association Committee on Vascular Lesions provided criteria for subdividing coronary atherosclerotic plaque progression into five phases with different lesion types corresponding to each phase. The basic thrust of this system is that some atherosclerotic lesions are "stable" and progress by gradually occluding the vessel lumen, whereas other lesions are "unstable" or complicated lesions and (even before there is any significant coronary occlusion) are prone to sudden plaque rupture and thrombus formation resulting in the acute coronary syndromes of unstable angina, myocardial infarction and even sudden death.

- Plaques that are unstable and prone to rupture are those with a core that is especially rich in deposited oxidized LDL and those with thin fibrous caps (Fig. 3-1).

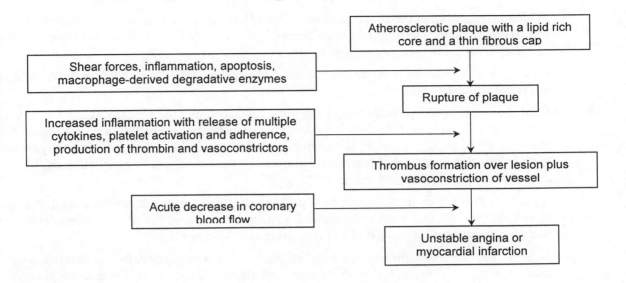

Fig 3-1 Pathogenesis of the Acute Coronary Syndromes

- Plaque disruption (erosions, fissuring, or rupture) occurs due to shear forces, inflammation with release of multiple inflammatory mediators, secretion of macrophage-derived degradative enzymes, and apoptosis of cells at the edges of the lesions.

- Exposure of the plaque substrate activates the clotting cascade and platelet activation results in the release of coagulants and exposure of platelet glycoprotein IIb/IIIa surface receptors resulting in further platelet aggregation and adherence.

- The resulting thrombus can form very quickly.

- Vessel obstruction is further exacerbated by the release of vasoconstrictors such as thromboxane A_2.

- The thrombus may break up before permanent myocyte damage has occurred (unstable angina) or it may cause prolonged ischemia with infarction of the heart muscle (myocardial infarction).

- Unstable angina:

  - Small fissuring or superficial erosion of the plaque leads to transient episodes of thrombotic vessel occlusion and vasoconstriction at the site of plaque damage.

  - This thrombus is labile and occludes the vessel for no more than 10 to 20 minutes with return of perfusion before significant myocardial necrosis occurs.

  - Careful pathologic examination frequently reveals some myocyte damage presumably due to distal embolization of the thrombus fragments.

  - Unstable angina presents as new onset angina, angina that is occurring at rest, or angina that is increasing in severity or frequency; patients may experience increased dyspnea, diaphoresis, and anxiety as the angina worsens (Braunwald Classification I-IV).

  - Those with unstable angina at rest have the greatest risk of subsequent infarction or death.

- Myocardial infarction (MI):
  - Plaque rupture occurs at the edge of the lesion in rest MI, or at an area of cap thinning in exertional MI, resulting in rapid thrombus formation and complete vessel occlusion.
  - Evidence suggests that the atherothrombotic events have an inflammatory component that contributes to platelet aggregation as evidenced by high levels of C-reactive protein in patients suffering from acute coronary ischemia.
  - Prolonged ischemia results in permanent damage to myocardial cells with loss of contractility and release of cellular enzymes.
  - If the thrombus breaks up before complete distal tissue necrosis has occurred, the infarction will involve only the myocardium directly beneath the endocardium, and will not be associated with the classic Q-wave tracing on the ECG (subendocardial or non-Q-wave MI). It is especially important to recognize this form of acute coronary syndrome because recurrent clot formation on the disrupted atherosclerotic plaque is likely.
  - If the thrombus lodges more permanently in the vessel, then the infarction will extend through the myocardium all the way from endocardium to epicardium resulting in severe cardiac dysfunction and the characteristic Q-wave on ECG (transmural or Q-wave MI).
  - Ischemic damage results in necrosis with infiltration of inflammatory cells and fibroblasts that lay down scar tissue (fibrosis) and result in permanent decreases in contractility and compliance.
  - Myocardial "stunning" may occur in the area around the infarcted tissue, a process in which myocytes lose their normal conductive and contractile function for prolonged periods even after perfusion has been restored. It is mediated by free radical-induced lipid peroxidation, enzyme defects (Na/K pump), and alterations in calcium homeostasis.
  - "Hibernating myocardium" is ischemic but not infarcted myocardium around the infarct area that has persistently impaired myocardial function due to reduced coronary blood flow (persistent ischemia).
    1) Myocytes may remain viable for months to years due to down-regulation of biochemical and physiologic activity to prolong myocyte survival (perfusion-contraction matching).
    2) Responds to reperfusion/revascularization (PTCA or surgery); calcium channel blockers may also improve function.
  - Myocardial "remodeling" is a process mediated in part by the renin/angiotensin/aldosterone (RAA) system that causes myocyte hypertrophy and abnormal contractile function in the areas surrounding the infarcted area; this process contributes to infarct expansion and the development of chronic congestive heart failure (CHF) (see Chapter 4).
  - During the ischemic episode, ventricular function is abnormal and ejection fraction falls with increases in ventricular end-diastolic volume (VEDV). If the coronary obstruction involves the perfusion to the left ventricle then pulmonary venous congestion ensues; if the right ventricle is ischemic then increases in systemic venous pressures occur.
  - Conduction disturbances with ischemia or infarction result in electrocardiogram (ECG) changes that are diagnostic in approximately 70% of patients; additional conductive abnormalities can result in bradycardia and heart block, tachyarrhythmias, ventricular fibrillation, or asystole.
  - Cardiogenic shock may occur if contractility is severely compromised, if there is rupture of the septal or ventricular wall, if there is infarction of the chordae tendinea with abrupt regurgitation of the mitral valve, or if there are arrhythmias.

PATIENT PRESENTATION

History

Previous coronary disease; family history of heart disease; hypertension; smoking; dyslipidemia; diabetes; previous episodes of dyspnea on exertion or edema; light-headed or syncopal episodes.

Symptoms

Substernal pressure/pain or chest tightness with or without radiation to the neck, jaw, left shoulder, or arm; dyspnea; nausea or vomiting; diaphoresis; light-headedness or loss of consciousness; onset of symptoms associated with exercise, cold exposure, or stress; pain relieved with rest versus prolonged and persistent.

Examination

Between ischemic episodes, the exam may be normal or reveal evidence of underlying risk factors such as hypertension, manifestations of dyslipidemia such as xanthelasma, corneal arcus, or diabetic manifestations such as intertrigo or neuropathy. There may be signs of atherosclerotic disease in the other arteries as evidenced by bruits, decreased pulses, or neurologic findings. Some patients will exhibit the signs of CHF from previous ischemic events (see Chapter 4). During acute ischemic episodes, the patient is usually anxious, tachycardic, tachypneic, with possible pulmonary rales, S_3, S_4, or murmurs. If there is cardiogenic shock, then hypotension with poor tissue perfusion occurs. Finally, acute arrhythmias may manifest with ectopic beats or the absence of a detectable pulse, shock, and loss of consciousness.

DIFFERENTIAL DIAGNOSIS

- Peptic ulcer disease with or without perforation
- Gastroesophageal reflux
- Pericarditis
- Costochondritis
- Aortic dissection
- Mitral valve prolapse
- Pulmonary embolus
- Other pulmonary disease
- Panic attack

KEYS TO ASSESSMENT

- **Acute chest pain**
    - Remember, elderly patients and diabetics may not have any of the classic symptoms and present with a feeling of unease or dyspnea only.
    - Rapid assessment is important while initiating supportive care measures.
    - The first decision is whether the patient is experiencing cardiac or noncardiac symptomatology, next if there is transient angina or MI. Symptoms correlated with a high likelihood of MI include symptoms less than 48 hours but more than 1 hour and pain radiating to the neck or left arm; symptoms correlated with low risk for MI include radiation of the pain to the abdomen or back and stabbing pain (versus pressure or heaviness).
    - If this is noncardiac pain, the physical exam may show evidence of primary lung or gastrointestinal disease, or pain with palpation of the rib cage consistent with costochondritis.

- Blood should be drawn immediately for complete blood count (CBC), coagulation parameters, electrolytes, creatinine phosphokinase MB (CPK-MB), and troponin I. (Troponin I is more sensitive and specific than CPK-MB for myocardial damage. If it is positive, there is some myocardial ischemia and the prognosis is worse; if it is negative, one still cannot "rule out" MI. The CPK-MB must be repeated at 4, 8, and 12 hours to "rule out" MI.)

- An ECG should be done immediately and, if possible, both with pain and after pain relief. ST segment elevation with T wave inversion is highly suggestive of MI. ST depression can be seen in transient ischemia, but remember that the ECG is neither sensitive (~30% will be nondiagnostic even with ischemia) nor specific. Bundle branch blocks make the interpretation of the ECG for ischemia more difficult and may themselves indicate myocardial damage. The presence of a new Q-wave is diagnostic for MI; many will not develop a Q-wave (non-Q-wave MI), which indicates that not all of the myocardium in the distribution of that artery has been infarcted and that the patient is at risk for recurrent infarction.

- If a patient presents in shock he or she may undergo immediate coronary catheterization.

- **Nonacute symptoms or MI "ruled out"**

  - Evaluation focuses on risk factors and character of the pain to determine likelihood that a history of chest pain was cardiac in origin.

  - If the history is consistent with cardiac pain and the symptoms occurred at rest, were more severe than in the past, or are occurring more frequently, then the diagnosis of unstable angina must be considered and the patient should be referred for immediate hospital evaluation.

  - If the history is consistent with cardiac pain but it is predictable, relieved with rest, and of normal severity and duration compared to any previous episodes, this most likely represents stable angina and the patient should undergo one of many possible diagnostic studies to determine the extent of coronary disease and the possible need for invasive therapy. Each of the following tests has been found to be useful in the evaluation of patients for coronary disease; the choice rests on the local availability of the test.

    1) Stress ECG with thallium; correlates with amount of myocardium at risk.

    2) Single photon emission computed tomography (SPECT) done at rest or with exercise is highly sensitive for coronary disease and has been correlated with prognosis.

    3) Dipyridamole, dobutamine, or arbutamine echocardiography is highly sensitive and specific for the detection of coronary disease.

    4) Coronary angiography should be considered if the noninvasive testing suggests significant coronary obstruction or myocardium at risk for ischemia.

KEYS TO MANAGEMENT

- **Prevention**

  - Exercise can decrease risk by as much as 45%; weight reduction by as much as 55%.

  - Smoking cessation.

  - Blood pressure control by lifestyle, diet, and medication can significantly decrease risk.

  - Diet: decreasing dietary fat and cholesterol decreases cardiac risk (see Chapter 2). Intake of increased fiber, fish oils, and garlic have all been suggested. Increasing antioxidants is still controversial, some studies show as much as a 40% decrease in coronary risk with the intake of 200 to 800 IU of vitamin E daily; other studies show no clear risk reduction with vitamin E, beta-carotene, or vitamin C. More studies are needed. Increasing folate decreases serum homocysteine and significantly lowers coronary risk. Finally, moderate alcohol intake has been shown to reduce cardiac risk.

- Pharmacologic
    1) Antiplatelet drugs, such as aspirin, ticlopidine, clopidogrel, or platelet glycoprotein receptor antagonists (GPIIb/IIIa antagonists) (see Chapter 2), significantly reduce risk.
    2) Cholesterol lowering drugs, especially the HMG-CoA reductase inhibitors, greatly reduce risk in patients with dyslipidemias and can cause regression of atherosclerotic lesions (see Chapter 2).
    3) Secondary prevention after MI includes beta-blockers, aspirin, and lipid lowering drugs; in patients with CHF following MI, the use of angiotensin converting enzyme (ACE) inhibitors, nitrates, and warfarin have been associated with decreased MI recurrence and mortality.

- **Stable angina**
    - Risk reduction and antithrombotic drugs are most important—treat hypertension, diabetes, and dyslipidemia; smoking cessation; and assess for contributing factors, such as anemia.
    - If noninvasive testing reveals three vessel or left main coronary disease, PTCA or coronary artery bypass grafting (CABG) is indicated.
    - If coronary disease is less severe, medical therapy has a good prognosis (although at least one study shows that quality of life was improved after PTCA or CABG in patients with mild to moderate coronary obstruction).
        1) Lifestyle changes: avoid excessive fatigue, modify early morning activities due to an increased risk of angina in the morning, eat several smaller meals, avoid anxiety-provoking situations, engage in stepped exercise program.
        2) Aspirin versus clopidogrel versus platelet GPIIb/IIIa antagonists.
        3) Sublingual nitrates or spray for episodes of pain or as prophylaxis against activities known to precipitate angina; topical or oral nitrates if angina occurs more than 3 to 4 times per week with nitrate-free intervals to avoid tolerance.
        4) Beta-blocker for most patients, especially if tachycardic or hypertensive; avoid in the elderly and patients with obstructive airways disease.
        5) Calcium channel blocker should be added to beta blockers if pain persists.
        6) New agents undergoing human trials include partial fatty acid oxidation (pFOX) inhibitors, such as ranolazine, that may be used in the management of stable angina.
    - If pain persists or worsens, then catheterization and possible PTCA with or without stenting or CABG (MIDCAB). If angina is refractory, consider percutaneous myocardial revascularization (PMR), transmyocardial laser revascularization (TMR), or biorevascularization.

- **Unstable angina**
    - Patients should be admitted to the hospital.
    - Aspirin is given immediately on admission; GP IIIa/IIb antagonists are being tried alone or with heparin and results have been positive.
    - Acute management with low molecular weight heparin, unfractionated heparin, direct thrombin inhibitors (hirudin, Hirulog), thrombolytics, or emergent PTCA reduce the risk of MI.
    - When stable, the patient should undergo noninvasive testing or catheterization for definitive diagnosis and to aid in selecting surgical or medical therapy.

- **Acute myocardial infarction**
    - Admit to the hospital.
    - Oxygen, intravenous (IV) access, support ventilation and circulation if indicated (CPR).

- Immediate administration of antithrombotic (aspirin, GPIIb/IIIa antagonists, etc.).

- Morphine and nitrates.

- If ECG is diagnostic for ischemia (>1 mm ST elevation in ≥2 leads or chest pain and ST depression in anterior precordial leads) and there are no contraindications, then administer intravenously (IV) thrombolytics plus heparin *or* perform emergent catheterization with percutaneous transluminal coronary angioplasty (PTCA) with or without coronary artery stenting and heparin (as effective if not more so than thrombolytics but requires experienced staff and proper support facilities).

- If contraindications to thrombolysis or nondiagnostic ECG but MI ruled in by enzymes, use combination therapy with nitrates, beta blockers, ACE inhibitors, and antithrombotics.

- In both non-Q-wave and Q-wave MI.

    1) IV nitrates should be used for refractory pain only.

    2) IV beta-blockers reduce mortality; they must be used cautiously to avoid CHF and bradycardia.

    3) ACE inhibitors given carefully post-MI reduce overall mortality by as much as 20%.

- Antiarrhythmics are not indicated prophylactically at this time; studies with amiodarone look promising.

- Prior to discharge, most patients should undergo noninvasive testing such as thallium or SPECT imaging to assess risk for recurrent ischemia and the need for angioplasty or coronary bypass grafting.

- Patient teaching prior to discharge is vital to recovery and risk reduction.

- After discharge, patients should be enrolled in a cardiac rehabilitation program.

Pathophysiology $\rightarrow$ Clinical Link

What is going on in the disease process that influences how the patient presents and how he or she should be managed?

What should you do now that you understand the underlying pathophysiology?

The spectrum of ischemic heart disease includes all of the stages in the pathogenesis of atherosclerosis and has the same risk factors, with superimposed threat of thrombosis.	Prevention of coronary artery disease rests on the reduction in risk factors for atherosclerosis plus antiplatelet drugs and/or anticoagulant drugs.
Ischemic myocardium produces lactic acid that stimulates the sympathetic nervous system.	Elderly patients and those with diabetes may not have pain with myocardial ischemia. The examiner must have a high index of suspicion in patients with risk factors.
Myocardial ischemia can be transient or prolonged with actual necrosis of heart muscle; myocyte death results in the release of the cardiac enzymes CPK-MB and troponin I.	Measurement of serum cardiac enzymes differentiates angina or noncardiac pain from true MI, but the serum levels of these markers may take hours to rise, thus delaying the definitive diagnosis.
Cardiac ischemia often results in decreased LV contractility with increased LVEDV and pulmonary venous congestion.	Dyspnea and transient or persistent CHF and pulmonary edema are common features of MI and carry a negative impact on prognosis.
Transient ischemia with exercise or stress occurs when there is a fixed but partial coronary obstruction such that demand exceeds supply for coronary perfusion.	Stable angina has predictable precipitating factors and is relieved with rest; lifestyle modification can reduce anginal symptoms.
MI occurs when a coronary atherosclerotic plaque ruptures and thrombus forms.	In patients without contraindications, the rapid administration of antiplatelet or thrombolytic drugs can restore perfusion, limit infarct size, and reduce mortality.
Unstable angina occurs when a coronary atherosclerotic plaque is beginning to crack and platelets begin sticking to the lesion.	Unstable angina is essentially one step from MI in its pathophysiology and must be treated aggressively to avoid MI.
Some of the effects of myocardial ischemia include remodeling and stunning; these have deleterious effects on LV function.	Treatment of ischemic disease with ACE inhibitors and beta-blockers may prevent future CHF.

SUGGESTED READING

Allen, K. B., Dowling, R. D., Fudge, T. L., Schoettle, G. P., Selinger, S. L., Gangahar, D. M., Angell, W. W., Petracek, M. R., Shaar, C. J., & O'Neill, W. W. (1999). Comparison of transmyocardial revascularization with medical therapy in patients with refractory angina. *New England Journal of Medicine, 341*(14), 1029-1036.

American Heart Association. (1999). 2000 heart and stroke statistical update. *American Heart Journal, 137*(5), 786-791.

Andreotti, F., Lanza, G. A., Sciahbasi, A., Fischetti, D., Sestito, A., De Cristofaro, R., & Maseri, A. (2001). Low-grade exercise enhances platelet aggregability in patients with obstructive coronary disease independently of myocardial ischemia. *American Journal of Cardiology, 87,* 16-20.

Antman, E. M., & Cohen, M. (1999). Newer antithrombin agents in acute coronary syndromes. *American Heart Journal, 138*(Suppl), S563-S569.

Antoniucci, D., Valenti, R., Santoro, G. M., Bolognese, L., Trapani, M., Moschi, G., & Fazzini, P. F. (1999). Primary coronary infarct artery stenting in acute myocardial infarction. *American Journal of Cardiology, 84*(5), 505-510.

Braunwald, E., Jones, R. H., & Mark, D. B. (1994). Diagnosing and managing unstable angina. Agency for Health Policy and Research. *Circulation, 90,* 613-622.

Brener, S. J. (2000). Unfractionated and low-molecular-weight heparins in acute coronary syndromes: Current recommendations. *Cleveland Clinic Journal of Medicine, 67,* 59-65.

British Cardiac Society Guidelines and Medical Practice Committee and Royal College of Physicians Clinical Effectiveness and Evaluation Unit. (2001). Guideline for the management of patients with acute coronary syndromes without persistent ECG ST segment elevation. *Heart, 85,* 133-142.

Burke, A. P., Farb, A., Malcom, G. T., Liang, Y., Smialek, J. E., & Virmani, R. (1999). Plaque rupture and sudden death related to exertion in men with coronary artery disease. *Journal of the American Medical Association, 281,* 921-926.

Buxton, A. E., Lee, K. L., Fisher, J. D., Josephson, M. E., Prystowsky, E. N., & Hafley, G. (1999). A randomized study of the prevention of sudden death in patients with coronary artery disease. Multicenter Unsustained Tachycardia Trial Investigators. *New England Journal of Medicine, 341*(25), 1882-1890.

Califf, R. M. (2000). Combination therapy for acute myocardial infarction: Fibrinolytic therapy and glycoprotein IIb/IIIa inhibition. *American Heart Journal, 139,* S33-S37.

Califf, R. M., & Cohn, J. N. (2000). Cardiac protection: Evolving role of angiotensin receptor blockers. *American Heart Journal, 139,* S15-S22.

Campbell, K. R., Ohman, E. M., Cantor, W., & Lincoff, A. M. (2000). The use of glycoprotein IIb/IIIa inhibitor therapy in acute ST-segment elevation myocardial infarction: Current practice and future trends. *American Journal of Cardiology, 85,* 32C-38C.

Crouch, M. A. (2000). Effective use of statins to prevent coronary heart disease. *American Family Physician, 63,* 309-320.

Danias, P. G. (2001). Stress testing and electron beam computed tomography for evaluation of patients with suspected coronary artery disease. *Journal of the American College of Cardiology, 37,* 334-335.

Davies, M. J. (2000). The pathophysiology of acute coronary syndromes. *Heart, 83,* 361-366.

Dhond, M. R. (2000). Cardiac troponins. *CVR&R, 21,* 20-25.

Duckers, H. J., & Nabel, E. G. (2000). Prospects for genetic therapy of cardiovascular disease. *Medical Clinics of North America, 84,* 199-213.

Dupuis, J., Tardif, J. C., Cernacek, P., & Theroux, P. (1999). Cholesterol reduction rapidly improves endothelial function after acute coronary syndromes. The RECIFE (reduction of cholesterol in ischemia and function of the endothelium) trial. *Circulation, 99*(25), 3227-3233.

Ferrari, R., Ceconi, C., Curello, S., Percoco, G., Toselli, T., & Antonioli, G. (1999). Ischemic preconditioning, myocardial stunning, and hibernation: Basic aspects. *American Heart Journal, 138*(2 Part 2 Suppl), S61-S68.

Fox, K. A. (2000). Coronary disease. Acute coronary syndromes: Presentation—Clinical spectrum and management. *Heart, 84,* 93-100.

Fuster, V., Fayad, Z., & Badimon, J. J. (1999). Acute coronary syndromes: Biology. *Lancet, 353*(Suppl II), 5-9.

Gerber, B. L., Wijns, W., Vanoverschelde, J. L. J., Heyndrickx, G. R., De Bruyne, B., Bartunek, J,. & Melin, J. A. (1999). Myocardial perfusion and oxygen consumption in reperfused noninfarcted dysfunctional myocardium after unstable angina. Evidence for myocardial stunning in humans. *Journal of the American College of Cardiology, 34*(7), 1939-1946.

Gersh, B. J. (1999). Optimal management of acute myocardial infarction at the dawn of the next millennium. *American Heart Journal, 138*(2 Pt 2), 188-202.

Gibson, C. M. (1999). Primary angioplasty compared with thrombolysis: New issues in the era of glycoprotein IIb/IIIa inhibition and intracoronary stenting. *Annals of Internal Medicine, 130*(10), 841-847.

Goncalves, L. M. (2000). Angiogenic growth factors: Potential new treatment for acute myocardial infarction. *Cardiovascular Research, 45,* 294-302.

Held, C., Hjemdahl, P., Hakan Wallen, N., Bjorkander, I., Forslund, L., Wiman, B., & Rehnqvist, N. (2000). Inflammatory and hemostatic markers in relation to cardiovascular prognosis in patients with stable angina pectoris. Results from the APSIS study. The Angina Prognosis Study in Stockholm. *Atherosclerosis, 148*(1), 179-188.

Johnson, P. A., Goldman, L., Sacks, D. B., Garcia, T., Albano, M., Bezai, M., Pedan, A., Cook, E. F., & Lee, T. H. (1999). Cardiac troponin T as a marker for myocardial ischemia in patients seen at the emergency department for acute chest pain. *American Heart Journal, 137*(6), 1137-1144.

Jurlander, B., Farhi, E. R., Banas, J. J., Keany, C. M., Balu, D., Grande, P., & Ellis, A. K. (2000). Coronary angiographic findings and troponin T in patients with unstable angina pectoris. *American Journal of Cardiology, 85*(7), 810-814.

Kario, K., & Pickering, T. G. (2000). Modification of high blood pressure after myocardial infarction. *Medical Clinics of North America, 84,* 1-21.

Kaul, S., & Shah, P. K. (2000). Low molecular weight heparin in acute coronary syndrome: Evidence for superior or equivalent efficacy compared with unfractionated heparin? *Journal of the American College of Cardiology, 35,* 1699-1712.

Kodama, K., Asakura, M., Ueda, Y., Yamaguchi, O., & Hirayama, A. (2000). The role of plaque rupture in the development of acute coronary syndrome evaluated by the coronary angioscope. *Internal Medicine, 39,* 333-335.

Kohler, H. P., & Grant, P. J. (2000). Plasminogen-activator inhibitor type 1 and coronary artery disease. *New England Journal of Medicine, 342,* 1792-1801.

Kuller, L. H. (2000). Hormone replacement therapy and coronary heart disease. A new debate. *Medical Clinics of North America, 84,* 181-198.

Lee, T. H., & Goldman, L. (2000). Evaluation of the patient with acute chest pain. *New England Journal of Medicine, 342,* 1187-1195.

Lincoff, A. M., Califf, R. M., & Topol, E. J. (2000). Platelet glycoprotein IIb/IIIa receptor blockade in coronary artery disease. *Journal of the American College of Cardiology, 35,* 1103-1115.

Lloyd-Jones, D. M., Larson, M. G., Beiser, A., & Levy, D. (1999). Lifetime risk of developing coronary heart disease. *Lancet, 353,* 89-92.

Losordo, D. W., Vale, P. R., & Isner, J. M. (1999). Gene therapy for myocardial angiogenesis. *American Heart Journal, 138*(2 Pt 2), 132-141.

Maggioni, A. P., & Latini, R. (1999). How to use ACE-inhibitors, beta-blockers, and newer therapies in AMI. *American Heart Journal, 138*(2 Pt 2), 183-187.

Naccarelli, G. V., Wolbrette, D. L., Patel, H. M., & Luck, J. C., (2000). Amiodarone: Clinical trials. *Current Opinion in Cardiology, 15*(1), 64-72.

Nakamura, M., Nishikawa, H., Mukai, S., Setsuda, M., Nakajima, K., Tamada, H., Suzuki, H., Ohnishi, T., Kakuta, Y., Nakano, T., & Yeung, A. C. (2001). Impact of coronary artery remodeling on clinical presentation of coronary artery disease: An intravascular ultrasound study. *Journal of the American College of Cardiology, 37,* 63-69.

Natarajan, M. K., Mehta, S., & Yusuf, S. (2000). Management of myocardial infarction: Looking beyond efficacy. *Journal of the American College of Cardiology, 35,* 380-381.

Noda, T., Minatoguchi, S., Fujii, K., Hori, M., Ito, T., Kanmatsuse, K., Matsuzaki, M., Miura, T., Nonogi, H., Tada, M., Tanaka, M., & Fujiwara, H. (1999). Evidence for the effect in human ischemic preconditioning: Prospective multicenter study for preconditioning in acute myocardial infarction. *Journal of the American College of Cardiology, 34*(7), 1966-1974.

Norris, R. M. (2000). The natural history of acute myocardial infarction. *Heart, 83,* 726-730.

Ornish, D., Scherwitz, L. W., Billings, J. H., et al. (1998). Intensive lifestyle changes for reversal of coronary heart disease. *Journal of the American Medical Association, 280,* 2001-2007.

Patel, V. B., & Topol, E. J. (1999). The pathogenesis and spectrum of acute coronary syndromes: From plaque formation to thrombosis. *Cleveland Clinic Journal of Medicine, 66*(9), 561-571.

Pfeffer, M. A. (2000). Enhancing cardiac protection after myocardial infarction: Rationale for newer clinical trials of angiotensin receptor blockers. *American Heart Journal, 139,* S23-S28.

Pope, J. H., Aufderheide, T. P., Ruthazer, R., Woolard, R. H., Feldman, J. A., Beshansky, J. R., Griffith, J. L., & Selker, H. P. (2000). Missed diagnoses of acute cardiac ischemia in the emergency department. *New England Journal of Medicine, 342*(16), 1163-1170.

Rauch, U., Osende, J. I., Fuster, V., Badimon, J. J., Fayad, Z., & Chesebro, J. H. (2001). Thrombus formation on atherosclerotic plaques: Pathogenesis and clinical consequences. *Annals of Intern Medicine, 134*(3), 224-238.

Rentrop, K. P. (2000). Thrombi in acute coronary syndromes: Revisited and revised. *Circulation, 101,* 1619-1626.

Ridker, P. M., Hennekens, C. H., Buring, J. E., & Rifai, N. (2000). C-reactive protein and other markers of inflammation in the prediction of cardiovascular disease in women. *New England Journal of Medicine, 342*(12), 836-843.

Reis, S. E., Costantino, J. P., Wickerham, D. L., Tan-Chiu, E., Wang, J., & Kavanah, M. (2001). Cardiovascular effects of tamoxifen in women with and without heart disease: Breast cancer prevention trial. National Surgical Adjuvant Breast and Bowel Project Breast Cancer Prevention Trial Investigators. *Journal of the National Cancer Institute, 93,* 16-21.

Rodriguez, A., Bernardi, V., Navia, J., Baldi, J., Grinfeld, L., Martinez, J., Vogel, D., Grinfeld, R., Delacasa, A., Garrido, M., Oliveri, R., Mele, E., Palacios, I., & O'Neill, W. (2001). Argentine randomized study: Coronary angioplasty with stenting versus coronary bypass surgery in patients with multiple-vessel disease (ERACI II): 30-day and one-year follow-up results. ERACI II Investigators. *Journal of the American College of Cardiology, 37,* 51-58.

Roe, M. T., & Moliterno, D. J. (1999). Emerging treatment of acute coronary syndromes with platelet glycoprotein IIB/IIIA inhibitors. *Journal of Thrombosis & Thrombolysis, 7*(3), 247-257.

Sanchis, J., Bodi, V., Insa, L. D., Berenguer, A., Chorro, F. J., Llacer, A., Lopez-Lereu, M. P., & Lopez-Merino, V. (1999). Predictors of early and late ventricular remodeling after acute myocardial infarction. *Clinical Cardiology, 22*(9), 581-586.

Shemesh, J., Weg, N., Tenenbaum, A., Apter, S., Fisman, E. Z., Stroh, C. I., Itzchak, Y., & Motro, M. (2000). Usefulness of spiral computed tomography (dual-slice mode) for the detection of coronary artery calcium in patients with chronic atypical chest pain, in typical angina pectoris, and in asymptomatic subjects with prominent atherosclerotic risk factors. *American Journal of Cardiology, 87,* 226-228.

Sheppard, R., & Eisenberg, M. J. (2001). Intracoronary radiotherapy for restenosis. *New England Journal of Medicine, 344,* 295-297.

Sutton, M. G., & Sharpe, N. (2000). Left ventricular remodeling after myocardial infarction: Pathophysiology and therapy. *Circulation, 101,* 2981-2988.

Theroux, P. (2000). Myocardial cell protection: A challenging time for action and a challenging time for clinical. *Circulation, 101,* 2874-2876.

Tomoda, H., & Aoki, N. (2001). Instability of coronary lesions in unstable angina assessed by C-reactive protein values following coronary interventions. *American Journal of Cardiology, 87,* 221-223.

Topol, E. J. (2000). Acute myocardial infarction: Thrombolysis. *Heart, 83,* 122-126.

Urano, H., Ikeda, H., Ueno, T., Matsumoto, T., Murohara, T., & Imaizumi, T. (2001). Enhanced external counterpulsation improves exercise tolerance, reduces exercise-induced myocardial ischemia and improves left ventricular diastolic filling in patients with coronary artery disease. *Journal of the American College of Cardiology, 37,* 93-99.

Verheugt, F. W. (1999). Acute coronary syndromes: Interventions. *Lancet, 353*(Suppl II), 16-19.

Vorchheimer, D. A., Badimon, J. J., & Fuster, V. (1999). Platelet glycoprotein IIb/IIIa receptor antagonists in cardiovascular disease. *Journal of the American Medical Association, 281*(15), 1407-1414.

White, H. D. (1999). Optimal treatment of patients with acute coronary syndromes and non-ST-elevation myocardial infarction. *American Heart Journal, 138*(Suppl), S105-S115.

Yamagishi, M., Terashima, M., Awano, K., Kijima, M., Nakatani, S., Daikoku, S., Ito, K., Yasumura, Y., & Miyatake. K. (2000). Morphology of vulnerable coronary plaque: Insights from follow-up of patients examined by intravascular ultrasound before an acute coronary syndrome. *Journal of the American College of Cardiology, 35*(1), 106-111.

Yousef, Z. R., Redwood, S. R., & Marber, M. S. (2000). Postinfarction left ventricular remodeling: Where are the theories and trials leading us? *Heart, 83,* 76-80.

Yusuf, S., Dagenais, G., Pogue, J., Bosch, J., & Sleight, P. (2000). Vitamin E supplementation and cardiovascular events in high-risk patients. The Heart Outcomes Prevention Study Investigators. *New England Journal of Medicine, 342,* 154-160.

Zaman, A. G., Helft, G., Worthley, S. G., Badimon, J. J. (2000). The role of plaque rupture and thrombosis in coronary artery disease. *Atherosclerosis. 149*(2), 251-266.

Case Study

Ischemic Heart Disease

INITIAL HISTORY
- 40-year-old male complaining of substernal chest pain that began approximately 90 minutes before he came to the emergency room.
- The pain has eased slightly but is still present; was 8/10 in severity, now 5/10.

Question 1   Based on this history alone, what is your differential diagnosis?

Question 2   What other symptoms would you like to ask him about?

ADDITIONAL HISTORY
- He can also feel the pain in his left shoulder.
- He also feels short of breath and somewhat sick to his stomach, but he has not vomited.
- He denies coughing, fever, or change in the nature of the pain with deep breathing.

Question 3   What risk factors would you like to ask him about?

ADDITIONAL HISTORY

- 40 pack/year history of smoking.
- His blood pressure has been a little elevated on his last 2 visits to his nurse practitioner at 148/92.
- He eats a lot of fatty foods but says his cholesterol doesn't change no matter what he eats; it was 242 last month.
- His father has angina that began at age 53.
- He denies diabetes.
- He exercises regularly and has not gained weight.

Question 4   What else would you like to know about his past medical history?

PAST MEDICAL HISTORY

- He says he has had a couple of episodes of shortness of breath while jogging but attributed it to "growing old."
- He has never been hospitalized except for one case of influenza complicated by pneumonia 3 years ago.
- He perceives himself as very healthy, is on no medications, and has no known allergies.

Question 5   Based on the history, now what is your differential diagnosis?

PHYSICAL EXAMINATION

- Alert, moderately anxious man in mild distress.
- T = 37 orally; P = 100 with occasional premature beat; RR = 24; BP = 160/98 in both arms sitting

HEENT, Skin, Neck

- Skin warm and diaphoretic without cyanosis.
- PERRLA, fundi benign, pharynx clear.
- Neck supple without thyromegaly, adenopathy, or bruits.
- <2 cm jugular venous distension.

Lungs
- Tachypneic, mild use of accessory muscles of respiration.
- No tenderness upon palpation of the chest wall.
- No dullness to percussion.
- Slight inspiratory crackles (rales) heard at both bases without egophony.
- No rubs.

Cardiac
- Tachycardia with occasional premature beat.
- Apical pulse at 5th intercostal space just lateral to the midclavicular line.
- Soft S_3, no S_4, no murmurs.
- No rubs.

Abdomen, Extremities, Neurological
- Abdomen with bowel sounds heard throughout; no organomegaly or tenderness; no bruits; rectal guaiac negative.
- Extremities with full and symmetrical pulses; slight bruit over left femoral artery; no pedal edema.
- Alert and oriented; neurologic exam in tact to cognition, strength, sensation, gait, and deep tendon reflexes.

Question 6   What are the pertinent positives and negatives on the exam and what might they mean?

Question 7   What diagnostics would you like to obtain now?

INITIAL DIAGNOSTICS
- ECG shows 4 mm ST elevation with T-wave inversion in the anterior precordial leads with occasional premature ventricular contraction.
- Oximetry shows O_2 saturation of 95%.
- Chest x-ray with borderline cardiomegaly and mild pulmonary congestion without acute infiltrates or pleural disease and no widening of the mediastinum.

Question 8   What do these initial diagnostic results indicate?

Question 9   What therapeutic interventions would you like to initiate while obtaining additional the diagnostic data?

INITIAL MANAGEMENT
- Patient is placed on nasal cannulae and an IV D_5W at KVO is started.
- He is given aspirin, 325 mg/PO.
- He receives 2 mg/IV morphine, 40 mg/IV furosemide, and topical nitrates.
- He is reassured and kept up-to-date with his diagnosis and care.

MORE DIAGNOSTICS
- Electrolytes and CBC normal.
- PT and PTT normal.
- CPK-MB normal.
- Troponin I normal.

Question 10   What now?

RE-EVALUATION OF THE PATIENT
- Pain is now 2/10 in severity, dyspnea is better.
- P = 98; RR = 20; BP = 148/92.
- Lungs are now clear.
- Cardiac with continued occasional PCV, S_3 is gone, no new murmurs.
- Repeat ECG with ST elevation now down to 2 mm and new Q-waves in anterior leads.

Question 11   What interventions should be considered now?

FURTHER MANAGEMENT
- Patient is given 2 mg morphine and the amount of topical nitrate is increased.
- Echocardiogram reveals wall motion abnormality of the anterior left ventricle; ejection fraction is now 55%.
- History reveals no contraindications to thrombolysis.

Question 12   What medications should be given now?

ADDITIONAL MANAGEMENT
- Patient receives thrombolytic therapy followed by heparin.
- He receives IV beta-blockers.
- His blood pressure normalizes and he has no more pain so no IV nitrates are given.
- His ECG normalized over time except for small Q-waves anteriorly.
- He is admitted to the CCU.

HOSPITAL COURSE

- Patient continues to do well without recurrence of chest pain or dyspnea.
- Telemetry reveals no more ectopy.
- Patient is started on an ACE inhibitor on day 3 post-MI.
- He undergoes SPECT evaluation and is found to have no additional myocardium at risk consistent with single-vessel disease and completed infarction.
- He is gradually ambulated and is ready for discharge by day 6.

Question 13   What should this patient be told and what medications should he be given before he is discharged?

4

Congestive Heart Failure

DEFINITION

- Congestive heart failure (CHF) is a pathophysiologic condition in which the heart is unable to generate an adequate cardiac output such that there is inadequate perfusion of tissues, and/or increased diastolic filling pressure of the left ventricle, such that pulmonary capillary pressures are increased.
- CHF refers to primary dysfunction of the left ventricle (LV).
- CHF may be systolic, diastolic, or both.
- Primary dysfunction of the right ventricle is associated most commonly with pulmonary disease (see Chapter 6) and is not considered congestive heart failure.

EPIDEMIOLOGY

- 1.5% to 2% of all adults in the United States are affected; 700,000 hospitalizations occur per year.
- The most common risk factor for the development of heart failure is age.
- CHF is the most common reason for the elderly to be admitted to the hospital (75% of patients admitted with CHF are between 65 and 75 years old).
- 44% of Medicare patients hospitalized for CHF will be readmitted within 6 months.
- There are 2 million outpatient visits per year for CHF; the costs are estimated at $10 billion annually.
- The 8-year survival overall for all classes of CHF is 30%; for severe CHF the 1-year mortality is 60%.
- The most important risk factor for CHF is coronary artery disease with ischemic heart disease. Hypertension is the second most important risk factor for CHF. Others include cardiomyopathy, arrhythmia, renal failure, diabetes, and valvular heart disease.

PATHOPHYSIOLOGY

- CHF results from a complex interaction between factors that affect the contractility, afterload, preload, or lusitropic function of the heart, and the subsequent neurohumoral and hemodynamic responses that seek to create circulatory compensation.
- Although the hemodynamic consequences of heart failure respond to standard pharmacologic interventions, there are critical neurohumoral interactions whose combined effect is to exacerbate and perpetuate the syndrome.
  - **Renin/angiotensin/aldosterone (RAA) system:** In addition to increasing peripheral resistance and circulating blood volume, angiotensin and aldosterone have been implicated in structural changes in the myocardium that are seen with ischemic injury and hypertensive hypertrophic cardiomyopathy. These changes include myocardial remodeling and sarcomere death, loss of the normal collagen matrix, and interstitial fibrosis. The resulting myocyte and sarcomere slippage, heart dilation, and scar formation with loss of normal myocardial compliance contribute to the hemodynamic and symptomatic features of CHF.

- **Sympathetic nervous system (SNS):** Epinephrine and norepinephrine cause increased peripheral resistance with increased work for the heart, tachycardia, increased oxygen consumption by the myocardium, and an increased risk for arrhythmias. The catecholamines also contribute to ventricular remodeling through direct toxicity to myocytes, the induction of myocyte apoptosis, and increased autoimmune responses.

- **Endogenous vasodilators, such as endothelin and nitric oxide, cardiac peptides, and natriuretic peptides:** The roles in CHF are being defined and the interventions are being tested.

- **Immune and inflammatory cytokines:** Tumor necrosis factor alpha (TNFα) and interleukin-6 (IL-6) contribute to ventricular remodeling with myocyte apoptosis, ventricular dilatation, and decreased contractility. Furthermore, They have been implicated in systemic effects such as weight loss and weakness seen in severe CHF (cardiac cachexia).

- The initial etiologic event influences the early responses of the myocardium, but as the syndrome progresses, common mechanisms emerge such that patients with advanced CHF share similar symptomatic presentations and respond to similar pharmacologic interventions irrespective of the initial cause of their CHF.

- Although many patients have both systolic and diastolic left ventricular dysfunction, these categories are best considered separately in order to understand their effects on circulatory homeostasis and their responses to various interventions.

   - **Systolic left ventricular dysfunction**

      1) **Diminished cardiac output** due to decreased contractility, increased afterload, or increased preload results in a decreased ejection fraction and an increased left ventricular end diastolic volume (LVEDV). This increases the end diastolic pressures in the left ventricle (LVEDP) and causes pulmonary venous congestion and pulmonary edema.

      2) **Decreased contractility (inotropy)** results from inadequate or uncoordinated myocardial function such that the LV cannot eject more than 60% of its end-diastolic volume (LVEDV). This causes a gradual increase in LVEDV (also called preload) resulting in an increase in LVEDP and pulmonary venous congestion. The most common cause of decreased contractility is ischemic heart disease, which not only results in actual necrosis of myocardial tissue, but also causes ischemic ventricular remodeling. Ischemic remodeling is a process mediated in part by angiotensin II (ANG II) that causes scarring and sarcomere dysfunction in the heart surrounding the area of ischemic injury. Cardiac arrhythmias and primary cardiomyopathies such as those caused by alcohol, infection, hemachromatosis, hyperthyroidism, drug toxicity and amyloidosis also cause decreased contractility. Decreased cardiac output leads to underperfusion of the systemic circulation and activation of the sympathetic nervous system and the RAA system, causing increased peripheral resistance and increased afterload.

      3) **Increased afterload** means there is increased resistance to LV ejection. This is usually due to the increased peripheral vascular resistance commonly seen in hypertension. It may also be due to aortic valvular stenosis. The LV responds to this increased work with myocardial hypertrophy, a response that increases LV muscle mass but at the same time increases LV demand for coronary perfusion. An energy-starved state is created that, in concert with ANG II and other neuroendocrine responses, causes deleterious changes in the myocytes such as fewer mitochondria for energy production, altered gene expression with production of abnormal contractile proteins (actin, myosin, and tropomyosin), interstitial fibrosis, and decreased myocyte survival. Over time, contractility begins to decline with decreased cardiac output and ejection fraction, increased LVEDV, and pulmonary congestion.

4) **Increased preload** means increased LVEDV, which can be caused directly by excess intravascular volume similar to that seen with an infusion of intravenous fluids or with renal failure. In addition, decreased ejection fraction caused by changes in contractility or afterload result in increased LVEDV and thus increased preload. As LVEDV increases, it stretches the heart, putting the sarcomeres at a mechanical disadvantage and thus decreasing contractility. This decreased contractility, resulting in a decreased ejection fraction, contributes further to the increased LVEDV, thus creating a viscous cycle of worsening heart failure.

5) Thus, a patient can enter this cycle of decreased contractility, increased afterload, and increased preload for a number of reasons (e.g., myocardial infarction [MI], hypertension, fluid overload) and will eventually develop all of the hemodynamic and neurohumoral features of CHF as one mechanism leads to the other (Fig. 4-1).

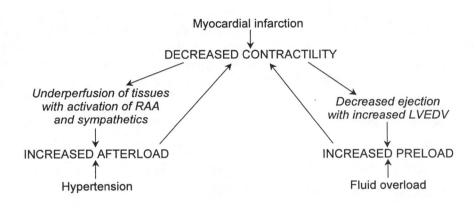

Fig. 4-1 The Self-Perpetuating Cycle of CHF

– Diastolic left ventricular dysfunction

1) It causes up to 40% of all cases of CHF.

2) It is defined as a condition with classic findings of congestive failure with abnormal diastolic but normal systolic function; pure diastolic dysfunction would be characterized by resistance to ventricular filling with an increase in LVEDP without an increase in LVEDV or a decrease in cardiac output.

3) The resistance to left ventricular filling results from abnormal relaxation (lusitropy) of the LV and can be caused by any condition that stiffens the ventricular myocardium such as ischemic heart disease resulting in scarring, hypertension resulting in hypertrophic cardiomyopathy, restrictive cardiomyopathy, valvular disease or pericardial disease.

4) Increases in heart rate allow less time for diastolic filling and exacerbate the symptoms of diastolic dysfunction. Therefore exercise intolerance is common.

5) Because treatment would require actually changing myocardial compliance, the effectiveness of currently available drugs is limited. Management currently is most successful with beta-blockers which improve lusitropic function, decrease heart rate, and improve symptoms. ACE inhibitors can help reverse hypertrophy and structural changes at the tissue level in patients with ischemic remodeling or hypertension.

PATIENT PRESENTATION

History

Previous myocardial infarction; risk factors for ischemic heart disease (smoking, hyperlipidemia, diabetes); hypertension; valvular disease; cardiomyopathy; pericardial disease; renal failure; excessive intravenous; recent high intake of salt.

Symptoms

Dyspnea especially on exertion; orthopnea; paroxysmal nocturnal dyspnea; cough; pedal edema; decreased urine output; fatigue; weight gain; chest pain. Patients are classified (New York Heart Association classes) based on the severity of symptoms; this classification scheme is correlated with prognosis.

Examination

Weight gain; tachypnea; tachycardia; murmurs; cyanosis; inspiratory crackles (rales); frothy sputum production; edema; cold, clammy skin; weak peripheral pulses; jugular venous distension; hepatojugular reflux; muscle wasting; *systolic dysfunction*: S_3, shift of apical pulse, hypotension during episodes of pulmonary edema; *diastolic dysfunction*: S_4, strong but nondisplaced apical pulse, hypertension during episodes of pulmonary edema; hepatosplenomegaly.

DIFFERENTIAL DIAGNOSIS

- CHF must be differentiated from the following:
  - Noncardiogenic pulmonary edema (acute respiratory distress syndrome [ARDS])
  - Chronic obstructive pulmonary disease (COPD)
  - Pneumonia
  - Asthma
  - Interstitial pulmonary fibrosis
  - Other primary lung diseases
- The underlying cause of the CHF must be established from the following:
  - Myocardial ischemia/infarction
  - Hypertensive hypertrophic cardiomyopathy
  - Valvular heart disease
  - Primary cardiomyopathy (idiopathic, alcohol, post infectious, amyloidosis, restrictive)
  - Pericardial disease
  - Fluid overload (iatrogenic versus renal failure)

KEYS TO ASSESSMENT

- CHF is a manifestation of an underlying cardiac insult; begin immediately to assess for the cause of LV dysfunction.
- A quick physical exam can often establish the diagnosis of CHF; therapeutic intervention can begin even as assessment progresses.
- Early electrocardiographic monitoring for ischemia or arrhythmias is vital.
- Obtain arterial blood gases immediately, then begin oxygen.
- Obtain serum electrolytes, blood urea nitrogen (BUN) and creatinine (Cr); complete blood count (CBC); and thyroid studies if age over 65 or atrial fibrillation.

- A chest x-ray may show cardiomegaly, pulmonary edema, and pleural effusions; the diagnosis of pericardial or valvular disease can often be made on the chest x-ray.

- Echocardiography (ECG) can estimate ejection fraction and cardiac output, demonstrate LV wall motion abnormalities consistent with ischemia, show hypertrophic cardiomyopathy, or diagnose valvular and pericardial disease.

- Emergent cardiac catheterization may be indicated in patients suspected of acute coronary artery disease and thrombosis.

- Hemodynamic monitoring (central venous catheter) remains controversial; current indications include the following:

  - Uncertainty about diagnosis.

  - Deteriorating course.

  - Lack of expected response to interventions.

  - High dose intravenous nitrates or inotropics indicated.

KEYS TO MANAGEMENT

- Acute CHF

  - Let the patient sit up if he/she is not hypotensive.

  - Oxygen: get arterial blood gas on room air quickly, then put on a mask at 60%; intubate if ventilatory failure or if the patient is progressively cyanotic and has decreasing mental status.

  - Treat myocardial ischemia if indicated (see Chapter 3).

  - Administer morphine, nitroglycerin, and IV diuretic (furosemide) if no significant hypotension.

  - Consider intravenous (IV) inotropics (dobutamine, dopamine)—use them early if hypotensive.

  - If necessary, switch to IV nitrates if there is a high peripheral vascular resistance (hypertensive). Nitroglycerin is safer than nitroprusside.

  - An intraaortic balloon pump is indicated if there is refractory hypotension (cardiogenic shock), refractory ischemia in preparation for emergency coronary bypass grafting (CABG), or acute mitral regurgitation in preparation for operative valvular repair or replacement.

  - Emergent coronary catheterization and balloon angioplasty or CABG is used in selected patients with ischemia.

- Chronic CHF

  - Definitive management of underlying cause is optimal.

  - Lifestyle modification with salt restriction, exercise, and education about monitoring symptoms (daily weights, dyspnea, edema, chest pain) is recommended.

  - Diuretics, inotropics, ACE inhibitors, and beta blockers are the mainstay of therapy for CHF.

    1) **Diuretics:** Furosemide remains the most commonly used diuretic along with bumetanide or torsemide. Diuretics clearly improve exercise intolerance and edema but electrolyte imbalance and adverse effects on serum lipids and glucose must be watched. Spironolactone has been shown to reduce mortality in severe CHF.

2) **Inotropics:**

a) Digoxin improves exercise tolerance, increases cardiac output, slows progression of CHF, decreases sympathetic and RAA activity, and improves quality of life in selected patients. May decrease mortality when used with angiotensin converting enzyme (ACE) inhibitors, however, mortality may be increased in patients for whom digoxin is subsequently discontinued. It is important to follow blood levels and avoid hypokalemia (arrhythmias).

b) Phosphodiesterase inhibitors (milrinone, amrinone, enoximone, piroximone) have short-term benefits to cardiac output and exercise tolerance; long-term safety is unclear, including increases in mortality, hypotension, and allergy.

c) Adrenergic agonists (intermittent IV dobutamine or xamoterol) have short- term benefits, but may cause increased mortality; oral levo-dopamine is being studied.

d) New inotropics, such as vesnarinone, flosequinan, and pimobendan, have shown promise but long-term safety has not yet been established.

3) **ACE inhibitors and angiotensin II receptor blockers** affect the hemodynamic and neurohumoral manifestations of CHF with improvements in symptoms and survival. Most are well tolerated except for first-dose hypotension, cough (especially with captopril), and risk of renal dysfunction in some patients.

4) **Beta-blockers** (carvedilol, metoprolol, bucindolol, labetalol) increase ejection fraction, decrease sympathetic tone with vasodilation and decreased myocardial oxygen consumption, and decrease ventricular remodeling. Carvedilol is emerging as the drug of choice with significant decreases in mortality and improvement symptoms. High dose beta-blockers can result in pulmonary edema; low dose causes clinical worsening for the first 4 to 10 weeks with improvement at about 10 to 12 weeks.

- Other agents:

1) Nitrates also improve hemodynamic and neurohumoral manifestations of CHF. They are associated with significant headache and tolerance requires intermittent dosing.

2) Calcium channel blockers (amlodipine, felodipine) may be useful in diastolic dysfunction and late-stage systolic dysfunction. First generation calcium blockers increase sympathetic activity and do not reduce mortality in CHF, however, these newer agents do not cause reflex tachycardia and may improve the neurohumoral, hemodynamic and symptomatic aspects of CHF.

3) Antiarrhythmics are generally not indicated despite the high incidence of sudden death in CHF; both beta-blockers and ACE inhibitors decrease ventricular ectopy. Amiodarone is the only antiarrhythmic that has been associated with decreased mortality. Implantable defibrillators should be considered in high-risk patients.

4) Anticoagulants are indicated if there is atrial fibrillation, valvular disease, or a known intraventricular thrombus.

- Sequential pacing can improve cardiac output in selected patients.

- Surgery for CHF includes heart transplant and cardiomyoplasty.

Pathophysiology → Clinical Link

What is going on in the disease process that influences how the patient presents and how he or she should be managed?

What should you do now that you understand the underlying pathophysiology?

CHF is a very common syndrome with age as the greatest risk factor along with underlying coronary or hypertensive heart disease.	A careful history and physical are important when evaluating elderly patients and those at risk for heart disease.
Acute congestive failure is a common complication of acute myocardial infarction, severe valvular disease, underlying fluid overload, and hypertensive crisis.	The management of acute CHF must include evaluation and therapy for the initiating process, not just for CHF.
Both hemodynamic and neurohumoral mechanisms contribute to the pathophysiology of CHF and to both acute and chronic symptoms.	These mechanisms contribute to the progression of CHF resulting in a significant mortality for patients with this syndrome. Treatment aimed at reversing these mechanisms provide not only short term relief of symptoms, but also improvements in morbidity and mortality over time.
Systolic LV dysfunction results in a vicious cycle of decreased contractility, increased afterload, and increased preload.	Once the full picture of CHF is established, most patients with systolic dysfunction will require inotropics, diuretics and vasodilators.
Diastolic LV dysfunction is common and results from decreased LV compliance and abnormal lusitropy. This usually results from the effects of hypertension and the RAA system.	Diastolic function should be suspected in symptomatic patients with normal ejection fraction; current treatment and prevention includes ACE inhibitors and beta blockers.
The hemodynamic and neurohumoral mechanisms of CHF include the RAA system and the SNS. Natriuretic factors and inflammatory and immune cytokines have also been implicated in CHF.	Management should include ACE inhibitors and beta-blockers. Experimental therapies for CHF include candotraxil (increases natriuretic factors), etanercept (TNFα blocker), and recombinant growth hormone.

Suggested Reading

Abraham, W. T. (2000). Beta-blockers: The new standard of therapy for mild heart failure. *Archives of Internal Medicine, 160,* 1237-1247.

Agnoletti, L., Curello, S., Bachetti, T., Malacarne, F., Gaia, G., Comini, L., Volterrani, M., Bonetti, P., Parrinello, G., Cadei, M., Grigolato, P. G., & Ferrari, R. (1999). Serum from patients with severe heart failure downregulates eNOS and is proapoptotic: Role of tumor necrosis factor-alpha. *Circulation, 100*(19), 1983-1991.

Albert, N. M. (1998). Advanced systolic heart failure: Emerging pathophysiology and current management. *Progress in Cardiovascular Nursing, 13*(3), 14-30.

Anonymous. (1999). Effect of metoprolol CR/XL in chronic heart failure: Metoprolol CR/XL randomised intervention trial in congestive heart failure (MERIT-HF). *Lancet, 353*(9169), 2001-2007.

Anonymous. (1997). The effect of digoxin on mortality and morbidity in patients with heart failure. The Digitalis Investigation Group. *New England Journal of Medicine, 336*(8), 525-533.

Baig, M. K., Mahon, N., McKenna, W. J., Caforio, A. L. P., Bonow, R. O., Francis, G. S., & Gheorghiade, M. (1999). The pathophysiology of advanced heart failure. *Heart & Lung, 28*(2), 87-101.

Belardinelli, R., Georgiou, D., Cianci, G., & Purcaro, A. (1999). Randomized, controlled trial of long-term moderate exercise training in chronic heart failure: Effects on functional capacity, quality of life, and clinical outcome. *Circulation, 99*(9), 1173-1182.

Bello, D., & Massie, B. M. (1998). The current role of amiodarone in patients with congestive heart failure. *Cleveland Clinic Journal of Medicine, 65*(9), 479-489.

Berry, C., & Clark, A. L. (2000). Catabolism in chronic heart failure. *European Heart Journal, 21,* 521-532.

Bonet, S., Agusti, A., Arnau, J. M., Vidal, X., Diogene, E., Galve, E., & Laporte, J. R. (2000). Beta-adrenergic blocking agents in heart failure—Benefits of vasodilating and nonvasodilating agents according to patients' characteristics: A meta-analyis of clinical trials. *Archives of Internal Medicine, 160*(5), 621-627.

Bristow, M. R. (2000). beta-adrenergic receptor blockade in chronic heart failure. *Circulation, 101,* 558-569.

Califf, R. M., & Cohn, J. N. (2000). Cardiac protection: Evolving role of angiotensin receptor blockers. *American Heart Journal, 139*(1 Pt 2), S15-S22.

Cohn, J. N. (2000). Heart failure: Future treatment approaches. *American Journal of Hypertension, 13,* 74S-78S.

Cohn, J. N., Ferrari, R., & Sharpe, N. (2000). Cardiac remodeling—Concepts and clinical implications: A consensus paper from an International Forum on Cardiac Remodeling. *Journal of the American College of Cardiology, 35,* 569-582.

Davila, D. F., Donis, J. H., Bellabarba, G., Torres, A., Casado, J., & Mazzei, D. D. (2000). Cardiac afferents and neurohormonal activation in congestive heart failure. *Medical Hypotheses, 54,* 242-253.

Davis, R. C., Hobbs, F. D., & Lip, G. Y. (2000). ABC of heart failure. History and epidemiology. *British Medical Journal, 320,* 39-42.

de Vries, R. J., van Veldhuisen, D. J., & Dunselman, P. H. (2000). Efficacy and safety of calcium channel blockers in heart failure: Focus on recent trials with second-generation dihydropyridines. *American Heart Journal, 139,* 185-194.

Diller, P. M., Smucker, D. R., David, B., & Graham, R. J. (1999). Congestive heart failure due to diastolic or systolic dysfunction. Frequency and patient characteristics in an ambulatory setting. *Archives of Family Medicine, 8*(5), 414-420.

Dries, D. L., & Stevenson, L. W. (2000). Brain natriuretic peptide as bridge to therapy for heart failure. *Lancet, 355,* 1112-1113.

Feldman, A. M., Combes, A., Wagner, D., Kadakomi, T., Kubota, T., Li, Y. Y., & McTiernan, C. (2000). The role of tumor necrosis factor in the pathophysiology of heart failure. *Journal of the American College of Cardiology, 35,* 537-544.

Gambassi, G., Lapane, K. L., Sgadari, A., Carbonin, P., Gatsonis, C., Lipsitz, L. A., Mor, V., & Bernabei, R. (2000). Effects of angiotensin-converting enzyme inhibitors and digoxin on health outcomes of very old patients with heart failure. SAGE Study Group. *Archives of Internal Medicine, 160*(1), 53-60.

Gandhi, S. K., Powers, J. C., Nomeir, A. M., Fowle, K., Kitzman, D. W., Rankin, K. M., & Little, W. C. (2001). The pathogenesis of acute pulmonary edema associated with hypertension. *New England Journal of Medicine, 344,* 17-22.

Gheorghiade, M., Cody, R. J., Francis, G. S., McKenna, W. J., Young, J. B., & Bonow, R. O. (2000). Current medical therapy for heart failure. *Heart & Lung, 29,* 16-32.

Ghio, S., Gavazzi, A., Campana, C., Inserra, C., Klersy, C., Sebastiani, R., Arbustini, E., Recusani, F., & Tavazzi, L. (2001). Independent and additive prognostic value of right ventricular systolic function and pulmonary artery pressure in patients with chronic heart failure. *Journal of the American College of Cardiology, 37,* 183-188.

Gomberg-Maitland, M., Baran, D. A., & Fuster, V. (2001). Guidelines for the primary care physician and the heart failure specialist. *Archives of Internal Medicine, 161,* 342-352.

Green, H. J., Duscha, B. D., Sullivan, M. J., Keteyian, S. J., & Kraus, W. E. (2001). Normal skeletal muscle Na(+)-K(+) pump concentration in patients with chronic heart failure. *Muscle & Nerve, 24,* 69-76.

Guazzi, M. (2000). Alveolar-capillary membrane dysfunction in chronic heart failure: Pathophysiology and therapeutic implications. *Clinical Science, 98,* 633-641.

Haji, S. A., & Movahed, A. (2000). Update on digoxin therapy in congestive heart failure. *American Family Physician, 62,* 409-416.

Harjai, K. J., Thompson, H. W., Turgut, T., & Shah, M. (2000). Simple clinical variables are markers of the propensity for readmission in patients hospitalized with heart failure. *American Journal of Cardiology, 87,* 234-237.

Hein, S., Kostin, S., Heling, A., Maeno, Y., & Schaper, J. (2000). The role of the cytoskeleton in heart failure. *Cardiovascular Research, 45,* 273-278.

Heindl, S., Dodt, C., Krahwinkel, M., Hasenfuss, G., & Andreas, S. (2001). Short term effect of continuous positive airway pressure on muscle sympathetic nerve activity in patients with chronic heart failure. *Heart, 85,* 185-190.

Herrera-Garza, E. H., Stetson, S. J., Cubillos-Garzon, A., Vooletich, M. T., Farmer, J. A., & Torre-Amione, G. (1999). Tumor necrosis factor-alpha—A mediator of disease progression in the failing human heart. *Chest, 115*(4), 1170-1174.

Lekuona, I., Laraudogoitia, E., Salcedo, A., & Sadaba, M. (2001). Congestive heart failure in a hypertensive patient (don't forget the stethoscope). *Lancet, 357,* 358.

Lindsay, S. J., Kearney, M. T., Prescott, R. J., Fox, K. A., & Nolan, J. (1999). Digoxin and mortality in chronic heart failure. UK heart investigation. *Lancet, 354*(9183), 1003.

Lonn, E., & McKelvie, R. (2000). Drug treatment in heart failure. *British Medical Journal, 320,* 1188-1192.

Mandinov, L., Eberli, F. R., Seiler, C., & Hess, O. M. (2000). Diastolic heart failure. *Cardiovascular Research, 45,* 813-825.

McMurray, J. J., & Stewart, S. (2000). Epidemiology, aetiology, and prognosis of heart failure. *Heart, 83,* 596-602.

Metra, M., Nodari, S., D'Aloia, A., Bontempi, L., Boldi, E., & Cas, L. D. (2000). A rationale for the use of beta-blockers as standard treatment for heart failure. *American Heart Journal, 139,* 511-521.

Millane, T., Jackson, G., Gibbs, C. R., & Lip, G. Y. (2000). ABC of heart failure. Acute and chronic management strategies. *British Medical Journal, 320,* 559-562.

Naccarelli, G. V., Wolbrette, D. L., Patel, H. M., & Luck, J. C. (2000). Amiodarone: Clinical trials. *Current Opinion in Cardiology, 15,* 64-72.

Niebauer, J., Volk, H-D., Kemp, P., et al. (1999). Endotoxin and immune activation in chronic heart failure: A prospective cohort study. *Lancet, 353,* 1838-1842.

Page, J., & Henry, D. (2000). Consumption of NSAIDs and the development of congestive heart failure in elderly patients—An underrecognized public health problem. *Archives of Internal Medicine, 160*(6), 777-784.

Parmley, W. W. (2000). Surviving heart failure: Robert L. Frye lecture. *Mayo Clinic Proceedings, 75*(1), 111-118.

Patel, A. R., Kuvin, J. T., Pandian, N. G., Smith, J. J., Udelson, J. E., Mendelsohn, M. E., Konstam, M. A., & Karas, R. H. (2001). Heart failure etiology affects peripheral vascular endothelial function after cardiac transplantation. *Journal of the American College of Cardiology, 37,* 195-200.

Pepper, G. S., & Lee, R. W. (1999). Sympathetic activation in heart failure and its treatment with beta-blockade. *Archives of Internal Medicine, 159*(3), 225-234.

Peters, R. W., & Gold, M. R. (2000). Pacing for patients with congestive heart failure and dilated cardiomyopathy. *Cardiology Clinics, 18,* 55-66.

Pitt, B., Zannad, F., Remme, W. J., Cody, R., Castaigne, A., Perez, A., Palensky, J., & Wittes, J. (1999). The effect of spironolactone on morbidity and mortality in patients with severe heart failure. Randomized Aldactone Evaluation Study Investigators. *New England Journal of Medicine, 341*(10), 709-717.

Polanczyk, C. A., Rohde, L. E., Dec, G. W., & DiSalvo, T. (2000). Ten-year trends in hospital care for congestive heart failure: Improved outcomes and increased use of resources. *Archives of Internal Medicine, 160*(3), 325-332.

Rich, M. W. (1999). Heart failure. *Cardiology Clinics, 17*(1), 123-135.

Roig, E., Perez-Villa, F., Morales, M., Jimenez, W., Orus, J., Heras, M., & Sanz, G. (2000). Clinical implications of increased plasma angiotensin II despite ACE inhibitor therapy in patients with congestive heart failure. *European Heart Journal, 21*(1), 53-57.

Sabbah, H. N. (2000). Apoptotic cell death in heart failure. *Cardiovascular Research, 45,* 704-712.

Schrier, R. W., & Abraham, W. T. (1999). Hormones and hemodynamics in heart failure. *New England Journal of Medicine, 341*(8), 577-585.

Singh, K., Communal, C., Sawyer, D. B., & Colucci, W. S. (2000). Adrenergic regulation of myocardial apoptosis. *Cardiovascular Research, 45,* 713-719.

Smit, A. J. (2000). Dopamine in heart failure and critical care. *Clinical & Experimental Hypertension (New York), 22,* 269-276.

Spargias, K. S., Hall, A. S., & Ball, S. G. (1999). Safety concerns about digoxin after acute myocardial infarction. *Lancet, 354*(9176), 391-392.

Spinale, F. G., Coker, M. L., Bond, B. R., & Zellner, J. L. (2000). Myocardial matrix degradation and metalloproteinase activation in the failing heart: A potential therapeutic target. *Cardiovascular Research, 46,* 225-238.

Stark, J. (1998). The interrelation between renal and cardiac function: Physiology and pathophysiology with a focus on congestive heart failure. *Critical Care Nursing Clinics of North America, 10*(4), 411-419.

Stevenson, L. W., Kormos, R. L., Bourge, R. C., Gelijns, A., Griffith, B. P., Hershberger, R. E., Hunt, S., Kirklin, J., Miller, L. W., Pae, W. E., Jr., Pantalos, G., Pennington, D. G., Rose, E. A., Watson, J. T., Willerson, J. T., Young, J. B., Barr, M. L., Costanzo, M. R., Desvigne-Nickens, P., Feldman, A. M., Frazier, O. H., Friedman, L., Hill, J. D., Konstam, M. A., McCarthy, P. M., Michler, R. E., Oz, M. C., Rosengard, B. R., Sapirstein, W., Shanker, R., Smith, C. R., Starling, R. C., Taylor, D. O., & Wichman, A. (2001). Mechanical cardiac support 2000: Current applications and future trial design. June 15-16, 2000; Bethesda, Maryland. *Journal of the American College of Cardiology, 37,* 340-370.

Torre-Amione, G., Vooletich, M. T., & Farmer, J. A. (2000). Role of tumour necrosis factor-alpha in the progression of heart failure: Therapeutic implications. *Drugs, 59,* 745-751.

Vasan, R. S., & Benjamin, E. J. (2001). Diastolic heart failure—No time to relax. *New England Journal of Medicine, 344,* 56-59.

Vasan, R. S., Larson, M. G., Benjamin, E. J., Evans, J. C., Reiss, C. K., & Levy, D. (1999). Congestive heart failure in subjects with normal versus reduced left ventricular ejection fraction: Prevalence and mortality in a population-based cohort. *Journal of the American College of Cardiology, 33*(7), 1948-1955.

Walker, C. A., Crawford, F. A., Jr., & Spinale, F. G. (2000). Myocyte contractile dysfunction with hypertrophy and failure: Relevance to cardiac surgery. *Journal of Thoracic & Cardiovascular Surgery, 119,* 388-400.

Walker, S., Levy, T. M., Coats, A. J., Peters, N. S., & Paul, V. E. (2000). Bi-ventricular pacing in congestive cardiac failure. Current experience and future directions. The Imperial College Cardiac Electrophysiology Group. *European Heart Journal, 21,* 884-889.

Westaby, S. (2000). Non-transplant surgery for heart failure. *Heart, 83,* 603-610.

Willenheimer, R., Rydberg, E., Cline, C., Broms, K., Hillberger, B., Oberg, L., & Erhardt, L. (2001). Effects on quality of life, symptoms and daily activity 6 months after termination of an exercise training programme in heart failure patients. *International Journal of Cardiology, 77,* 25-31.

Williams, R. S. (1999). Apoptosis and heart failure. *New England Journal of Medicine, 341*(10), 759-760.

Young J. (2000). Heart failure: Highlights from new consensus guidelines. *Cleveland Clinic Journal of Medicine, 67*(1), 13-16.

Zuccala, G., Onder, G., Pedone, C., Cocchi, A., Carosella, L., Cattel, C., Carbonin, P. U., & Bernabei, R. (2001). Cognitive dysfunction as a major determinant of disability in patients with heart failure: Results from a multicentre survey. On behalf of the GIFA (SIGG-ONLUS) Investigators. *Journal of Neurology, Neurosurgery & Psychiatry, 70*(1), 109-112.

Case Study*

Congestive Heart Failure

INITIAL HISTORY

- 66-year-old white male.
- Increasing shortness of breath over last month.
- Noticed feet and ankles swelling by end of the day.
- Has occasional episodes of chest tightness.
- Has been waking up in the middle of the night with acute shortness of breath.
- Feels tired most of the time.

Question 1   Based on this information, what is your differential diagnosis?

PAST MEDICAL/SURGICAL HISTORY

- History of transmural anterior wall; MI 7 years ago.
- 3-vessel coronary artery bypass graft surgery 7 years ago.
- 15-year history of hypertension.

SOCIAL HISTORY

- 2 pack/day smoker for 40 years; quit after bypass surgery.
- No alcohol or recreational drugs.
- Works as a janitor at a local elementary school.
- Married with 2 children.

FAMILY HISTORY

- Father had MI at age 50 and died at age 70 with MI.
- Mother had hypertension, diabetes, and died after a CVA at age 82.
- One brother, age 58, with hypertension who had a coronary stent placed at age 57.

CURRENT MEDICATIONS

- SL NTG 1/150 prn
- Metoprolol 50 mg bid
- ASA 1 daily

*Juanita Reigle contributed this case study.

Question 2 How has this additional information helped you focus your differential?

PHYSICAL EXAMINATION

- BP = 110/60 (sitting); AP 104; RR = 24 (increases with minimal activity, such as walking to exam room); T = 37.2 orally; WT = 82 kg.

HEENT, Skin, Neck

- Funduscopic exam normal.
- Skin is pale; cool extremities.
- Neck supple, no bruits over carotid arteries.
- No thyromegaly, no adenopathy.
- + jugular venous distension (JVD); increased 6 cm above sternal angle at 45 degrees.

Lungs

- Bibasilar crackles that do not clear with cough.

Cardiac

- Point of maximal impulse (PMI) displaced laterally.
- Normal S_1 S_2.
- + S_3 at apex.
- II/VI blowing holosystolic murmur at apex, radiating to axilla.

Abdomen, Extremities, Neurological

- Liver percusses to 12 cm in midclavicular line; no bruits.
- 2+ pitting edema in feet and ankles extending to midcalf bilaterally.
- 2+ radial pulses, 1+ dorsalis pedis, and 1+ posterior tibial pulses bilaterally; cool skin.
- Alert and oriented.
- Cranial nerves intact, sensory intact.
- Deep tendon reflexes (DTR) 2+ and symmetrical; strength 4/5 throughout.

Question 3 What findings on the physical exam support the diagnosis of heart failure?

Question 4 What studies would you initiate while preparing your interventions?

Question 5 What therapies would you initiate immediately while awaiting results of the laboratory studies?

LABORATORY RESULTS

- NA = 134 nmol/L WBC = 7800 mm^3
- K = 3.6 nmol/LHCT = 40 %
- BUN = 48 mg/dL HGB = 13.2 g/dL
- Cr = 1.9 mg/dLPLT = 219,000 mm^3
- GLU = 97 mg/dL
- CA = 8.6 mg/dL ALB = 3.2 g/dL
- MG = 2.2 mg/dL TSH = 0.64 μU/ml
- ALK PHOS = 60 U/L T4 = 1.4 μg/dL
- AST = 15 U/L
- pH = 7.34; PaCO$_2$ = 48 mmHg; PaO$_2$ = 90 mmHg (room air)

CHEST X-RAY AND READING

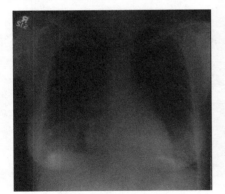 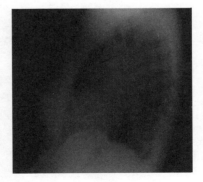

- Cardiomegaly
- Bilateral small pleural effusions (right > left)
- Perihilar infiltrates
- +Kerley B lines

ELECTROCARDIOGRAM

- Sinus tachycardia.
- Possible left atrial enlargement.
- Poor R wave progression V1-V3.
- No evidence of acute ischemia.
- Left ventricular hypertrophy (LVH) with strain.

Question 6   What additional therapies would you initiate based on the laboratory values?

EMERGENCY ROOM COURSE

- Pt diuresis 2500 cc clear yellow urine after administration of a loop diuretic.
- Bibasilar crackles diminish.
- Weight now 81.5 kg.

Question 7   Should this patient be prescribed spironolactone?

Question 8   What additional diagnostic and laboratory tests should be scheduled for further follow up?

Question 9   What discharge medications should be prescribed?

Question 10   What patient teaching should occur before discharge?

5

Asthma

DEFINITION

- "A *chronic inflammatory disorder* of the airways in which many cells and cellular elements play a role, in particular, mast cells, eosinophils, T lymphocytes, macrophages, neutrophils, and epithelial cells. In susceptible individuals, this inflammation causes *recurrent episodes* of wheezing, breathlessness, chest tightness, and coughing, particularly at night or in the early morning. These episodes are usually associated with widespread but variable *airflow obstruction that is often reversible* either spontaneously or with treatment. The inflammation also causes an associated increase in the existing *bronchial hyperresponsiveness to a variety of stimuli.* Subbasement membrane *fibrosis* may occur in some patients with asthma and these changes contribute to persistent abnormalities in lung function" (Second Expert Panel on the Management of Asthma; National Heart, Lung, and Blood Institute; 1997; p. 8).

- Asthma classification in the United States (according to the National Heart Lung and Blood Institute of the National Institutes of Health) is based on clinical severity (mild intermittent, mild persistent, moderate persistent, and severe persistent) (Table 5-1).

Table 5-1 Asthma Classification

Disease Category	Symptoms	Nocturnal Symptoms	Daily Medical for Long-term Control	Medical for Quick Relief
	Continual symptoms Limited physical activity Frequent exacerbations	Frequently	**Two daily medications** Antiinflammatory agent (high-dose inhaled glucocorticoid) **and** Long-acting bronchodilator (inhaled or oral β$_2$-agonist or theophylline) **and** Oral glucocorticoid	Short-acting inhaled β$_2$-agonist Daily use or increasing use indicates need for additional long-term therapy
STEP 3 Moderate persistent	Daily symptoms Daily use of inhaled short-acting β$_2$-agonist Exacerbations affect activity Exacerbations at least twice weekly and may last for days	More frequently than once weekly	**One or two daily medications** Antiinflammatory agent (medium-dose inhaled glucocorticoid) **and/or** Medium-dose inhaled glucocorticoid plus long-acting bronchodilator	Short-acting inhaled β$_2$-agonist Daily use or increasing use indicates need for additional long-term therapy
STEP 2 Mild persistent	Symptoms more frequent than twice weekly but less than once a day Exacerbations may affect activity	More frequently than once weekly	**One daily medication** Antiinflammatory agent (low-dose inhaled glucocorticoid, cromolyn, or nedocromil) **or** Sustained-release theophylline ***Note:*** Leukotriene modifiers may be considered for patients at least 12 years old.	Short-acting inhaled β$_2$-agonist Daily use or increasing use indicates need for additional long-term therapy
STEP 1 Mild intermittent	Symptoms no more frequent than twice weekly Asymptomatic and with normal PEFR between exacerbations Exacerbations brief (hours to days) Intensity of exacerbations varies	No more frequently than twice monthly	No daily medication	Short-acting inhaled β$_2$-agonist Used more than twice weekly indicates need to initiate long-term therapy

EPIDEMIOLOGY

- Approximately 5% of adults and 8% of children in the United States have asthma. It is estimated that 15 million people in the United States have asthma. There has been a significant increase in asthma incidence and mortality during recent decades, especially in minority populations.

- Risk factors

    - Over 20 genetic abnormalities have been linked to asthma including those for interleukin-4 (IL-4), inflammatory cytokines, interferon gamma (INFγ), beta adrenergic receptors, 5-lipoxygenase, and leukotriene C4 synthetase.

    - Allergen exposure (even during fetal life via transplacental leakage) increases the risk of asthma in genetically predisposed individual by shifting the immune system toward humoral (antibody-mediated) immunity. The most common allergens are dust mites, dog or cat dander, and cockroaches as the major causes of year-round symptoms; pollens and grasses for seasonal symptoms.

    - Urban residence with exposure to ozone, nitrogen and sulfur dioxide, carbon monoxide, tire debris, and particles from the combustion of fuels has been linked to increased asthma risk.

    - Occupational exposures such as dusts, chemicals and irritants have also been linked to asthma.

    - Recurrent respiratory viral infections (especially RSV) in childhood can increase the subsequent risk for asthma, and viruses are the most common cause of acute exacerbations of asthma. Viral infections cause inflammation and injury to lower respiratory airways (exposes sensory nerves) by inducing the release of a wide variety of inflammatory cytokines.

    - Gastroesophageal reflux disease (GERD) and allergic rhinitis have been linked to asthma risk.

PATHOPHYSIOLOGY

- **Inflammatory mechanisms in asthma**

    - Allergens are presented to the immune system by macrophages resulting in the activation of CD4 cells (T helper) which produce interleukins (especially IL-2, interferons, IL-4, IL-5, and IL-8). These cytokines activate other cells of inflammation including B lymphocytes, polymorphonucleocytes (PMN), eosinophils, and macrophages (Fig. 5-1).

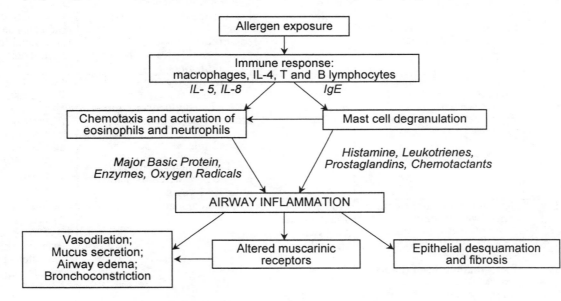

Fig. 5-1 Inflammatory Mechanisms in Asthma

- B cells produce IgE which attaches to receptors on the mast cells and results in mast cell degranulation; irritants can directly stimulate mast cell degranulation.

- Mast cell degranulation releases multiple mediators such as histamine, leukotrienes, prostaglandins, and inflammatory cell chemotactants causing intense airway inflammation.

- This inflammation causes bronchoconstriction, mucus secretion, and mucosal edema resulting in an acute attack..

- Eosinophils, lymphocytes, PMN, and macrophages cause direct tissue injury as well stimulate the release of toxic neuropeptides that can cause further desquamation of the bronchial epithelium leading to increased bronchial hyperresponsiveness.

- Inflammatory cytokines also alter muscarinic receptor function leading to increased levels of acetylcholine which causes bronchial smooth muscle contraction and mucus secretion.

- In allergic disease, there may be a late asthmatic response (LAR)—eosinophils release neuropeptides and lymphocytes are further activated resulting in a recurrence of bronchoconstriction at 4 to 12 hours after the initial attack.

- Evidence is mounting that untreated asthma can lead to long-term desquamation of the bronchial epithelium with increasing bronchial hyperresponsiveness and eventual scarring of the airways with permanent airway obstruction, i.e., airway remodeling (chronic airways obstruction CAO).

- **Pathophysiology of an acute asthma attack** (Fig. 5-2)

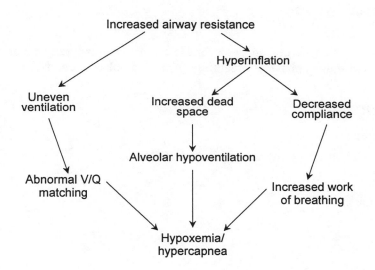

Fig. 5-2 Pathophysiology of Asthma Attack

- These pathophysiologic events produce airway obstruction that is worse with expiration.

- Airway obstruction leads to V/Q mismatch and hypoxemia early.

- Air trapping puts the respiratory muscles at a mechanical disadvantage with increased work of breathing that can eventually result in decreased ventilation and hypercapnia.

- Thus, most patients with acute symptoms start out with rapid respirations, hypoxemia, and a respiratory alkalosis, but persistent airway obstruction leads to shallow inefficient ventilation and respiratory acidosis.

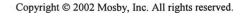

– Infants have greater peripheral airway resistance, fewer collateral channels of ventilation, further extension of airway smooth muscle into the peripheral airways, less elastic recoil, and mechanical disadvantage of the diaphragm. Edematous airways result in relatively greater obstruction to airflow with severe air trapping and hyperinflation, atelectasis, and decreased ventilation. Progression to respiratory failure can be rapid, close monitoring is critical.

PATIENT PRESENTATION

History

Allergic reactions, especially in children; allergic rhinitis and eczematous rashes are particularly common; *recurrent respiratory infections* such as "bronchitis" or "pneumonia" may be complications of asthma, or may represent misdiagnoses of asthma attacks; *episodic dyspnea and chest tightness,* initially may be related to allergic reactions or infections, but careful history can often bring out *exercise limitation; episodic audible wheezing,* worse during expiration but may be inspiratory in severe episodes; *recurrent cough*, airway inflammation may present with cough, especially at night or after exercise; *assess severity*, continuous versus intermittent symptoms; frequency of episodic symptoms; degree of exercise or activity limitation; presence and frequency of nocturnal symptoms.

Symptoms

Intermittent dry cough, wheezing, chest tightness, dyspnea often after a predictable stimulus (allergen, cold exposure, smoke, etc.); may be associated with rhinitis, postnasal drainage, pharyngitis, sputum production, or viral prodromal symptoms.

Examination

Anxiety, cyanosis, tachypnea, tachycardia, accessory muscle use, chest hyperexpansion; expiratory wheezing with prolonged expiratory phase of breathing; increased pulsus paradoxus.

DIFFERENTIAL DIAGNOSIS

- Bronchitis or bronchiolitis
- Exacerbation of chronic obstructive pulmonary disease (COPD)
- Pneumonia
- Allergic rhinitis and sinusitis
- Pneumonitis
- Anaphylaxis
- Foreign body
- Upper airway obstruction
- Congestive heart failure
- Pulmonary embolus
- Bronchogenic carcinoma
- Bronchopulmonary aspergillosis

KEYS TO ASSESSMENT

Assessment Between Attacks (diagnostic or to assess severity [see Table 5-1])

- Between attacks, the patient will often have a completely normal exam or there may be evidence of allergic rhinitis or rashes.

- Peak flow: once the diagnosis of asthma has been established, it is important to determine the "personal best" peak expiratory flow rate (PEFR).
    - Record the PEFR at home 2 to 4 times daily for 2 to 3 weeks, best if done in the early afternoon with the same meter each time.
    - Used to monitor response to therapy and to help with patient decision-making about management.
- Spirometry:
    - A reduction in forced expiratory volume in one second (FEV_1) of greater than 20% with acute attack or methacholine challenge.
    - A greater than 12% increase in FEV_1 after short-acting bronchodilator.
- Sputum stain may reveal the presence of eosinophils or mucoid casts.
- Allergy skin testing or radioallergosorbent testing (RAST) for patients with persistent asthma, recognized initiators for attacks, or other allergic symptoms.

Assessment of Acute Attack

- Level of consciousness, cyanosis.
- Respiratory rate, heart rate, blood pressure.
- Use of accessory muscles, lung expansion, expiratory phase, wheezing.
- Peak flow is used for monitoring the severity of airflow obstruction and contributes to management decisions; often a peak flow of <50% of predicted indicates the need for hospital admission.
- Pulsus paradoxus: drop in systolic blood pressure with inspiration of greater than 10 mmHg.
- Oximetry is adequate for assessment of oxygenation in patients who fall into the mild or moderate severity of exacerbation category, however is not adequate in more severe cases in that it does not test $PaCO_2$.
- Arterial blood gases: indicated in severe attacks and when oxygen saturation falls to <91%.
    - Calculate the A-a gradient.
    - Expect respiratory alkalosis and mild hypoxemia.
    - Normalization of arterial pH and carbon dioxide ($PaCO_2$) may indicate impending respiratory failure.
- Chest x-ray:
    - Only indicated if pneumothorax, pneumonia, or other complications are suspected.
    - May appear completely normal except for hyperexpansion.
    - Mucus plugging or infiltrates may be visible.
- Sputum: assess for evidence of bacterial infection.
- CBC and electrolyte analysis may reveal anemia, evidence of infection, or changes in potassium, magnesium, and phosphate.
- Electrocardiogram (ECG) is indicated in patients over 50 years of age or any with a history of cardiac disease; patients should be monitored while undergoing emergency treatment.

KEYS TO MANAGEMENT

- **Prevention and nonpharmacologic management:**
    - Treat any chronic sinusitis or gastroesophageal reflux disease.
    - Limit allergen or irritant exposure.

- Home peak flow monitoring.
- Consider immunotherapy in the atopic patient.
- Treat infections early.
- Annual influenza vaccine.
- Patient education.

- **Chronic:** management based on clinical severity (see Table 5-1).
    - In all patients, except those with mild intermittent symptoms (require use of a β-agonist inhaler less than twice per week), antiinflammatories are crucial for preventing long-term airway damage.
    - Inhaled steroids are safe and effective as first line antiinflammatory agents.
    - Recommend starting antiinflammatory therapy (inhaled corticosteroids) early, even in young children; latest studies suggest there is no growth retardation or other problems with inhaled steroids and that they are more effective than cromolyn in children.
    - The new leukotriene receptor antagonists may be used as first line drugs for mild to moderate persistent asthma but their efficacy is not as clearly proven as with inhaled steroids.
        1) Efficacy of leukotriene receptor antagonists: increase FEV_1 10% to 15% (half as much as with inhaled steroids) and provide a 40% to 60% reduction in exercise-induced bronchospasm, a 25% to 35% improvement in daytime and nocturnal asthma symptom scores, and a 30% to 60% decrease in exacerbation rates.
        2) Indications for leukotriene receptor antagonists: especially effective in exercise-induced and aspirin-sensitive asthma, mild to moderate asthma who fail to respond to inhaled steroids, moderate to severe asthma who have side effects to high-dose steroids, and patients with poor compliance with inhaled steroids due to improper technique or physical limitations.
    - β-agonists have been found to be safe and effective when used properly; new long-acting drugs (salmeterol) provide consistent control of symptoms.
    - Ipratropium may be additive but is controversial in the United States.
    - "Quick relief" drugs are used in addition to the antiinflammatory and long-acting beta$_2$-agonists, and for acute exacerbations.
    - Consider theophylline if symptoms persist or the patient has nighttime attacks.
    - Use oral steroids as a last resort; leukotriene receptor antagonists may allow for decreased oral steroid dependence.
    - Peak flows lowest at 0400; for nocturnal symptoms, consider evening medication dosing.
    - Other treatments/experimental:
        1) Cromones: cromolyn sodium (Intal) or nedocromil sodium (Tilade); decrease mast cell degranulation, improve response to inhaled antigen, aspirin, exercise, and cold air.
        2) Cyclosporin or methotrexate: only for severe steroid resistant asthma, side effects!
        3) Anti-immunoglobulin E (rhuMAb- E25): monoclonal IgG antibody to IgE blocks both the early and late phase response to allergen challenge; improves symptoms and FEV_1.
        4) Specific cytokine blockers: antibodies to IL-4, IL-5; interleukin production inhibitors (CCR-3); many others being studied.
    - Refer to asthma specialist for moderate to severe asthma.

- **Acute:** β-agonists remain the mainstay of therapy; steroids are crucial for treating the inflammatory process.
    - Must initiate management promptly without delaying for diagnostic tests.
    - Start oxygen; consider intubation at the first sign of hypercapnia.
    - Inhaled short-acting β-agonists by metered dose inhaler (MDI) or continuous nebulizer.
    - Prednisone orally (IV steroids indicated only if cannot take orally or life-threatening attack).
    - Consider ipratropium MDI or nebulized as adjunctive therapy.
    - Antibiotics, mucolytics, aggressive hydration, or chest physical therapy are not recommended.
    - Monitor needed for admission and late asthmatic response (4 to 8 hrs).

Pathophysiology $\rightarrow$ Clinical Link

What is going on in the disease process that influences how the patient presents and how he or she should be managed?

What should you do now that you understand the underlying pathophysiology?

Over 20 genetic abnormalities have been identified that are associated with asthma. The most frequently cited abnormality is one associated with an increase in IL-4.	$\rightarrow$ A family history of asthma and allergy is important, and new therapies are geared toward blocking IL-4 which is a key component of genetic predisposition in asthma.
Allergen exposure is a risk factor for both the development of asthma and for initiating acute attacks.	$\rightarrow$ History of exposure, skin testing, reduction in allergen exposure, and consideration for immunotherapy are all important in asthma assessment and management.
Respiratory viruses play a role in the natural history of asthma	$\rightarrow$ The role of vaccination and antivirals is being evaluated; use of steroid bursts during acute viral respiratory infections is being explored.
Mast cells release inflammatory mediators that cause bronchoconstriction, edema, and sputum production.	$\rightarrow$ Management must include antiinflammatories such as steroids and leukotriene receptor blockers as well as bronchodilators.
Eosinophils and neuropeptides cause the late asthmatic response.	$\rightarrow$ Recurrent symptoms can occur after 4 to 8 hours and the patient must be monitored during this time.
A combination of inflammatory mediators, neuropeptides, and immune responses lead to epithelial desquamation and chronic inflammation.	$\rightarrow$ Antiinflammatories MUST be used accurately and chronically to treat attack and to prevent long-term airway hyperresponsiveness and scarring.
Inflammatory mediators induce increased acetylcholine release which is a bronchoconstrictor.	$\rightarrow$ There are additive effects of inhaled anticholinergics (ipratropium) that may improve Beta agonist bronchodilation.
V/Q mismatch and hypoxemia with hypocapnia early but increased work of breathing may lead to hypercapnia and sudden respiratory failure.	$\rightarrow$ Arterial blood gases should be monitored carefully; oximetry is NOT adequate alone because it does not measure $PaCO_2$.

Suggested Reading

Abramson, M. J., Puy, R. M., & Weiner, J. M. (2000). Allergen immunotherapy for asthma. *Cochrane Database of Systematic Reviews [computer file]*, CD001186.

Anonymous. (2000). Long-term effects of budesonide or nedocromil in children with asthma. The Childhood Asthma Management Program Research Group. *New England Journal of Medicine, 343*(15), 1054-1063.

Ball, T. M., Castro-Rodriguez, J. A., Griffith, K. A., Holberg, C. J., Martinez, F. D., & Wright, A. L. (2000). Siblings, day-care attendance, and the risk of asthma and wheezing during childhood. *New England Journal of Medicine, 343*(8), 538-543.

Barnes, N. C. (2000). Effects of antileukotrienes in the treatment of asthma. *American Journal of Respiratory & Critical Care Medicine, 161,* S73-S76.

Beasley, R., Crane, J., Lai, C. K., & Pearce, N. (2000). Prevalence and etiology of asthma. *Journal of Allergy & Clinical Immunology, 105,* S466-S472.

Becker, A. B. (2000). Is primary prevention of asthma possible? *Pediatric Pulmonology, 30,* 63-72.

Blumenthal, M. N. (2000). Genetics of asthma and allergy. *Allergy & Asthma Proceedings, 21,* 55-59.

Bousquet, J., Jeffery, P. K., Busse, W. W., Johnson, M., & Vignola, A. M. (2000). Asthma. From bronchoconstriction to airways inflammation and remodeling. *American Journal of Respiratory & Critical Care Medicine, 161,* 1720-1745.

Braun, A., Lommatzsch, M., & Renz, H. (2000). The role of neurotrophins in allergic bronchial asthma. *Clinical & Experimental Allergy, 30,* 178-186.

Bresciani, M., Paradis, L., Des, R. A., Vernhet, H., Vachier, I., Godard, P., Bousquet, J., & Chanez, P. (2001). Rhinosinusitis in severe asthma. *Journal of Allergy & Clinical Immunology, 107,* 73-80.

Celli, B. R. (2000). The importance of spirometry in COPD and asthma: Effect on approach to management. *Chest, 117,* 15S-19S.

Chapman, K. R., Walker, L., Cluley, S., & Fabbri, L. (2000). Improving patient compliance with asthma therapy. *Respiratory Medicine, 94,* 2-9.

Chassany, O., & Fullerton, S. (2000). Meta-analysis of ipratropium bromide in adults with acute asthma. *American Journal of Medicine, 108*(7), 596-597.

Cochrane, M. G., Bala, M. V., Downs, K. E., Mauskopf, J., & Ben Joseph, R. H. (2000). Inhaled corticosteroids for asthma therapy: Patient compliance, devices, and inhalation technique. *Chest, 117,* 542-550.

Colavita, A., Reinach, A., & Peters, S. (2000). Contributing factors to the pathobiology of asthma. The Th1/Th2 paradigm. *Clinics in Chest Medicine, 21,* 263-277.

Crain, E. F., & Gershel, J. C. (2000). Emergency care of asthma. *Respiratory Care Clinics of North America, 6,* 135-154.

Creticos, P. S. (2000). The consideration of immunotherapy in the treatment of allergic asthma. *Journal of Allergy & Clinical Immunology, 105,* S559-S574.

Crombie, I. K., Wright, A., Irvine, L., Clark, R. A., & Slane, P. W. (2001). Does passive smoking increase the frequency of health service contacts in children with asthma? *Thorax, 56,* 9-12.

Dauletbaev, N., Rickmann, J., Viel, K., Buhl, R., Wagner, T. O., & Bargon, J. (2001). Glutathione in induced sputum of healthy individuals and patients with asthma. *Thorax, 56,* 13-18.

Djukanovic, R. (2000). Asthma: A disease of inflammation and repair. *Journal of Allergy & Clinical Immunology, 105,* S522-S526.

Dupre, D., Audrezet, M. P., & Ferec, C. (2000). Atopy and a mutation in the interleukin-4 receptor gene. *New England Journal of Medicine, 343*(1), 69-70.

Fahy, J. V. (2000). Reducing IgE levels as a strategy for the treatment of asthma. *Clinical & Experimental Allergy, 30*(Suppl 1), 16-21.

Fireman, P. (2000). Rhinitis and asthma connection: Management of coexisting upper airway allergic diseases and asthma. *Allergy & Asthma Proceedings, 21,* 45-54.

Fogarty, A., & Britton, J. (2000). The role of diet in the aetiology of asthma. *Clinical & Experimental Allergy, 30,* 615-627.

Fuhlbrigge, A. L., Kitch, B. T., Paltiel, A. D., Kuntz, K. M., Neumann, P. J., Dockery, D. W., & Weiss, S. T. (2001). FEV(1) is associated with risk of asthma attacks in a pediatric population. *Journal of Allergy & Clinical Immunology, 107,* 61-67.

Gereda, J. E., Leung, D. Y., Thatayatikom, A., Streib, J. E., Price, M. R., Klinnert, M. D., & Liu, A. H. (2000). Relation between house-dust endotoxin exposure, type 1 T-cell development, and allergen sensitization in infants at high risk of asthma. *Lancet, 355*(9216), 1680-1683.

Gern, J. E. (2000). Viral and bacterial infections in the development and progression of asthma. *Journal of Allergy & Clinical Immunology, 105,* S497-S502.

Gibson, P. G., Henry, R. L., & Coughlan, J. L. (2000). Gastro-esophageal reflux treatment for asthma in adults and children. *Cochrane Database of Systematic Reviews [computer file],* CD001496.

Gosset, P., Lamblin-Degros, C., Tillie-Leblond, I., Charbonnier, A. S., Joseph, M., Wallaert, B., Kochan, J. P., & Tonnel, A. B. (2001). Modulation of high-affinity IgE receptor expression in blood monocytes: Opposite effect of IL-4 and glucocorticoids. *Journal of Allergy & Clinical Immunology, 107,* 114-122.

Hamid, Q. A., & Minshall, E. M. (2000). Molecular pathology of allergic disease: I: Lower airway disease. *Journal of Allergy & Clinical Immunology, 105*(1 Pt 1), 20-36.

Hammarquist, C., Burr, M. L., & Gotzsche, P. C. (2000). House dust mite control measures for asthma. *Cochrane Database of Systematic Reviews [computer file]*, CD001187.

Harper, D. S., Cox, R., Summers, D., Butler, W., & Hagan, L. (2001). Tobacco hypersensitivity and environmental tobacco smoke exposure in a pediatric population. *Annals of Allergy, Asthma, & Immunology, 86*, 59-61.

Havinga, W. (2001). Risk of asthma. *Lancet, 357*, 313-314.

Henriksen, A. H., Holmen, T. L., & Bjermer, L. (2001). Sensitization and exposure to pet allergens in asthmatics versus non-asthmatics with allergic rhinitis. *Respiratory Medicine, 95*, 122-129.

Hirst, S. J. (2000). Airway smooth muscle as a target in asthma. *Clinical Experimental Allergy, 30*(Suppl 1), 54-59.

Holgate, S. T., & Sampson, A. P. (2000). Antileukotriene therapy. *American Journal of Respiratory & Critical Care Medicine, 161*, S147-S153.

Holt, P. G., & Sly, P. D. (2000). Prevention of adult asthma by early intervention during childhood: Potential value of new generation immunomodulatory drugs. *Thorax, 55*, 700-703.

Homer, R., & Elias, J. (2000). Consequences of long-term inflammation. Airway remodeling. *Clinics in Chest Medicine, 21*, 331-343.

Horiuchi, T., & Castro, M. (2000). The pathobiologic implications for treatment. Old and new strategies in the treatment of chronic asthma. *Clinics in Chest Medicine, 21*, 381-393.

Htut, T., Higenbottam, T. W., Gill, G. W., Darwin, R., Anderson, P. B., & Syed, N. (2001). Eradication of house dust mite from homes of atopic asthmatic subjects: A double-blind trial. *Journal of Allergy & Clinical Immunology, 107*, 55-60.

Jones, A. P. (2000). Asthma and the home environment. *Journal of Asthma, 37*, 103-124.

Joos, G. F., Germonpre, P. R., & Pauwels, R. A. (2000). Neural mechanisms in asthma. *Clinical & Experimental Allergy, 30*(Suppl 1), 60-65.

Kraft, M. (2000). The role of bacterial infections in asthma. *Clinics in Chest Medicine, 21*, 301-313.

Laitinen, L. A., Altraja, A., Karjalainen, E. M., & Laitinen, A. (2000). Early interventions in asthma with inhaled corticosteroids. *Journal of Allergy & Clinical Immunology, 105*, S582-S585.

Lemanske, R. F., Jr. (2000). Inflammatory events in asthma: An expanding equation. *Journal of Allergy & Clinical Immunology, 105*, S633-S636.

Litonjua, A. A., Carey, V. J., Burge, H. A., Weiss, S. T., & Gold, D. R. (2001). Exposure to cockroach allergen in the home is associated with incident doctor-diagnosed asthma and recurrent wheezing. *Journal of Allergy & Clinical Immunology, 107*, 41-47.

Mandelberg, A., Tsehori, S., Houri, S., Gilad, E., Morag, B., & Priel, I. E. (2000). Is nebulized aerosol treatment necessary in the pediatric emergency department? *Chest, 117*(5), 1309-1313.

Manser, R., Reid, D., & Abramson, M. (2000). Corticosteroids for acute severe asthma in hospitalized patients. *Cochrane Database of Systematic Reviews [computer file]*, CD001740.

Mash, B., Bheekie, A., & Jones, P. W. (2000). Inhaled vs oral steroids for adults with chronic asthma. *Cochrane Database of Systematic Reviews [computer file]*, CD002160.

Matricardi, P. M., Rosmini, F., Riondino, S., Fortini, M., Ferrigno, L., Rapicetta, M., & Bonini, S. (2000). Exposure to foodborne and orofecal microbes versus airborne viruses in relation to atopy and allergic asthma. *British Medical Journal, 320*(7232), 412-417.

McDowell, K. M. (2000). Pathophysiology of asthma. *Respiratory Care Clinics of North America, 6*, 15-26.

McFadden E., & Hejal, R. (2000). The pathobiology of acute asthma. *Clinics in Chest Medicine, 21*, 213-223.

McFadden, E. R., Jr. (2000). Natural history of chronic asthma and its long-term effects on pulmonary function. *Journal of Allergy & Clinical Immunology, 105*, S535-S539.

Meltzer, E. O. (2000). Role for cysteinyl leukotriene receptor antagonist therapy in asthma and their potential role in allergic rhinitis based on the concept of "one linked airway disease." *Annals of Allergy, Asthma, & Immunology, 84*, 176-185.

Menzies-Gow, A., & Robinson, D. S. (2000). Eosinophil chemokines and their receptors: An attractive target in asthma? *Lancet, 355*(9217), 1741-1743.

Muro, S. Minshall, E., & Qutayba, A. (2000) The pathology of chronic asthma. *Clinics in Chest Medicine, 21*, 225-244.

Nafstad, P., Magnus, P., & Jaakkola, J. J. (2000). Early respiratory infections and childhood asthma. *Pediatrics, 106*(3), E38.

Nelson, H. S. (2000). The importance of allergens in the development of asthma and the persistence of symptoms. *Journal of Allergy & Clinical Immunology, 105*, S628-S632.

Ober, C., & Moffatt, M. (2000). Contributing factors to the pathobiology. The genetics of asthma. *Clinics in Chest Medicine, 21*, 245-261.

Pearce, N., Douwes, J., & Beasley, R. (2000). Is allergen exposure the major primary cause of asthma? *Thorax, 55*, 424-431.

Platts-Mills, T. A., Rakes, G., & Heymann, P. W. (2000). The relevance of allergen exposure to the development of asthma in childhood. *Journal of Allergy & Clinical Immunology, 105*, S503-S508.

Plotnick, L. H., & Ducharme, F. M. (2000). Combined inhaled anticholinergic agents and beta-2-agonists for initial treatment of acute asthma in children. *Cochrane Database of Systematic Reviews [computer file]*, CD000060.

CHAPTER 5 Asthma **79**

Redington, A. E. (2000). Fibrosis and airway remodelling. *Clinical & Experimental Allergy, 30*(Suppl 1), 42-45.

Reicin, A., White, R., Weinstein, S. F., Finn, A. F., Jr., Nguyen, H., Peszek, I., Geissler, L., & Seidenberg, B. C. (2000). Montelukast, a leukotriene receptor antagonist, in combination with loratadine, a histamine receptor antagonist, in the treatment of chronic asthma. *Archives of Internal Medicine, 160*(16), 2481-2488.

Reinke, L. F., & Hoffman, L. (2000). Asthma education: A partnership. *Heart & Lung, 29*(3), 225-236.

Richter, J. E. (2000). Gastroesophageal reflux disease and asthma: The two are directly related. *American Journal of Medicine, 108*(Suppl 4a), 153S-158S.

Rosenwasser, L. J. (2000). New immunopharmacologic approaches to asthma: Role of cytokine antagonism. *Journal of Allergy & Clinical Immunology, 105,* S586-S591.

Rowe, B. H., Spooner, C., Ducharme, F. M., Bretzlaff, J. A., & Bota, G. W. (2000). Early emergency department treatment of acute asthma with systemic corticosteroids. *Cochrane Database of Systematic Reviews [computer file], CD002178.*

Salvi, S. S., & Babu, K. S. (2000). Treatment of allergic asthma with monoclonal anti-IgE antibody. *New England Journal of Medicine, 342*(17), 1292-1293.

Sampson, A. P. (2000). The role of eosinophils and neutrophils in inflammation. *Clinical & Experimental Allergy, 30*(Suppl 1), 22-27.

Schuh, S., Reisman, J., Alshehri, M., Dupuis, A., Corey, M., Arseneault, R., & Canny, G. (2000). A comparison of inhaled fluticasone and oral prednisone for children with severe acute asthma. *New England Journal of Medicine, 343*(10), 689-694.

Second Expert Panel on the Management of Asthma; National Heart, Lung, and Blood Institute. (1997). *Highlights of the Expert Panel report 2: Guidelines for the diagnosis and management of asthma.* Bethesda, MD: National Institutes of Health (Pub. No. HIN 97-4051A).

Silkoff, P. E., Robbins, R. A., Gaston, B., Lundberg, J. O., & Townley, R. G. (2000). Endogenous nitric oxide in allergic airway disease. *Journal of Allergy & Clinical Immunology, 105,* 438-448.

Silverman, R. (2000) Treatment of acute asthma. *Clinics in Chest Medicine, 21,* 361-379.

Stephens, M. B. (2000). Is there a clinical difference in outcomes when beta-agonist therapy is delivered through metered-dose inhaler (MDI) with a spacing device compared with standard nebulizer treatments in acutely wheezing children? *Journal of Family Practice, 49*(8), 760-761.

Suissa, S., Ernst, P., Benayoun, S., Baltzan, M., & Cai, B. (2000). Low-dose inhaled corticosteroids and the prevention of death from asthma. *New England Journal of Medicine, 343*(5), 332-336.

Tuffaha, A., Gern, J., & Lemanski, R. (2000). The role of respiratory viruses in acute and chronic asthma. *Clinics in Chest Medicine, 21,* 289-300.

Vignola, A. M., Chanez, P., Bonsignore, G., Godard, P., & Bousquet, J. (2000). Structural consequences of airway inflammation in asthma. *Journal of Allergy & Clinical Immunology, 105,* S514-S517.

Wills-Karp, M. (2001). IL-12/IL-13 axis in allergic asthma. *Journal of Allergy & Clinical Immunology, 107,* 9-18.

Wong, C. A., Walsh, L. J., Smith, C. J., Wisniewski, A. F., Lewis, S. A., Hubbard, R., Cawte, S., Green, D. J., Pringle, M., & Tattersfield, A. E. (2000). Inhaled corticosteroid use and bone-mineral density in patients with asthma. *Lancet, 355*(9213), 1399-1403.

Case Study

Asthma

INITIAL HISTORY

- 15-year-old girl presents to the emergency department complaining of chest tightness and dyspnea.
- She was mowing the lawn when these symptoms developed.
- She describes a prodrome of rhinorrhea and tearing that began soon after she went outside, followed by the chest symptoms.
- She felt no better after going inside.
- It is now 1 hour later.

Question 1   What is your differential diagnosis based on the information you have now?

Question 2   What other questions would you like to ask now?

ADDITIONAL HISTORY

- History of asthma since childhood; mother and brother also have asthma.
- Allergic to grass, ragweed, cats.
- She has a cough productive of clear phlegm that comes and goes.
- She has used a "blue" inhaler when needed for the past 6 months, as often as twice a day.
- No other medical history.

Question 3   Now what do you think about her history?

PHYSICAL EXAMINATION

- Alert but anxious teenager; in some respiratory distress; using accessory muscle of respiration.
- T = 37 orally; P = 105 beats/min and regular; RR = 30 breaths/min and labored; BP = 115/68 mmHg sitting.

HEENT, Skin, Neck

- Conjunctiva inflamed and edematous, tearing; fundi without lesions; nasal mucosa edematous, clear discharge; pharynx with clear postnasal drainage.
- Skin flushed and pink; diaphoretic; supple.
- No adenopathy; no thyromegaly, no bruits.

Lungs

- Chest expansion somewhat limited; diaphragms percuss low in posterior chest with 2 cm movement bilaterally.
- Prolonged expiratory phase with expiratory wheezes heard throughout all lung fields.
- Scattered coarse rhonchi; no rales or egophony.

Cardiac

- Heart sounds distant; tachycardia but regular.
- Slight systolic ejection murmur (SEM) LLSB without radiation; no gallops or clicks.

Abdomen, Extremities, Neurological

- Abdomen nondistended; bowel sounds present and not hyperactive; liver percusses 2 cm below RCM but overall size 8 cm; no tenderness or masses.
- Extremities clammy but good capillary refill at 3 seconds; no edema; no clubbing.
- Alert, oriented but anxious; cranial nerves intact; strength 5/5 throughout; DTR 2+ and symmetrical; sensory intact to touch.

Question 4   What studies would you initiate now while preparing your interventions?

Question 5   What therapies would you initiate immediately while awaiting results of the lab studies?

LABORATORY RESULTS
- pH = 7.55, PaO_2 = 65, $PaCO_2$ = 30 (RA); peak flow = 200 (<50% of predicted); electrolytes normal
- HCT = 37%, WBC = 5500, PLTS = 340,000
- ECG = sinus tachycardia

Question 6   What is her A-a gradient?

EMERGENCY ROOM COURSE
- The patient becomes increasingly dyspneic despite nebulizer and O_2.
- She is also becoming more anxious and confused.

PHYSICAL EXAM NOW
- P = 110 and regular; RR = 40 and labored; BP = 130/90.
- Lungs with inspiratory and expiratory wheezes; early cyanosis.
- Extremities cold and clammy; no longer alert or oriented.

REPEAT LAB STUDIES
- pH = 7.35, PaO_2 = 45, $PaCO_2$ = 42 (40% mask)
- Peak flow = cannot cooperate
- Heart monitor = sinus tachycardia

Question 7   What do you think is happening? Why is she more dyspneic? What does her lung exam suggest? Why are her extremities cold? Why is her color changing? Why is she confused? What do her blood gases mean?

Question 8   What interventions should be initiated now?

RESPONSE TO THERAPY
- Gradual return of respiratory rate to 35, pulse to 100; color improves; more alert.
- Lungs with expiratory wheezes only; peak flow = 180.
- pH = 7.48, PaO_2 = 90, $PaCO_2$ = 32 (60% mask).

Question 9   Now what should be done and what can the patient expect?

HOSPITAL COURSE
- Patient does well with normalization of labs.
- Tired but breathing normally after 3 days.
- Discharged on 4th day.

Question 10   What instructions and medications should this patient go home with? What should the chronic pharmacologic management of her asthma be?

Question 11   What steps can she take to prevent future attacks?

6

Chronic Obstructive Pulmonary Disease

DEFINITION

- Chronic obstructive pulmonary disease (COPD) is a syndrome characterized by abnormal tests of expiratory airflow that do not change markedly over periods of several months of observation.
- Pathologic lung changes are consistent with emphysema or chronic bronchitis.
    - **Emphysema:** reduced elastic recoil and disintegration of alveolar walls with bulla formation, expiratory airway collapse with air trapping and hyperinflation.
    - **Chronic bronchitis:** chronic cough productive of phlegm for at least 3 months per year for at least 2 consecutive years.
- Airflow limitation is worse during expiration (as measured by the forced expiratory volume in one second [FEV_1]) and does not show major reversibility in response to pharmacological agents.
- COPD may also include chronic asthmatic bronchitis which has a reversible component to the airflow limitation but progresses and becomes less reversible.

EPIDEMIOLOGY

- Fourth leading cause of death in the United States. It is estimated that over 16 million people in the U.S. and 20% of people in the industrialized world have symptomatic COPD.
- Risk factors
    - Smoking accounts for >90% of the risk for COPD and approximately 15% of smokers get COPD. Some smokers are considered "susceptible" and develop very rapid declines in lung function. Environmental smoke exposure has been linked to decreased lung function and increased risk of obstructive lung diseases in children.
    - There is an increased risk for COPD for first-degree relatives who smoke. In less than 1% of persons with COPD, there is an inherited α1-antitrypsin gene defect that causes early onset of emphysema.
    - Recurrent childhood respiratory infections are associated with a lower maximal attained level of pulmonary function and an increased risk for development of COPD as an adult. Chronic respiratory infections, such as with adenovirus and chlamydia, may play a role in the development of COPD.
    - Occupational dust exposure (gold, cadmium, coal) is as an independent risk factor for COPD.
    - Air pollution and urban living are associated with an increased risk for COPD morbidity.
- **Emphysema:** reduced elastic recoil resulting in expiratory airway collapse and hyperinflation; disintegration of alveolar walls and bulla formation.
    - In the lung, there is a normal balance between proteases that promote lung remodeling (elastases) and antiproteases that inhibit lung remodeling (antielastases such as alpha$_1$-antitrypsin) (Fig. 6-1, next page).

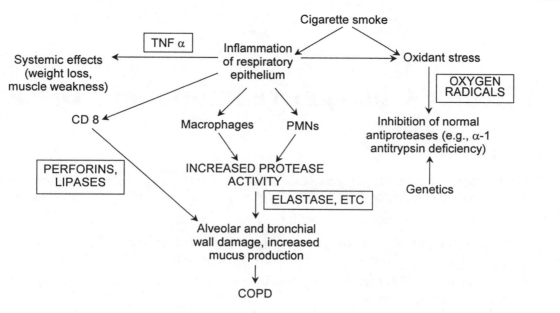

Fig. 6-1 Pathogenesis of Emphysema

- Cigarette smoke results in oxidant stress (production of toxic oxygen radicals) that inhibits the activity of the normal antiproteases.

- Inflammation of the respiratory epithelium, and the associated activity of T cytotoxic lymphocytes (CD8), macrophages, and polymorphonucleocytes (PMNs), results in increased protease (elastase) activity and direct damage to the lung.

- This imbalance between proteases and antiproteases results in alveolar and bronchial wall damage and increased mucus production.

- Production of inflammatory cytokines such as tumor necrosis factor α (TNF α) results in systemic symptoms such as weight loss and muscle weakness.

- Airway collapse during expiration with airtrapping leads to hyperexpansion of the lung and chest wall putting the muscles of respiration at a mechanical disadvantage and increasing the work of breathing. This leads to decreased tidal volume and hypercapnia.

- Loss of alveolar surface area and abnormalities of the alveolar capillary barrier lead to decreased gas exchange and result in hypoxemia.

• **Chronic bronchitis:** chronic cough productive of phlegm for at least 3 months per year for at least 2 consecutive years.

- Goblet cells in the airway mucosa are increased with hypertrophy and hyperplasia of submucosal glands and production of copious amounts of tenacious sputum. Microorganisms (especially bacteria) can adhere and grow with persistent colonization of the airways and cause recurrent infectious exacerbations.

- The associated epithelial inflammation and smooth muscle hypertrophy lead to scarring.

• **Both emphysema and chronic bronchitis.**

- COPD (both chronic bronchitis and emphysema) results in expiratory airway obstruction and ventilation/perfusion (V/Q) mismatch.

– Expiratory airway obstruction and airtrapping put the respiratory muscles at a mechanical disadvantage with increased work of breathing.

  1) Shallow rapid breathing is inefficient.

  2) Muscle weakness worsens ventilation.

– Ventilation/perfusion mismatch leads to hypoxemia.

– Thus, most patients will develop a mixed hypoxemia and hypercapnia.

– Chronic hypercapnia can lead to decreased sensitivity of the respiratory center such that the patient becomes insensitive to changes in $PaCO_2$, and thus dependent on the chemoreception of low PaO_2 as the main stimulus to breathing. Supplemental oxygen may eliminate this stimulus resulting in decreased ventilatory response and additional carbon dioxide retention.

– Diffuse pulmonary damage with hypoxemia and hypercapnia results in widespread pulmonary arteriolar vasoconstriction and increased pulmonary artery pressures. The right ventricle responds poorly to this increased workload and may dilate and fail with increased pressures being transmitted to the systemic venous circulation and resultant peripheral edema (*cor pulmonale).*

– Superimposed infection and bronchospasm result in acute exacerbations with worsening gas exchange.

PATIENT PRESENTATION

History

Active or passive smoking history; occupational history; recurrent respiratory infections; progressive exercise limitation; family history (especially if in nonsmoker); weight loss; sputum production.

Symptoms

Progressive dyspnea on exertion; paroxysmal nocturnal dyspnea; pedal edema; productive cough; wheezing, pedal edema or abdominal fullness (cor pulmonale).

Examination

Decreased level of consciousness and cyanosis during severe exacerbations; tachypnea; increased anterior-posterior chest diameter (barrel chest); use of accessory muscles of breathing, low diaphragms on percussion; decreased breath sounds; prolonged expiratory phase of breathing; expiratory wheezing and coarse crackles; clubbing, cyanosis, and pedal edema (advanced disease).

DIFFERENTIAL DIAGNOSIS

- Asthma
- Acute bronchitis
- Pneumonia
- Bronchiectasis
- Congestive heart failure
- Pulmonary fibrosis
- Recurrent pulmonary emboli

KEYS TO ASSESSMENT

- It is crucial to assess acuteness of onset of symptoms and deviation from "baseline."
- New pedal edema may indicate worsening hypoxemia/hypercapnia and *cor pulmonale.*

- Spirometry, all results are compared to "predicted" values based on gender, age, and height.
  - Decreased FEV_1 (forced expiratory volume in first second of expiration).
  - Decrease in FEV_1 greater than any decrease in FVC (forced vital capacity); decreased FEV_1/FVC ratio (<70%).
  - Decreased FEF_{25-75} (forced expiratory flow during middle 50% of total expiratory volume).
  - No significant improvement with bronchodilator treatment (<20%).
  - Specialized pulmonary function testing includes the DLCO and oxygen desaturation with exercise.
- High resolution spiral computed tomography can diagnose COPD with high sensitivity.
- Arterial blood gases (ABG) are useful for evaluating the severity of pulmonary dysfunction in both the stable COPD patient (establish baseline values) and during acute exacerbations.
  - Look for both hypercapnia and hypoxemia (oximetry is inadequate for these patients in that it does not indicate the $PaCO_2$).
  - Acidosis is a clear indicator of acute hypercapnia.
  - Severe hypoxemia should not be tolerated even in the patient with long-standing advanced COPD; institution of oxygen therapy requires close monitoring of ABG for increasing hypercapnia, and ventilation may be required.
- Chest x-ray is often normal until late-stage disease but is useful for documenting infection.
  - Expect flattened diaphragms, increased retrosternal space, enlarged pulmonary arteries, bullae, and scarring in emphysema.
  - Look closely for pneumothorax or acute infiltrates.
- Sputum stain and culture is useful for the diagnosis of chronic bronchitis and for evaluating acute exacerbations of COPD.
  - Look for polymorphonucleocytes and bacteria on gram stain.
  - The most common microorganisms include *H. influenzae, M. catarrhalis*, and *S. pneumoniae*; in patients with advanced disease, consider *P. aeruginosa*.

KEYS TO MANAGEMENT

- Prevention and nonpharmacologic treatment
  - **Smoking cessation:** many modalities available, including hypnosis, nicotine replacements (nasal, oral, dermal), buspirone, and support groups.
    1) Causes some prompt improvement in pulmonary function.
    2) Slows the rate of lung function decline over years.
    3) Reduces number of infectious complications and exacerbations.
    4) Often associated with an increase in cough and anxiety during first few weeks.
    5) Frequent follow-up contacts between the provider and the patient improves the chances for long-term smoking cessation.
  - **Oxygen therapy:** in an acute exacerbation with severe hypoxemia, oxygen is vital to sustain life; in patients with sustained hypoxemia and cor pulmonale, home oxygen therapy improves exercise tolerance and survival.
  - **Nutrition:** low body weight is correlated with decreased respiratory muscle strength and increased mortality; dietary supplements and rapid institution of supplemental feeding if hospitalized is crucial.

- **Vaccination:** regular influenza and pneumococcal.

- **Rehabilitation:** some techniques are more effective than others but all are potentially helpful; breathing control techniques, chest physical therapy, exercise training, respiratory muscle training, occupational therapy.

- **Education:** studies show patients instructed about their disease and the implications of treatment can better understand, recognize, and treat the symptoms of their disease.

- **Psychological support:** anxiety, depression and fatigue are common in patients with COPD; evidence is strong that participation in a rehabilitation program with education, exercise, and relaxation techniques was more effective in reducing anxiety than is psychotherapy.

- **Referral for possible surgery:** several techniques are now available for carefully selected patients, including lung volume reduction surgery, bullectomy, and lung transplant, resulting in improved dyspnea and pulmonary function testing.

- Chronic pharmacotherapy

  - **Ipratropium:** the first-line drug for stable COPD (instead of beta$_2$-agonists) due to its more prolonged effectiveness with few side effects and some evidence that it may slow the progression of disease; it should be used regularly rather than prn; new longer acting agents, such as tiotropium, may improve adherence.

  - **Inhaled Beta$_2$-agonists:** now considered second-line drugs that can be used to supplement ipratropium (combination inhalers are available); long-acting drugs (e.g., salmeterol) may result in significant improvement in symptoms, especially through the night.

  - **Theophylline:** controversial benefit:risk ratio; may be useful at night for sustained relief during sleep; serum levels and potential drug interactions should be monitored carefully.

  - **Steroids:** unlike in asthma, antiinflammatory drugs are not necessary for airway protection in COPD and only about 20% of patients will improve with steroids, thus a therapeutic trial should be conducted only in severe COPD and the drug discontinued if there is no measurable improvement in FEV$_1$ in 2 weeks. In steroid responsive patients, a trial of inhaled steroids should be considered.

- Management of acute exacerbation

  - Rapid assessment of status, obtain IV access.

  - Begin oxygen, give patient enough to relieve significant hypoxemia (goal of PaO$_2$ $\geq$55 mmHg) but watch for increasing hypercapnia (oximetry is not adequate for full assessment and management); consider noninvasive mechanical ventilation.

  - Begin beta$_2$-agonist by continuous nebulizer or q 20 minutes; metered dose inhalers can also be used.

  - Give ipratropium 2 puffs 5 minutes after first beta$_2$-agonist dose.

  - **Antibiotics:** some studies show no benefit of antibiotics for acute exacerbations unless there is evidence of infection (fever, leukocytosis, purulent sputum, new infiltrate on x-ray), however, other more recent articles suggest they should be used in all acute exacerbations; more trials are pending.

  - Consider theophylline; some still give for all acute exacerbations, others only use it if the patient is already on theophylline with sub therapeutic level.

  - **Steroids:** recent studies show significant improvement in outcomes in hospitalized patients with acute exacerbations of COPD, the only significant complication was hyperglycemia.

Pathophysiology $\rightarrow$ Clinical Link

What is going on in the disease process that influences how the patient presents and how he or she should be managed?

What should you do now that you understand the underlying pathophysiology?

Pathophysiology		Clinical Link
A small minority of patients have a genetic deficiency of the antielastase α_1-antitrypsin as the cause of early-onset emphysema.	$\rightarrow$	A careful examination of family history and genetic testing is indicated in patients with early onset COPD symptoms, especially if there is a minimal smoking history.
Cigarette smoke results in bronchial epithelial inflammation and toxic oxygen radical destruction of antielastases which, in turn, lead to damage to alveoli and bronchi.	$\rightarrow$	Smoking cessation is vital to slow disease progression but will not normalize lung function.
Damage to bronchial mucosa and the elastin in bronchial walls results in expiratory airway obstruction due to either loss of airway elasticity, increased mucous production, or both.	$\rightarrow$	Patients with both emphysema and chronic bronchitis present with dyspnea, prolonged expiration and wheezing.
Expiratory obstruction with airtrapping, increased work of breathing, and uneven ventilation result in decreased minute volume and ventilation/perfusion mismatching, especially during late stage disease and acute exacerbations.	$\rightarrow$	Mixed hypercapnia and hypoxemia are common in COPD. Evaluation of arterial blood gases helps determine the severity of disease at "baseline" and contributes to appropriate management decisions during acute exacerbations.
Chronic hypercapnia results in reliance on hypoxic ventilatory drive to maintain adequate ventilation.	$\rightarrow$	Oxygen therapy is vital, but patients must be monitored for decreased minute volume and hypercapnia; some may need mechanical ventilation.
Ipratropium may slow the progression of disease in COPD.	$\rightarrow$	Ipratropium (and the newer long acting agents) are the first line pharmacologic choice for COPD.
Bronchoconstriction is a relatively minor component of the disease process in COPD.	$\rightarrow$	Pharmacotherapy is less effective and must be balanced against the risk of side effects. Nonpharmacologic therapy should include smoking cessation, rehabilitation, patient education, psychological support, nutrition, and possible referral for surgery.

Suggested Reading

Anonymous. (1999). Skeletal muscle dysfunction in chronic obstructive pulmonary disease. A statement of the American Thoracic Society and European Respiratory Society. *American Journal of Respiratory & Critical Care Medicine, 159*(4 Pt 2), S1-40.

Anonymous. (2000). Chronic obstructive pulmonary disease. Stopping smoking can make a huge difference for people with this lung condition. *Mayo Clinic Health Letter,* (Suppl), 1-8.

Appleton, S., Smith, B., Veale, A., & Bara, A. (2000). Long-acting beta2-agonists for chronic obstructive pulmonary disease. *Cochrane Database of Systematic Reviews [computer file],* CD001104.

Aubry, M. C., Wright, J. L., & Myers, J. L. (2000). The pathology of smoking-related lung diseases. *Clinics in Chest Medicine, 21,* 11-35.

Barnes, P. J. (1999). Genetics and pulmonary medicine. 9. Molecular genetics of chronic obstructive pulmonary disease. *Thorax, 54*(3), 245-252.

Barnes, P. J. (2000). Chronic obstructive pulmonary disease. *New England Journal of Medicine, 343,* 269-280.

Barnes, P. J. (2000). Mechanisms in COPD: Differences from asthma. *Chest, 117,* 10S-14S.

Barnes, P. J. (2000). The pharmacological properties of tiotropium. *Chest, 117,* 63S-66S.

Bellamy, D. (2000). Progress in the management of COPD. *Practitioner, 244,* 24-28.

Bernard, S., Whittom, F., Leblanc, P., Jobin, J., Belleau, R., Berube, C., Carrier, G., & Maltais, F. (1999). Aerobic and strength training in patients with chronic obstructive pulmonary disease. *American Journal of Respiratory & Critical Care Medicine, 159*(3), 896-901.

Calverley, P., & Bellamy, D. (2000). The challenge of providing better care for patients with chronic obstructive pulmonary disease: The poor relation of airways obstruction? *Thorax, 55,* 78-82.

Calverley, P. M. (2000). COPD: Early detection and intervention. *Chest, 117,* 365S-371S.

Casaburi, R. (2000). Skeletal muscle function in COPD. *Chest, 117,* 267S-271S.

Chang, H. W. (2001). The severity of pulmonary emphysema investigated with fractal analysis: Regional dependence. *Journal of Nuclear Medicine, 42,* 177-178.

Coakley, R. J., Taggart, C., O'Neill, S., & McElvaney, N. G. (2001). Alpha1-antitrypsin deficiency: Biological answers to clinical questions. *American Journal of the Medical Sciences, 321,* 33-41.

Criner, G. J. (2000). Effects of long-term oxygen therapy on mortality and morbidity. *Respiratory Care, 45,* 105-118.

Dahl, M., Nordestgaard, B. G., Lange, P., Vestbo, J., & Tybjaerg-Hansen, A. (2001). Molecular diagnosis of intermediate and severe alpha(1)-antitrypsin deficiency: MZ individuals with chronic obstructive pulmonary disease may have lower lung function than MM individuals. *Clinical Chemistry, 47,* 56-62.

Dorinsky, P. M., Reisner, C., Ferguson, G. T., Menjoge, S. S., Serby, C. W., & Witek, T. J. J. (1999). The combination of ipratropium and albuterol optimizes pulmonary function reversibility testing in patients with COPD. *Chest, 115*(4), 966-971.

Ferguson, G. T. (2000). Recommendations for the management of COPD. *Chest, 117,* 23S-28S.

Ferguson, G. T., Enright, P. L., Buist, A. S., & Higgins, M. W. (2000). Office spirometry for lung health assessment in adults: A consensus from the National Lung Health Education Program. *Respiratory Care, 45,* 513-530.

Gallefoss, F., Bakke, P. S., & Rsgaard, P. K. (1999). Quality of life assessment after patient education in a randomized controlled study on asthma and chronic obstructive pulmonary disease. *American Journal of Respiratory & Critical Care Medicine, 159*(3), 812-817.

Gompertz, S., Bayley, D. L., Hill, S. L., & Stockley, R. A. (2001). Relationship between airway inflammation and the frequency of exacerbations in patients with smoking related COPD. *Thorax, 56,* 36-41.

Hensley, M., Coughlan, J. L., & Gibson, P. (2000). Lung volume reduction surgery for diffuse emphysema. *Cochrane Database of Systematic Reviews[computer file],* CD001001.

Heunks, L. M., & Dekhuijzen, P. N. (2000). Respiratory muscle function and free radicals: From cell to COPD. *Thorax, 55,* 704-716.

Hirschmann, J. V. (2000). Do bacteria cause exacerbations of COPD? *Chest, 118,* 193-203.

Hogg, J. C. (2000). Latent adenoviral infection in the pathogenesis of emphysema: The Parker B. Francis Lectureship. *Chest, 117,* 282S-285S.

Keenan, S. P., Gregor, J., Sibbald, W. J., Cook, D., & Gafni, A. (2000). Noninvasive positive pressure ventilation in the setting of severe, acute exacerbations of chronic obstructive pulmonary disease: More effective and less expensive. *Critical Care Medicine, 28,* 2094-2102.

King, G. G., Muller, N. L., & Pare, P. D. (1999). Evaluation of airways in obstructive pulmonary disease using high-resolution computed tomography. *American Journal of Respiratory & Critical Care Medicine, 159*(3), 992-1004.

Lacasse, Y., Ferreira, I., Brooks, D., Newman, T., & Goldstein, R. S. (2001). Critical appraisal of clinical practice guidelines targeting chronic obstructive pulmonary disease. *Archives of Internal Medicine, 161,* 69-74.

Loppow, D., Schleiss, M. B., Kanniess, F., Taube, C., Jorres, R. A., & Magnussen, H. (2001). In patients with chronic bronchitis a four week trial with inhaled steroids does not attenuate airway inflammation. *Respiratory Medicine, 95,* 115-121.

MacNee, W. (2000). Oxidants/antioxidants and COPD. *Chest, 117,* 303S-317S.

MacNee, W., & Donaldson, K. (2000). Exacerbations of COPD: Environmental mechanisms. *Chest, 117,* 390S-397S.

Mahler, D. A., Donohue, J. F., Barbee, R. A., Goldman, M. D., Gross, N. J., Wisniewski, M. E., Yancey, S. W., Zakes, B. A., Rickard, K. A., & Anderson, W. H. (1999). Efficacy of salmeterol xinafoate in the treatment of COPD. *Chest, 115*(4), 957-965.

McNicholas, W. T. (2000). Impact of sleep in COPD. *Chest, 117,* 48S-53S.

Nadel, J. A. (2000). Role of neutrophil elastase in hypersecretion during COPD exacerbations, and proposed therapies. *Chest, 117,* 386S-389S.

Niewoehner, D. E., Erbland, M. L., Deupree, R. H., Collins, D., Gross, N. J., Light, R. W., Anderson, P., & Morgan, N. A. (1999). Effect of systemic glucocorticoids on exacerbations of chronic obstructive pulmonary disease. Department of Veterans Affairs Cooperative Study Group. *New England Journal of Medicine, 340*(25), 1941-1947.

O'Brien, G. M., Furukawa, S., Kuzma, A. M., Cordova, F., & Criner, G. J. (1999). Improvements in lung function, exercise, and quality of life in hypercapnic COPD patients after lung volume reduction surgery. *Chest, 115*(1), 75-84.

O'Donohue, W. J., Jr., & Bowman, T. J. (2000). Hypoxemia during sleep in patients with chronic obstructive pulmonary disease: Significance, detection, and effects of therapy. *Respiratory Care, 45,* 188-191.

Petty, T. L. (2000). Scope of the COPD problem in North America: Early studies of prevalence and NHANES III data: Basis for early identification and intervention. *Chest, 117,* 326S-331S.

Rennard, S. I., & Daughton, D. M. (2000). Smoking cessation. *Chest, 117,* 360S-364S.

Ringbaek, T. (2001). Supplemental oxygen in COPD. *Thorax, 56,* 86.

Rodriguez-Roisin, R. (2000). Toward a consensus definition for COPD exacerbations. *Chest, 117,* 398S-401S.

Roland, M., Bhowmik, A., Sapsford, R. J., Seemungal, T. A., Jeffries, D. J., Warner, T. D., & Wedzicha, J. A. (2001). Sputum and plasma endothelin-1 levels in exacerbations of chronic obstructive pulmonary disease. *Thorax, 56,* 30-35.

Sestini, P., & Ram, F. S. (2000). Short-acting beta 2 agonists for stable chronic obstructive pulmonary disease. *Cochrane Database of Systematic Reviews [computer file],* CD001495.

Sethi, J. M., & Rochester, C. L. (2000). Smoking and chronic obstructive pulmonary disease. *Clinics in Chest Medicine, 21,* 67-86.

Sethi, S. (2000). Bacterial infection and the pathogenesis of COPD. *Chest, 117,* 286S-291S.

Smith, J. A., Redman, P., & Woodhead, M. A. (1999). Antibiotic use in patients admitted with acute exacerbations of chronic obstructive pulmonary disease. *European Respiratory Journal, 13*(4), 835-838.

Snider, G. L. (2000). Clinical relevance summary: Collagen vs elastin in pathogenesis of emphysema; cellular origin of elastases; bronchiolitis vs emphysema as a cause of airflow obstruction. *Chest, 117,* 244S-246S.

Steiner, M. C., & Morgan, M. D. (2001). Enhancing physical performance in chronic obstructive pulmonary disease. *Thorax, 56,* 73-77.

Stehbens, W. E. (2000). Proteinase imbalance versus biomechanical stress in pulmonary emphysema. *Experimental & Molecular Pathology, 69,* 46-62.

Stick, S. (2000). Pediatric origins of adult lung disease. 1. The contribution of airway development to paediatric and adult lung disease. *Thorax, 55,* 587-594.

Stockley, R. A. (2000). New approaches to the management of COPD. *Chest, 117,* 58S-62S.

Takeyama, K., Jung, B., Shim, J. J., Burgel, P. R., Dao-Pick, T., Ueki, I. F., Protin, U., Kroschel, P., & Nadel, J. A. (2001). Activation of epidermal growth factor receptors is responsible for mucin synthesis induced by cigarette smoke. *American Journal of Physiology—Lung Cellular & Molecular Physiology, 280,* L165-L172.

Vestbo, J., Sorensen, T., Lange, P., Brix, A., Torre, P., & Viskum, K. (1999). Long-term effect of inhaled budesonide in mild and moderate chronic obstructive pulmonary disease: A randomised controlled trial. *Lancet, 353*(9167), 1819-1823.

Voelkel, N. F., & Tuder, R. (2000). COPD: Exacerbation. *Chest, 117,* 376S-379S.

Voelkel, N. F. (2000). Raising awareness of COPD in primary care. *Chest, 117,* 372S-375S.

Wedzicha, J. A. (2000). Oral corticosteroids for exacerbations of chronic obstructive pulmonary disease. *Thorax, 55*(Suppl 1), S23-S27.

Wouters, E. F. (2000). Nutrition and metabolism in COPD. *Chest, 117,* 274S-280S.

Yamaguchi, K., & Matsubara, H. (2000). Computed tomographic diagnosis of chronic obstructive pulmonary disease. *Current Opinion in Pulmonary Medicine, 6,* 92-98.

Case Study

Chronic Obstructive Pulmonary Disease

INITIAL HISTORY
- 58-year-old female presents to the clinic complaining of shortness of breath that has increased slowly for years.
- Symptoms have become worse in recent months; last 2 days much worse now with productive cough.
- Now also complaining of new-onset ankle swelling.

Question 1   What other questions would you like to ask?

ADDITIONAL HISTORY
- 60-pack-year smoking history; quit 5 years ago.
- Sputum is yellow in color; no blood.
- No fever, chills, or chest pain.
- Usually brings up only scant white sputum in the A.M.
- No weight loss.
- No history of heart disease.

Question 2   What would you like to ask about the past medical history?

PAST MEDICAL HISTORY
- Has been fairly healthy in the past.
- No TB or asbestos exposure; no occupational exposures.
- No allergies.
- Occasional bronchitis treated as an outpatient with antibiotics.
- No history of asthma.
- Family history positive for heart disease (brother in 50s).

Question 3 What is the differential diagnosis at this time?

PHYSICAL EXAMINATION
- Alert, mild dyspnea with climbing on the exam table
- Afebrile
- P = 95; RR = 28; BP = 135/85, no orthostatic changes
- No cyanosis
- No rashes

HEENT, Neck
- PERRL, fundi without hemorrhages or exudates.
- Yellowed teeth.
- Nares clear; pharynx clear.
- Pursed lip breathing.
- Mild jugular venous distension.
- Shotty anterior cervical adenopathy.

Lungs
- Using accessory muscles at rest.
- Barrel chest; decreased diaphragmatic excursion bilaterally.
- Percussion hyperresonant; decreased breath sounds throughout.
- Prolonged expiration with expiratory wheezes with rhonchi in all lung fields.
- No supraclavicular or axillary adenopathy.

Cardiac
- Regular rate rhythm with occasional premature beat; mild precordial heave.
- Normal S_1, loud S_2, no S_3 or S_4.

Abdomen, Extremities
- Liver palpable, span 12 cm at the right midclavicular line.
- Spleen palpable.
- No masses or tenderness.
- No cyanosis or clubbing.
- 2+ bilateral pitting pedal edema.

Neurologic
- Alert, oriented
- Cranial nerves intact.
- Strength, sensation, deep tendon reflexes intact and symmetrical.
- Gait steady.

Question 4 What are the important positive and negative findings on exam and what might they mean?

Question 5 What laboratory tests would you order at this time?

LABORATORY

- Serum chemistries normal except bicarbonate = 38; calcium normal.
- HCT = 49%; WBC = 9,000, normal differential.
- Liver function tests normal.
- Sputum = occasional epithelial cell, scattered epithelial cells; PMNs and GM+ diplococci seen.

Question 6 What do these laboratory results tell you?

ARTERIAL BLOOD GAS RESULTS
- pH = 7.38; $PaCO_2$ = 56; PaO_2 = 54 on room air

Question 7 What is the A-a gradient?

SPIROMETRY RESULTS

- Forced expiratory volume in 1 second (FEV_1) = 1.67 L/sec (45% of predicted)
- Forced vital capacity (FVC) = 4.10 L (85% of predicted)
- FEV_1/FVC = 37 (predicted = 72)

Question 8   What do these spirometry results indicate?

CHEST X-RAY AND READING

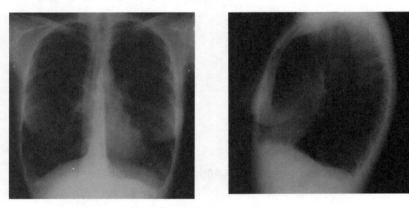

- Hyperinflation with flattened diaphragms.
- Increased anterior-posterior diameter and retrosternal space.
- Diffuse scarring and bullae especially in the lower lobes.
- No acute infiltrates.

Question 9   What is the pathophysiology behind these chest x-ray findings?

Question 10   What are the key elements of management for this patient?

7

Pneumonia

DEFINITION

- Although the term "pneumonia" can be used to describe a large number of diseases that cause pulmonary parenchymal consolidation, it is most commonly used to refer to infections of the lower respiratory tract.

- Infectious causes may be viral, bacterial, fungal, protozoal, or parasitic.

- May be community-acquired (CAP), nursing home acquired (NHAP), or nosocomial.

EPIDEMIOLOGY

- Sixth leading cause of death in the U.S.

- Advanced age, immunocompromise, reduced forced expiratory volume in 1 second (FEV_1), and high alcohol intake are the greatest risk factors in the general population.

- Other risk factors include altered consciousness, smoking, underlying lung disease, endotracheal intubation, malnutrition, airway obstruction, and immobilization.

- Overall incidence of CAP is 3% per year in people >65 years old; mortality ranges from 5% to >30% depending on the etiologic microorganism. The most common bacterial infections include *S. pneumoniae, H. influenza, M. pneumoniae, C. pneumoniae*, and *M. catarrhalis*; influenza is a common viral CAP.

- NHAP is commonly caused by the same microorganisms as CAP (unless patient was recently discharged from the hospital) but, due to the advanced age of the patient, has a 13% mortality rate.

- Nosocomial pneumonia is the second most common nosocomial infection but has the greatest mortality (overall 20% to 50% mortality). It is the most common infection in intensive care units (ICUs) where ventilator associated pneumonia (VAP) occurs in 9% to 68% of patents. If VAP occurs within the first 48 hours of hospitalization, community acquired microorganisms are most common; if late in onset, then *staphylococcus aureus* and *pseudomonas aeruginosa* are most common.

PATHOPHYSIOLOGY

- Aspiration of microorganisms that colonize the oropharyngeal secretions is the most common route of infection. Other routes of inoculation include inhalation, hematogenous spread from remote sites of infection, and direct extension from contiguous sites of infection.

- The upper airway is the first line of defense against infection, however, the clearance of microorganisms by saliva, mucociliary expulsion, and secretory IgA can be inhibited by many diseases, immunocompromise, smoking, and endotracheal intubation.

- The lower airway defenses include cough, gag reflex, mucociliary expulsion, surfactant, macrophage and polymorphonucleocyte (PMN) phagocytosis, and cellular and humoral immunity. These defenses are inhibited by altered consciousness, smoking, abnormal mucous production (e.g., cystic fibrosis or chronic bronchitis), immunocompromise, intubation and prolonged bedrest.

- The alveolar macrophage is the primary defender against inasion of the lower respiratory tract and it daily clears the airways of aspirated microorganisms without initiating significant inflammation.

- If the number or virulence of the microorganisms is too great, the macrophage will recruit PMNs and initiate the inflammatory cascade with release of numerous cytokines including leukotrienes, tumor necrosis factor (TNF), interleukins, oxygen radicals, and proteases.

- This inflammation leads to alveolar filling with ventilation/perfusion mismatching and hypoxemia. Widespread apoptosis of lung cells occurs, this helps to eradicate intracellular microorganisms such as tuberculosis or chlamydia, but also contributes to the pathologic process of lung damage.

- The infection and inflammation may remain localized to the lung or may cause bacteremia resulting in meningitis or endocarditis, the systemic inflammatory response syndrome (SIRS), and/or sepsis.

- Virulence factors of various microorganisms can influence the pathophysiology and clinical course of disease. Streptococcus pneumoniae (pneumococcus) provides an excellent example (Fig. 7-1).

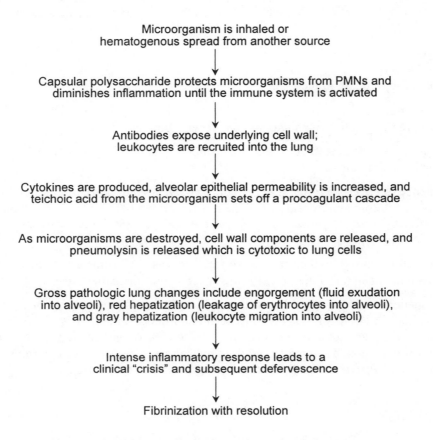

Microorganism is inhaled or
hematogenous spread from another source

↓

Capsular polysaccharide protects microorganisms from PMNs and
diminishes inflammation until the immune system is activated

↓

Antibodies expose underlying cell wall;
leukocytes are recruited into the lung

↓

Cytokines are produced, alveolar epithelial permeability is increased, and
teichoic acid from the microorganism sets off a procoagulant cascade

↓

As microorganisms are destroyed, cell wall components are released, and
pneumolysin is released which is cytotoxic to lung cells

↓

Gross pathologic lung changes include engorgement (fluid exudation
into alveoli), red hepatization (leakage of erythrocytes into alveoli),
and gray hepatization (leukocyte migration into alveoli)

↓

Intense inflammatory response leads to a
clinical "crisis" and subsequent defervescence

↓

Fibrinization with resolution

Fig. 7-1 Pathogenesis of Pneumococcal Pneumonia

PATIENT PRESENTATION

History

Age; altered consciousness; immunocompromise; smoking; underlying lung disease; prolonged bedrest; recent hospitalization; intubation.

Symptoms

Upper respiratory prodrome (headache, rhinitis, postnasal drainage); cough; sputum production with discoloration; dyspnea; pleuritic chest pain; hemoptysis; fever; rigors; myalgias.

Examination

Fever; tachypnea; tachycardia; decreased level of consciousness; cyanosis; use of accessory muscles of respiration; splinting; dullness to percussion; inspiratory crackles (rales); egophony; whispered pectoriloquy; increased tactile fremitus; pleural friction rub; tenacious and/or discolored sputum.

DIFFERENTIAL DIAGNOSIS

- Acute or chronic bronchitis
- Noninfectious pneumonitis
- Pulmonary embolus
- Asthma, COPD
- Congestive heart failure
- Acute respiratory distress syndrome

KEYS TO ASSESSMENT

- Look for source of infection, aspiration; assess for septic shock (hypotension, poor tissue perfusion).
- Arterial blood gases:
  - Indicated if the patient is in respiratory distress or has significant underlying lung disease.
  - Expect hypoxemia with respiratory alkalosis in patient without underlying lung disease.
- White blood cell (WBC) count with differential.
- Electrolytes and liver function tests may be useful in patients with an atypical presentation or severe symptoms (e.g., patients with *legionella pneumophila*).
- Sputum
  - Gram stain is indicated in all inpatients; numerous PMNs consistent with bacterial infection; microorganisms may be preliminarily identified by staining characteristics and shape.
  - Sputum culture is indicated in patients who are hospitalized or have been recently discharged, or who present with severe or unusual symptoms.
- Chest x-ray:
  - Currently recommended in all patients with a history and physical exam suggestive of pneumonia.
  - Expect lobar or patchy infiltrates; look for air bronchograms.
- Blood cultures are indicated in hospitalized patients.
- Bronchoscopy with biopsy may be necessary in high risk patients who do not respond to empiric therapy.

KEYS TO MANAGEMENT

Prevention

- Isolation precautions for immunocompromised patients.
- Patient positioning to prevent aspiration.
- For prevention of VAP.
    - Avoid large gastric volumes.
    - Oral intubation rather than nasal.
    - Careful maintenance of ventilator circuits.
    - Continuous subglottic suctioning.
    - Postural oscillation/rotation.
    - Sucralfate rather than H2 blockers for ulcer prophylaxis (still controversial).
    - Chlorhexidine oral rinse.

Management of Acute Infection

- Oxygen and hydration if indicated.
- Consider respiratory isolation.
- Hospital admission indicated if:
    - Age over 65, homeless, hospitalized for pneumonia in the past year.
    - Pulse >140/minute, respiratory rate >30/minute, hypotension.
    - Temperature >38.3°F.
    - Altered mental status, cyanosis.
    - Immunosuppression, comorbid condition.
    - High-risk microorganism (e.g., recent nosocomial pseudomonas infection).
    - WBC <4000 or >30,000/μL.
    - Partial pressure of oxygen in arterial blood (PaO_2) <60 or $PaCO_2$ >50.
    - Chest x-ray with multiple lobes involved or rapid progression.
- Deep breathing and cough, chest physical therapy (PT) if available.
- Antibiotics for bacterial, parasitic, or fungal pneumonia (not viral).
    - Most often empiric coverage is used in outpatients; sputum gram stain may guide therapy with inpatients but therapy may need to be altered when cultures with sensitivities become available (48 to 72 hours).
    - Choice of empiric antibiotic varies based on outpatient versus inpatient, age, patient risk factors, and patient presentation; common empiric antibiotic choices are listed in Table 7-1.

**Table 7-1 Empiric Therapy for Community Acquired
Pneumonia According to the Infectious Disease Society of America, 1998**

Type of Patient	Patient Presentation	Empiric Antiobotic
Outpatient	Immunocompetent	Macrolide, fluoroquinolone, or doxycycline
	Suspected PCN-resistant *S. pneumoniae*	Fluoroquinolone
	Aspiration	Amoxicillin/clavulanate
	Age 18 to 40	Doxycycline
Hospitalized	General medical ward	Beta lactam with macrolide or fluoroquinolone
	ICU	Same as general medical ward
	Lung disease	Antipseudomonal penicillin with macrolide, or fluoroquinolone with aminoglycoside
	Aspiration	Fluoroquinolone with clindamycin

Pathophysiology → Clinical Link

What is going on in the disease process that influences how the patient presents and how he or she should be managed?

What should you do now that you understand the underlying pathophysiology?

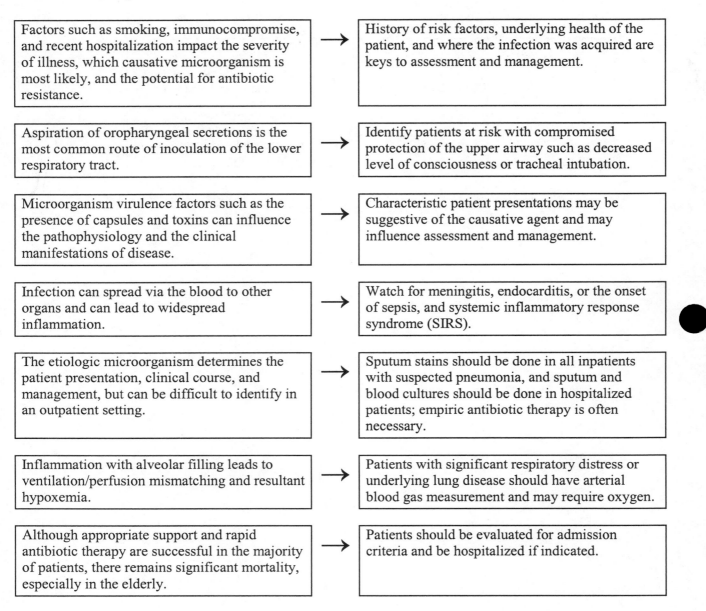

Pathophysiology	Clinical Link
Factors such as smoking, immunocompromise, and recent hospitalization impact the severity of illness, which causative microorganism is most likely, and the potential for antibiotic resistance.	→ History of risk factors, underlying health of the patient, and where the infection was acquired are keys to assessment and management.
Aspiration of oropharyngeal secretions is the most common route of inoculation of the lower respiratory tract.	→ Identify patients at risk with compromised protection of the upper airway such as decreased level of consciousness or tracheal intubation.
Microorganism virulence factors such as the presence of capsules and toxins can influence the pathophysiology and the clinical manifestations of disease.	→ Characteristic patient presentations may be suggestive of the causative agent and may influence assessment and management.
Infection can spread via the blood to other organs and can lead to widespread inflammation.	→ Watch for meningitis, endocarditis, or the onset of sepsis, and systemic inflammatory response syndrome (SIRS).
The etiologic microorganism determines the patient presentation, clinical course, and management, but can be difficult to identify in an outpatient setting.	→ Sputum stains should be done in all inpatients with suspected pneumonia, and sputum and blood cultures should be done in hospitalized patients; empiric antibiotic therapy is often necessary.
Inflammation with alveolar filling leads to ventilation/perfusion mismatching and resultant hypoxemia.	→ Patients with significant respiratory distress or underlying lung disease should have arterial blood gas measurement and may require oxygen.
Although appropriate support and rapid antibiotic therapy are successful in the majority of patients, there remains significant mortality, especially in the elderly.	→ Patients should be evaluated for admission criteria and be hospitalized if indicated.

Suggested Reading

Afessa, B., & Green, B. (2000). Bacterial pneumonia in hospitalized patients with HIV infection: The pulmonary complications, ICU support, and prognostic factors of hospitalized patients with HIV (PIP) study. *Chest, 117,* 1017-1022.

Almirall, J., Bolibar, I., Balanzo, X., & Gonzalez, C. A. (1999). Risk factors for community-acquired pneumonia in adults: A population-based case-control study. *European Respiratory Journal, 13*(2), 349-355.

Barie, P. S. (2000). Importance, morbidity, and mortality of pneumonia in the surgical intensive care unit. *American Journal of Surgery, 179,* 2S-7S.

Bartlett, J. (2000). Treatment of community-acquired pneumonia. *Chemotherapy, 46*(Suppl 1), 24-31.

Baughman, R. P. (1999). The lung in the immunocompromised patient. Infectious complications part 1. *Respiration, 66*(2), 95-109.

Behnia, M., Robertson, K. A., & Martin, W. J. (2000). Lung infections: Role of apoptosis in host defense and pathogenesis of disease. *Chest, 117,* 1771-1777.

Bernstein, J. M. (1999). Treatment of community-acquired pneumonia—IDSA guidelines. Infectious Diseases Society of America. *Chest, 115*(3 Suppl), 9S-13S.

Blot, S., Vandewoude, K., Hoste, E., & Colardyn, F. (2000). Tracheal colonization in pneumonia *Chest, 117,* 1216.

Bowton, D. L. (1999). Nosocomial pneumonia in the ICU—Year 2000 and beyond. *Chest, 115*(3 Suppl), 28S-33S.

Campbell, G. D. J. (1999). Commentary on the 1993 American Thoracic Society guidelines for the treatment of community-acquired pneumonia. *Chest, 115*(3 Suppl), 14S-18S.

Cazzola, M., Blasi, E., & Allegra, L. (2001). Critical evaluation of guidelines for the treatment of lower respiratory tract bacterial infections. *Respiratory Medicine, 95,* 95-108.

Cook, D., De, J. B., Brochard, L., & Brun-Bruisson, C. (1998). Influence of airway management on ventilator-associated pneumonia: Evidence from randomized trials. *Journal of the American Medical Association, 279*(10), 781-787.

Cunha, B. A. (2001). Community-acquired pneumonia. Diagnostic and therapeutic approach. *Medical Clinics of North America, 85,* 43-77.

Cunha, B. A. (2001). Nosocomial pneumonia. Diagnostic and therapeutic considerations. *Medical Clinics of North America, 85,* 79-114.

Ephgrave, K. S., Kleiman-Wexler, R., Pfaller, M., Booth, B. M., Reed, D., Werkmeister, L., & Young, S. (1998). Effects of sucralfate vs antacids on gastric pathogens: Results of a double-blind clinical trial. *Archives of Surgery, 133*(3), 251-257.

Eron, L. J., & Passos, S. (2001). Early discharge of infected patients through appropriate antibiotic use. *Archives of Internal Medicine, 161,* 61-65.

Ewig, S., Seifert, K., Kleinfeld, T., Goke, N., & Schafer, H. (2000). Management of patients with community-acquired pneumonia in a primary care hospital: A critical evaluation. *Respiratory Medicine, 94,* 556-563.

Fagon, J. Y., Chastre, J., Wolff, M., Gervais, C., Parer-Aubas, S., Stephan, F., Similowski, T., Mercat, A., Diehl, J. L., Sollet, J. P., & Tenaillon, A. (2000). Invasive and noninvasive strategies for management of suspected ventilator-associated pneumonia. A randomized trial. *Annals of Internal Medicine, 132,* 621-630.

Farr, B. M. (1997). Prognosis and decisions in pneumonia. *New England Journal of Medicine, 336*(4), 288-289.

Fine, M. J., Auble, T. E., Yealy, D. M., Hanusa, B. H., Weissfeld, L. A., Singer, D. E., Coley, C. M., Marrie, T. J., & Kapoor, W. N. (1997). A prediction rule to identify low-risk patients with community-acquired pneumonia. *New England Journal of Medicine, 336*(4), 243-250.

Gant, V., & Parton, S. (2000). Community-acquired pneumonia. *Current Opinion in Pulmonary Medicine, 6,* 226-233.

Gleason, P., Wishwa, N., Stone, R., Lave, J., Obrosky, S., Shulz, R., Singer, D., Coley, C., Marrie, T., & Fine, M. (1997). Medical outcomes and antimicrobial costs with the use of the American Thoracic Society guidelines for outpatients with community-acquired pneumonia. *Journal of the American Medical Association, 278*(4), 32-39.

Harwell, J. I., & Brown, R. B. (2000). The drug-resistant pneumococcus: Clinical relevance, therapy, and prevention. *Chest, 117,* 530-541.

Heyland, D. K., Cook, D. J., Griffith, L., Keenan, S. P., & Brun-Buisson, C. (1999). The attributable morbidity and mortality of ventilator-associated pneumonia in the critically ill patient. The Canadian Critical Trials Group. *American Journal of Respiratory & Critical Care Medicine, 159*(4 Pt 1), 1249-1256.

Heyland, D. K., Cook, D. J., Marshall, J., Heule, M., Guslits, B., Lang, J., & Jaeschke, R. (1999). The clinical utility of invasive diagnostic techniques in the setting of ventilator-associated pneumonia. Canadian Critical Care Trials Group. *Chest, 115*(4), 1076-1084.

Hilbert, G., Gruson, D., Vargas, F., Valentino, R., Gbikpi-Benissan, G., Dupon, M., Reiffers, J., & Cardinaud, J. P. (2001). Noninvasive ventilation in immunosuppressed patients with pulmonary infiltrates, fever, and acute respiratory failure. *New England Journal of Medicine, 344,* 481-487.

Hixson, S., Sole, M. L., & King, T. (1998). Nursing strategies to prevent ventilator-associated pneumonia. *AACN Clinical Issues, 9*(1), 76-90, quiz 145-146.

Holmes, A., Jacklin, A., Impallomeni, M., & Rogers, T. R. (1999). Community-acquired pneumonia [letter; comment]. *Lancet, 353*(9163), 1528-1529.

Ibrahim, E. H., Ward, S., Sherman, G., & Kollef, M. H. (2000). A comparative analysis of patients with early-onset vs late-onset nosocomial pneumonia in the ICU setting. *Chest, 117,* 1434-1442.

Jones, R. N., Croco, M. A., Kugler, K. C., Pfaller, M. A., & Beach, M. L. (2000). Respiratory tract pathogens isolated from patients hospitalized with suspected pneumonia: Frequency of occurrence and antimicrobial susceptibility patterns from the SENTRY antimicrobial surveillance program (United States and Canada, 1997). *Diagnostic Microbiology & Infectious Disease, 37,* 115-125.

Kollef, M. H. (1999). The prevention of ventilator-associated pneumonia. *New England Journal of Medicine, 340*(8), 627-634.

Lange, M. (2000). Community-acquired pneumonia: An approach to antimicrobial therapy. *Allergy & Asthma Proceedings, 21,* 33-38.

Mandell, L. A., & Campbell, G. D. J. (1998). Nosocomial pneumonia guidelines: An international perspective. *Chest, 113*(3 Suppl), 188S-193S.

Markowicz, P., Wolff, M., Djedaini, K., Cohen, Y., Chastre, J., Delclaux, C., Merrer, J., Herman, B., Veber, B., Fontaine, A., & Dreyfuss, D. (2000). Multicenter prospective study of ventilator-associated pneumonia during acute respiratory distress syndrome. Incidence, prognosis, and risk factors. ARDS Study Group. *American Journal of Respiratory & Critical Care Medicine, 161,* 1942-1948.

Mascellino, M. T., Delogu, G., Pelaia, M. R., Ponzo, R., Parrinello, R., & Giardina, A. (2001). Reduced bactericidal activity against *Staphylococcus aureus* and *Pseudomonas aeruginosa* of blood neutrophils from patients with early adult respiratory distress syndrome. *Journal of Medical Microbiology, 50,* 49-54.

McCracken, G. H., Jr. (2000). Etiology and treatment of pneumonia. *Pediatric Infectious Disease Journal, 19,* 373-377.

Meehan, T. P., Chua-Reyes, J. M., Tate, J., Prestwood, K. M., Scinto, J. D., Petrillo, M. K., & Metersky, M. L. (2000). Process of care performance, patient characteristics, and outcomes in elderly patients hospitalized with community-acquired or nursing home-acquired pneumonia. *Chest, 117,* 1378-1385.

Metlay, J., Kapoor, W., & Fine, M. (1997). Does this patient have community-acquired pneumonia: Diagnosing pneumonia by history and physical examination. *Journal of the American Medical Association, 278*(17), 1440-1445.

Miyashita, N., Niki, Y., Matsushima, T., & Okimoto, N. (2000). Community-acquired *Chlamydia pneumoniae* pneumonia. *Chest, 117,* 615-616.

Morehead, R. S., & Pinto, S. J. (2000). Ventilator-associated pneumonia. *Archives of Internal Medicine, 160,* 1926-1936.

Moss, P. J., & Finch, R. G. (2000). The next generation: Fluoroquinolones in the management of acute lower respiratory infection in adults. *Thorax, 55,* 83-85.

Mouton, C. P., Bazaldua, O. V., Pierce, B., & Espino, D. V. (2001). Common infections in older adults. *American Family Physician, 63,* 257-268.

Muder, R. R. (2000). Management of nursing home-acquired pneumonia: Unresolved issues and priorities for future investigation. *Journal of the American Geriatrics Society, 48,* 95-96.

Mushatt, D. M. (2000). Advances in antimicrobial therapy for respiratory tract infections. *Current Opinion in Pulmonary Medicine, 6,* 250-253.

Nelson, J. D. (2000). Community-acquired pneumonia in children: Guidelines for treatment. *Pediatric Infectious Disease Journal, 19,* 251-253.

Nelson, S., Mason, C. M., Kolls, J., & Summer, W. R. (1995). Pathophysiology of pneumonia. *Clinics in Chest Medicine, 16*(1), 1-12.

Niederman, M. S. (1998). Community-acquired pneumonia: A North American perspective. *Chest, 113*(3 Suppl), 179S-182S.

Ruimy, R., Genauzeau, E., Barnabe, C., Beaulieu, A., Tibayrenc, M., & Andremont, A. (2001). Genetic diversity of *Pseudomonas aeruginosa* strains isolated from ventilated patients with nosocomial pneumonia, cancer patients with bacteremia, and environmental water. *Infection & Immunity, 69,* 584-588.

Schaad, U. B. (1999). Antibiotic therapy of childhood pneumonia. *Pediatric Pulmonology—Supplement, 18,* 146-149.

Sinaniotis, C. A. (1999). Community-acquired pneumonia: Diagnosis and treatment. *Pediatric Pulmonology—Supplement, 18,* 144-145.

Torres, A., & El Ebiary, M. (2000). Bronchoscopic BAL in the diagnosis of ventilator-associated pneumonia. *Chest, 117,* 198S-202S.

Vanhems, P., Lepape, A., Savey, A., Jambou, P., & Fabry, J. (2000). Nosocomial pulmonary infection by antimicrobial-resistant bacteria of patients hospitalized in intensive care units: Risk factors and survival. *Journal of Hospital Infection, 45,* 98-106.

Ward, M. A. (2000). Lower respiratory tract infections in adolescents. *Adolescent Medicine, 11,* 251-262.

Waterer, G. W., Baselski, V. S., & Wunderink, R. G. (2001). Legionella and community-acquired pneumonia: A review of current diagnostic tests from a clinician's viewpoint. *American Journal of Medicine, 110,* 41-48.

Wipf, J. E., Lipsky, B. A., Hirschmann, J. V., Boyko, E. J., Takasugi, J., Peugeot, R. L., & Davis, C. L. (1999). Diagnosing pneumonia by physical examination: Relevant or relic? *Archives of Internal Medicine, 159*(10), 1082-1087.

Case Study

Pneumonia

INITIAL HISTORY
- 63-year-old female bank manager presents to the clinic in November.
- 1-week history of upper respiratory symptoms; 2-day history of increasing fever, malaise, nausea.
- Cough productive yellow sputum.
- Right-sided pleuritic chest pain.

Question 1   What other questions would you like to ask?

ADDITIONAL HISTORY
- No rashes, headache, or vomiting; no hemoptysis; some friends recently ill.
- Nonsmoker; denies HIV risk (husband died 10 years ago; has not been sexually active since his death).
- Negative past medical history.
- No allergies.
- Usual childhood immunizations; had a flu shot this year.

Question 2   What is your differential diagnosis based on the history?

PHYSICAL EXAMINATION
- Alert, flushed, coughing, and using accessory muscles; in moderate respiratory distress.
- T = 39.2 orally; P = 100 and regular; RR = 32; BP = 110/80, no orthostatic changes.
- Skin warm, moist, and flushed without rashes.

HEENT, Neck
- PERRLA, fundi without lesions; nares slightly flared, purulent drainage visible; ears with slight serous fluid seen behind both tympanic membranes.
- Pharynx erythematous with purulent postnasal drainage, no tonsillar exudate, mucus membranes moist; neck with mild anterior cervical adenopathy.

Lungs
- Normal chest configuration; mild use of accessory muscles; decreased expansion (splinting) over right chest and increased fremitus.
- Inspiratory rales, egophony, and whispered pectoriloquy at right anterior axillary line; clear left lung, right upper and right lower lobes.

Cardiac, Abdomen, Extremities, Neurological
- Regular rate and rhythm, tachycardiac with I/VI SEM left lower sternal border.
- Abdomen soft, nontender, no organomegaly, bowel sounds present.
- Extremities warm and flushed without cyanosis or edema, no clubbing.
- Alert and oriented; strength, sensation, and deep tendon reflexes 2+ and symmetrical.

Question 3   What are the significant findings on physical exam and what might they mean?

Question 4   What laboratories should now be obtained?

LABORATORY

- ABG: pH = 7.56, $PaCO_2$ = 26, PaO_2 = 90 on room air; HCT 42%; WBC 15,000; 5% bands, 83% segs, 10% lymphs, 3% monos, 1% eos; LFT normal.
- Sputum with TNTC (too numerous to count) polymorphonucleocytes and multiple gram + diplococci.

Question 5   What is the A-a gradient?

Question 6   What do the rest of the laboratories indicate?

CHEST X-RAY

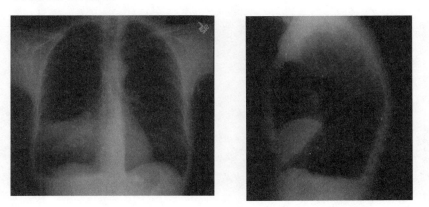

Question 7   What are the major findings on the chest x-ray?

Question 8 What are the possible diagnoses now?

Question 9 How should this patient be managed?

8

Lung Cancer

DEFINITION

- Malignant neoplasms arising from the bronchial epithelium.

- In 1999 the World Health Organization developed a pathologic classification scheme for lung tumors that includes over 100 subcategories, but generally, lung cancer can be classified as nonsmall cell lung carcinoma (NSCLC, 85% of all lung cancers) and small cell lung carcinoma (SCLC, 15% of all lung cancers).

- NSCLC can be further divided into three subtypes.

    - Adenocarcinoma (including bronchoalveolar carcinoma)

    - Squamous cell carcinoma

    - Large cell undifferentiated carcinoma

EPIDEMIOLOGY

- Number 1 cancer killer of men and women in the United States (>177,000 cases and 159,000 deaths in 1999) and in the world.

- Lung cancer deaths in African Americans and women continue to increase; women in the United States have the highest incidence of lung cancer of all women in the world.

- Incidence is highest in men >70 years old and women 50 to 60 years old.

- Clearly some heritable risk: first degree relatives who smoke have a 2.5 fold increase in risk over those with no family history; possible inherited lack of enzymes that detoxify smoke carcinogens (ex. glutathione S-transferase M1 gene).

- 80% to 90% of lung cancer is caused by cigarette smoking; smoking rates in US males are on the decline but rates in women and young people continue to increase (smoking rates among US college students is now estimated at over 25%).

- Other risks include air pollution, radiation, radon, and industrial exposure (e.g., asbestos, arsenic, sulfur dioxide, formaldehyde, silica, nickel).

- The risk of environmental tobacco smoke (passive smoking) has been estimated to be between 1.4 and 3.0 times the unexposed risk, especially if exposed as children.

- Airflow obstruction as in chronic obstructive pulmonary disease (COPD) is an important indicator of increased risk for lung cancer.

- Overall 5 year survival is 14% in whites and 11% in blacks in the United States.

PATHOPHYSIOLOGY

- Cigarette smoke contains an estimated 60 carcinogens (including benzene, nitrosamines [NNK], and oxidants) which can cause DNA mutations (Fig. 8-1).

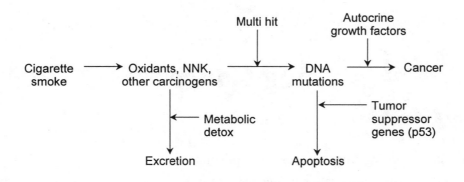

Fig. 8-1 Pathogenesis of Lung Cancer

- It is proposed that lung cancer occurs in those smokers who lack the ability to adequately metabolically detoxify these carcinogens.

- A lung tumor results from many exposures to carcinogens rather than one initiating event ("multi-hit"); it is estimated that it takes between 10 and 20 genetic mutations to create a tumor. Some of the more common mutations that have been identified include:
  - Deletion of the short arm of chromosome #3.
  - Activation of oncogenes (jun, fos, ras and myc).
  - Inactivation of tumor suppressor genes (p53, RB, DKN2).

- In bronchi exposed to carcinogens, dysplastic cells become carcinoma in situ, then bronchogenic carcinoma.

- Cancer cells produce autocrine growth factors (e.g., epithelial growth factor, tissue growth factor, gastrin-releasing peptide, insulin-like growth factor) that promote tumor growth.

- The type of lung cancer depends on the cell of origin.
  - Nonsmall cell lung carcinoma (NSCLC):
    1) Adenocarcinoma arises from glandular cells in bronchial epithelium and is often peripheral in location; metastasizes early.
       a) Most common type of lung cancer, especially in women.
       b) Includes bronchiolar-alveolar carcinoma which arises from the smallest bronchioles and alveolar septae; often appears as an infiltrate rather than a mass on x-ray; is not associated with smoking.
    2) Squamous arises from squamous bronchial epithelium and is often central in location; it is a frequent cause of occult cancer and metastasizes late.
    3) Large cell is probably either adenocarcinoma or squamous in origin, but the cancer is so anaplastic that the cell of origin cannot be identified; aggressive tumor with early metastasis.
  - Small cell lung carcinoma (SCLC) arises from neuroendocrine cells in bronchi; it is a very aggressive tumor and has usually metastasized by the time of diagnosis.

PATIENT PRESENTATION

- 90% are asymptomatic and are discovered incidentally.

History

History of smoking; family history; asbestos exposure; other industrial exposures; pulmonary radiation; history of COPD.

Symptoms

Result from tumor invasion of specific sites or systemic reaction; endobronchial: cough, hemoptysis, dyspnea, atelectasis, postobstructive pneumonia; peripheral (pleura and chest wall): chest pain, pleural effusions; regional spread: dysphagia, stridor, chest pain, syncope, face and arm pain or swelling, hoarseness; metastasis: pain in involved organs, edema, bone pain, seizures, headache; endocrine (paraneoplastic): hyerpigmentation, centripetal obesity, syncope; constitutional: weight loss, anorexia, weakness, fever.

Examination

Weight loss and cachexia, fever, stridor, vocal cord paralysis, dullness to percussion; localized wheeze, crackles that do not clear with antibiotics, adenopathy (supraclavicular, axillary); decreased strength or sensation in arm, and focal neurologic findings.

DIFFERENTIAL DIAGNOSIS

- Benign lung tumors (hematomas, granulomas)
- Other primary tumor metastatic to the lung (breast, prostate, colon, testicular, etc.)
- COPD
- Pneumonia
- Tuberculosis
- Inhaled foreign body
- Endocrine disorder

KEYS TO ASSESSMENT

- Most cancers remain occult until late stage (only 15% of NSCLC found at stage I, 44% at stage IV).
- Screening is controversial but there is increasing evidence that high-risk individuals (>40 years old, >30 pack years smoking, airway obstruction, and symptoms) benefit. Screening includes x-ray (plain film versus spiral computed tomography) and sputum cytology. Tumors caught early have a much-improved prognosis in response to treatment.
- Hemoptysis in the absence of bronchitis, pneumonia, or sinus infection must be evaluated for possible bronchogenic cancer.
- A history of COPD increases the risk of cancer; pulmonary function testing is important.
- Patients may present with a pneumonia that doesn't clear with antibiotics. Smokers always need follow-up after treatment for pneumonia or bronchitis.
- Patients may present with what appears to be an endocrine disorder (e.g., Cushing syndrome, syndrome of inappropriate antidiuretic hormone [SIADH]). The underlying cancer is often found late.
- A supraclavicular node is never normal.
- The chest x-ray is the simplest diagnostic modality. A solitary pulmonary nodule is common, and the appearance of the nodule on the x-ray can help determine whether it is malignant or not (high risk lesions are not densely calcified and have spiculations). Unfortunately, chest x-ray has a relatively low sensitivity and can miss a significant number of small tumors. The x-ray should be evaluated for evidence of hilar or mediastinal adenopathy, pleura disease (effusions) and lesions in the bone.

- Sputum cytology may be diagnostic, however, sensitivity has been estimated to be 20% to 30% overall; sensitivity is improved using monoclonal antibody and specialized staining techniques.

- Bronchoscopy can often visualize and allow for biopsy if the tumor is endobronchial and relatively proximal; new techniques allow for fluorescence bronchoscopy and photodynamic therapy which can identify early lesions and allow for local treatment. Endoscopic ultrasound can be used to define the size and depth of the lesion.

- Computed tomography (CT) with fine-needle aspiration of the tumor is used for small and peripheral lesions that are not likely to be seen via bronchoscopy.

- Serum laboratories results may include pancytopenia from marrow involvement, electrolyte imbalances due to endocrine disorders (ex. hypercalcemia), and elevation of liver enzymes.

- Once the diagnosis of lung cancer has been made, a careful staging work-up is crucial for appropriate choice of management.

  - Mediastinoscopy or positron emission tomography (PET) to evaluate for mediastinal involvement (PET can also be used to evaluate the primary tumor).

  - CT or magnetic resonance imagery (MRI) to evaluate for metastases to abdomen and bone (also consider bone scan).

  - Bone marrow biopsy is indicated for SCLC (likelihood of bone marrow metastases).

  - Head CT to evaluate for brain metastases in SCLC (present in 10% at time of diagnosis).

- Staging:

  - Nonsmall cell: TNM system for the evaluation of tumor size, nodal involvement, or metastases; determines resectability and prognosis; independent of cell type.

  - Small cell: extensive metastatic work up to find the few (<15%) that have "limited disease."

- Performance status testing (e.g., Karnofsky scale) is used to assess for operability and prognosis; ventilation/perfusion lung scanning can help to assess viability of tumor-involved lobe.

- Specific hormone markers are becoming increasingly useful for following the cancer once the diagnosis is made, and are being evaluated for screening (ex. cytokeratin 19, CYFRA 21-1, neuron specific enolase [NSE], and tissue polypeptide antigen [TPA]).

KEYS TO MANAGEMENT

- **Prevention**

  - Smoking cessation is the only truly effective preventative measure, although risk may never return to normal (half of all new lung cancer diagnoses are in former smokers).

  - A diet high in fruits and vegetables has been shown to reduce cancer risk.

  - Antioxidants have had mixed results. Some studies have shown that retinoids and vitamin E levels can reduce risk, however, some studies have shown a significant increase in risk of cancer in smokers taking beta-carotene.

  - Other experimental chemoprevention methods: N-acetylcysteine and antiinflammatory drugs

- **General management**

  - A tissue diagnosis is important to planning care; NSCLC and SCLC are treated differently.

  - Once the diagnosis is established, a well-informed patient can best choose if and what kind of therapy is appropriate.

  - Maximizing nutrition and watching for depression and anxiety helps prepare the patient for treatment. Cancer cachexia is a major contributor to morbidity; drugs that may be helpful include metoclopramide, tetrahydrocannabinol, megestrol, and steroids.

- **Surgery**
  - In all types, lung cancer is a surgical disease if at all possible. Complete resection of the tumor is the best hope for cure.
  - The aggressiveness of the planned surgery is dependent on the patient's operability as well as the tumor's resectability. Optimizing the patient's strength and stamina preoperatively is important.
  - In NSCLC, relatively healthy patients may be surgical candidates even if they are stage III; in SCLC, very few tumors are found to be resectable.
  - Surgical procedures range from thoracoscopic wedge resection to lobectomy to lung resection with mediastinal dissection.

- **Chemotherapy**
  - Chemotherapy, especially if used for advanced stage tumors, can improve survival in NSCLC.
  - SCLC responds dramatically to chemotherapy with tumor responses of 75% to 80% with a marked increase in survival time (ex. increases median survival from less than 3 months to 7 to 10 months in extensive disease), however, relapse is inevitable in most patients.
  - The most commonly used drug regimens include cisplatin in combination with Adriamycin, cyclophosphamide, vincristine, etoposide; carboplatin, irinotecan, topotecan, paclitaxel, docetaxel, edatrexate, gemcitabine, ifosfamide, or vinorelbine.

- **Radiation**
  - NSCLC responds fairly well in terms of palliative care but there is little hope for cure.
  - SCLC responds well to radiation but the extension of survival time is not as good as with chemotherapy. Prophylactic cranial irradiation can reduce relapse in the brain but is associated with considerable toxicity and little survival benefit.

- **Others**
  - Laser therapy through the bronchoscope can be palliative especially in patients with significant hemoptysis.
  - Photodynamic therapy.
  - Endobronchial brachytherapy.
  - Biologic response modifiers (monoclonal antibodies to growth factors, interleukins).
  - Gene therapy (transfecting with p53, antisense therapy, tumor vaccines).

Pathophysiology $\rightarrow$ Clinical Link

What is going on in the disease process that influences how the patient presents and how he or she should be managed?

What should you do now that you understand the underlying pathophysiology?

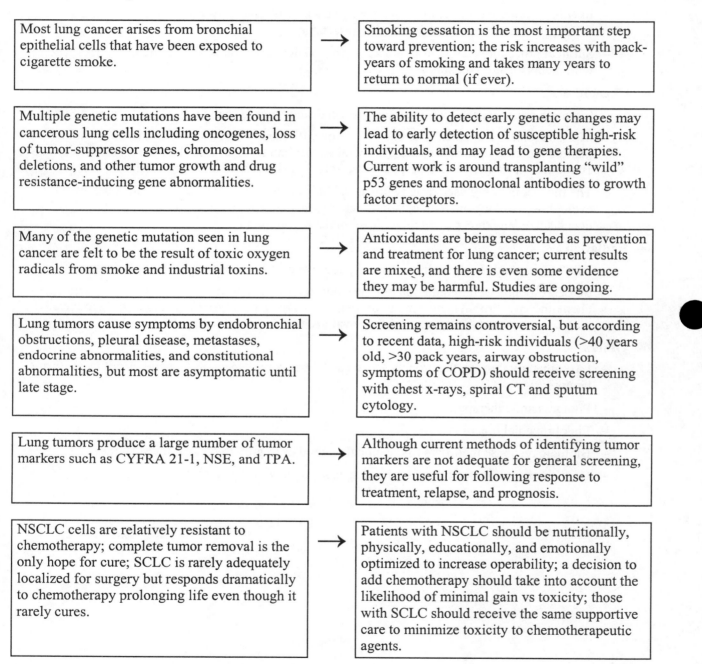

Pathophysiology	Clinical Link
Most lung cancer arises from bronchial epithelial cells that have been exposed to cigarette smoke.	Smoking cessation is the most important step toward prevention; the risk increases with pack-years of smoking and takes many years to return to normal (if ever).
Multiple genetic mutations have been found in cancerous lung cells including oncogenes, loss of tumor-suppressor genes, chromosomal deletions, and other tumor growth and drug resistance-inducing gene abnormalities.	The ability to detect early genetic changes may lead to early detection of susceptible high-risk individuals, and may lead to gene therapies. Current work is around transplanting "wild" p53 genes and monoclonal antibodies to growth factor receptors.
Many of the genetic mutation seen in lung cancer are felt to be the result of toxic oxygen radicals from smoke and industrial toxins.	Antioxidants are being researched as prevention and treatment for lung cancer; current results are mixed, and there is even some evidence they may be harmful. Studies are ongoing.
Lung tumors cause symptoms by endobronchial obstructions, pleural disease, metastases, endocrine abnormalities, and constitutional abnormalities, but most are asymptomatic until late stage.	Screening remains controversial, but according to recent data, high-risk individuals (>40 years old, >30 pack years, airway obstruction, symptoms of COPD) should receive screening with chest x-rays, spiral CT and sputum cytology.
Lung tumors produce a large number of tumor markers such as CYFRA 21-1, NSE, and TPA.	Although current methods of identifying tumor markers are not adequate for general screening, they are useful for following response to treatment, relapse, and prognosis.
NSCLC cells are relatively resistant to chemotherapy; complete tumor removal is the only hope for cure; SCLC is rarely adequately localized for surgery but responds dramatically to chemotherapy prolonging life even though it rarely cures.	Patients with NSCLC should be nutritionally, physically, educationally, and emotionally optimized to increase operability; a decision to add chemotherapy should take into account the likelihood of minimal gain vs toxicity; those with SCLC should receive the same supportive care to minimize toxicity to chemotherapeutic agents.

Suggested Readings

Antonia, S. J., & Sotomayor, E. (2000). Gene therapy for lung cancer. *Current Opinion in Oncology, 12,* 138-142.

Belani, C. P. (2000). Combined modality therapy for unresectable stage III non-small cell lung cancer: New chemotherapy combinations. *Chest, 117,* 127S-132S.

Berman, C. G., & Clark, R. A. (2000). Positron emission tomography in initial staging and diagnosis of persistent or recurrent disease. *Current Opinion in Oncology, 12,* 132-137.

Bogot, N. R., & Shaham, D. (2000). Semi-invasive and invasive procedures for the diagnosis and staging of lung cancer. II. Bronchoscopic and surgical procedures. *Radiologic Clinics of North America, 38,* 535-544.

Bungay, H. K., Davies, R. J., & Gleeson, F. V. (2001). CT scanning in lung cancer. *Thorax, 56,* 84.

Bunn, P. A., Jr., & Kelly, K. (2000). New combinations in the treatment of lung cancer: A time for optimism. *Chest, 117,* 138S-143S.

Bunn, P. A., Jr., Soriano, A., Johnson, G., & Heasley, L. (2000). New therapeutic strategies for lung cancer: Biology and molecular biology come of age. *Chest, 117,* 163S-168S.

Christiani, D. C. (2000). Smoking and the molecular epidemiology of lung cancer. *Clinics in Chest Medicine, 21,* 87-93.

De Ruysscher, D., & Vansteenkiste, J. (2000). Chest radiotherapy in limited-stage small cell lung cancer: Facts, questions, prospects. *Radiotherapy & Oncology, 55,* 1-9.

Deslauriers, J., & Gregoire, J. (2000). Clinical and surgical staging of non-small cell lung cancer. *Chest, 117,* 96S-103S.

Deslauriers, J., & Gregoire, J. (2000). Surgical therapy of early non-small cell lung cancer. *Chest, 117,* 104S-109S.

Goldsmith, S. J., & Kostakoglu, L. (2000). Nuclear medicine imaging of lung cancer. *Radiologic Clinics of North America, 38,* 511-524.

Green, M. C., Murray, J. L., & Hortobagyi, G. N. (2000). Monoclonal antibody therapy for solid tumors. *Cancer Treatment Reviews, 26,* 269-286.

Gruidl, M. E., & Shaw Wright, G. L. (2000). Potential biomarkers for the early detection of lung cancer. *Journal of Thoracic Imaging, 15,* 13-20.

Grunenwald, D. H. (2000). Surgery for advanced stage lung cancer. *Seminars in Surgical Oncology, 18,* 137-142.

Henschke, C. I., & Yankelevitz, D. F. (2000). CT screening for lung cancer. *Radiologic Clinics of North America, 38,* 487-495.

Hanaoka, T., Nakayama, J., Mukai, J., Irie, S., Yamanda, T., & Sato, T. A. (2001). Association of smoking with apoptosis-regulated proteins (Bcl-2, bax and p53) in resected non-small-cell lung cancers. *International Journal of Cancer, 91,* 267-269.

Hirao, T., Nelson, H. H., Ashok, T. D., Wain, J. C., Mark, E. J., Christiani, D. C., Wiencke, J. K., & Kelsey, K. T. (2001). Tobacco smoke-induced DNA damage and an early age of smoking initiation induce chromosome loss at 3p21 in lung cancer. *Cancer Research, 61,* 612-615.

Hoffman, P. C., Mauer, A. M., & Vokes, E. E. (2000). Lung cancer. *Lancet, 355,* 479-485.

Hyer, J. D., & Silvestri, G. (2000). Diagnosis and staging of lung cancer. *Clinics in Chest Medicine, 21,* 95-106.

Johnson, D. H. (2000). Locally advanced, unresectable non-small cell lung cancer: New treatment strategies. *Chest, 117,* 123S-126S.

Junker, K., Wiethege, T., & Muller, K. M. (2000). Pathology of small-cell lung cancer. *Journal of Cancer Research & Clinical Oncology, 126,* 361-368.

Kelly, K. (2000). New chemotherapy agents for small cell lung cancer. *Chest, 117,* 156S-162S.

Kennedy, T. C., Miller, Y., & Prindiville, S. (2000). Screening for lung cancer revisited and the role of sputum cytology and fluorescence bronchoscopy in a high-risk group. *Chest, 117,* 72S-79S.

Khuri, F. R., & Lippman, S. M. (2000). Lung cancer chemoprevention. *Seminars in Surgical Oncology, 18,* 100-105.

Kozin, S. V., Boucher, Y., Hicklin, D. J., Bohlen, P., Jain, R. K., & Suit, H. D. (2001). Vascular endothelial growth factor receptor-2-blocking antibody potentiates radiation-induced long-term control of human tumor xenografts. *Cancer Research, 61,* 39-44.

Lau, C. L., & Harpole, D. H., Jr. (2000). Noninvasive clinical staging modalities for lung cancer. *Seminars in Surgical Oncology, 18,* 116-123.

Lee, R. B. (2000). Surgical palliation of airway obstruction resulting from lung cancer. *Seminars in Surgical Oncology, 18,* 173-182.

Marom, E. M., Erasmus, J. J., & Patz, E. F. (2000). Lung cancer and positron emission tomography with fluorodeoxyglucose. *Lung Cancer, 28,* 187-202.

Mehta, M. P. (2000). The contemporary role of radiation therapy in the management of lung cancer. *Surgical Oncology Clinics of North America, 9,* 539-561.

Miettinen, O. S. (2000). Screening for lung cancer. *Radiologic Clinics of North America, 38,* 479-486.

Montuenga, L. M., & Mulshine, J. L. (2000). New molecular strategies for early lung cancer detection. *Cancer Investigation, 18,* 555-563.

Nakajima, E., Hirano, T., Konaka, C., Ikeda, N., Kawate, N., Ebihara, Y., & Kato, H. (2001). K-ras mutation in sputum of primary lung cancer patients does not always reflect that of cancerous cells. *International Journal of Oncology, 18,* 105-110.

Non-small Cell Lung Cancer Collaborative Group. (2000). Chemotherapy for non-small cell lung cancer. *Cochrane Database of Systematic Reviews [computer file]* CD002139.

Patz, E. F., Jr. (2000). Imaging bronchogenic carcinoma. *Chest, 117,* 90S-95S.

Pfeifer, G. P. (2000). p53 mutational spectra and the role of methylated CpG sequences. *Mutation Research, 450,* 155-166.

Pignatelli, B., Li, C. Q., Boffetta, P., Chen, Q., Ahrens, W., Nyberg, F., Mukeria, A., Bruske-Hohlfeld, I., Fortes, C., Constantinescu, V., Ischiropoulos, H., & Ohshima, H. (2001). Nitrated and oxidized plasma proteins in smokers and lung cancer patients. *Cancer Research, 61,* 778-784.

Porter, J. C., & Spiro, S. G. (2000). Detection of early lung cancer. *Thorax, 55*(Suppl 1), S56-S62.

Prochazka, A. V. (2000). New developments in smoking cessation. *Chest, 117,* 169S-175S.

Reif, M. S., Socinski, M. A., & Rivera, M. P. (2000). Evidence-based medicine in the treatment of non-small-cell lung cancer. *Clinics in Chest Medicine, 21,* 107-120.

Rom, W. N., Hay, J. G., Lee, T. C., Jiang, Y., & Tchou-Wong, K. M. (2000). Molecular and genetic aspects of lung cancer. *American Journal of Respiratory & Critical Care Medicine, 161,* 1355-1367.

Rosell, R., & Felip, E. (2000). Role of multimodality treatment for lung cancer. *Seminars in Surgical Oncology, 18,* 143-151.

Shaham, D. (2000). Semi-invasive and invasive procedures for the diagnosis and staging of lung cancer. I. Percutaneous transthoracic needle biopsy. *Radiologic Clinics of North America, 38,* 525-534.

Shields, P. G., & Harris, C. C. (2000). Cancer risk and low-penetrance susceptibility genes in gene-environment interactions. *Journal of Clinical Oncology, 18,* 2309-2315.

Shin, S. W., Breathnach, O. S., Linnoila, R. I., Williams, J., Gillespie, J. W., Kelley, M. J., & Johnson, B. E. (2001). Genetic changes in contralateral bronchioloalveolar carcinomas of the lung. *Oncology, 60,* 81-87.

Sone, S., Li, F., Yang, Z. G., Honda, T., Maruyama, Y., Takashima, S., Hasegawa, M., Kawakami, S., Kubo, K., Haniuda, M., & Yamanda, T. (2001). Results of three-year mass screening programme for lung cancer using mobile low-dose spiral computed tomography scanner. *British Journal of Cancer, 84,* 25-32.

Stevens, C. W., Lee, J. S., Cox, J., & Komaki, R. (2000). Novel approaches to locally advanced unresectable non-small cell lung cancer. *Radiotherapy & Oncology, 55,* 11-18.

Toloza, E. M., Roth, J. A., & Swisher, S. G. (2000). Molecular events in bronchogenic carcinoma and their implications for therapy. *Seminars in Surgical Oncology, 18,* 91-99.

Uramoto, H., Nakanishi, R., Fujino, Y., Imoto, H., Takenoyama, M., Yoshimatsu, T., Oyama, T., Osaki, T., & Yasumoto, K. (2001). Prediction of pulmonary complications after a lobectomy in patients with non-small cell lung cancer. *Thorax, 56,* 59-61.

Wright, G. S., & Gruidl, M. E. (2000). Early detection and prevention of lung cancer. *Current Opinion in Oncology, 12,* 143-148.

Yip, D., & Harper, P. G. (2000). Predictive and prognostic factors in small cell lung cancer: Current status. *Lung Cancer, 28,* 173-185.

Zochbauer-Muller, S., Fong, K. M., Virmani, A. K., Geradts, J., Gazdar, A. F., & Minna, J. D. (2001). Aberrant promoter methylation of multiple genes in non-small cell lung cancers. *Cancer Research, 61*(1), 249-255.

Zorn, G. L., III, & Nesbitt, J. C. (2000). Surgical management of early stage lung cancer. *Seminars in Surgical Oncology, 18,* 124-136.

Case Study

Lung Cancer

INITIAL HISTORY

- 52-year-old female smoker with a history of emphysema comes in for routine yearly check-up.
- Over the past year, she has experienced a mild increase in her chronic dyspnea with a dramatic worsening over the past 4 months.
- She has begun coughing more frequently.

Question 1   Based on this limited history, what is your differential diagnosis?

Question 2   What questions about her symptoms would you like to ask this patient?

ADDITIONAL HISTORY

- She is now dyspneic on walking to her bathroom and back.
- She denies change in her chronic production of scant white sputum.
- She denies fever.
- She denies hemoptysis.
- She has had increasing discomfort in her left chest with deep breathing and cough.
- She denies substernal chest pain, palpitations, or edema.
- She admits to a 10 pound weight loss over the past year.

Question 3 What questions about her past medical history would you like to ask?

PAST MEDICAL HISTORY

- 60 pack/year smoker.
- Emphysema diagnosed 5 years ago managed with inhaled beta agonist and ipratropium.
- Last pulmonary function testing was at the time of emphysema diagnosis; she doesn't know results.
- Had pneumonia 3 years ago treated at home.
- Seen in the emergency room with bronchitic exacerbation of her emphysema last year.
- Has never had angina or congestive heart failure (CHF) symptoms.
- Has no allergies.
- Is on no other medications.
- Had influenza vaccine last year and pneumococcal vaccine 2 years ago.

PHYSICAL EXAMINATION

- Alert thin woman looking older than stated age in mild respiratory distress, became dyspneic moving from chair to exam table.
- T = 37 orally; P = 90 and regular; RR = 22 and mildly labored; BP = 124/74.
- Pursed-lip breathing, no cyanosis.

HEENT, Skin, Neck

- PERRLA, pharynx clear, pursed-lip breathing.
- No rashes.
- No thyromegaly or bruits.

Lungs

- Increase in anteroposterior (AP) diameter.
- Use of accessory muscles of respiration.
- Chest tympanic without dullness.
- Diaphragms low with decreased excursion bilaterally.
- Scattered wheezes without crackles or rhonchi.
- No rubs.

Cardiac

- Apical pulse felt at 5th intercostal space at the midclavicular line.
- Regular rate and rhythm; no murmurs or gallops.

Abdomen, Extremities, Neurological

- Bowel sounds present, no masses, tenderness, or organomegaly.
- No edema, pulses full, no bruits.
- Cognition intact; strength, sensation, and reflexes normal and symmetrical; gait steady.

Question 4   What are the pertinent positives and negatives on the exam and what might they mean?

Question 5   How has your differential diagnosis changed?

Question 6   What tests would be indicated now?

INITIAL DIAGNOSTICS

- Arterial blood gases: pH = 7.42, $PaCO_2$ = 48, PaO_2 = 68 on room air.
- Electrocardiogram (ECG) reveals sinus tachycardia without evidence of ischemia.
- Pulmonary function testing reveals forced expiratory volume in 1 second (FEV_1) = 55% of predicted.

CHEST X-RAY AND READING

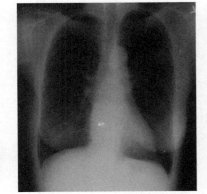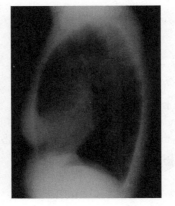

- Small, peripheral, noncalcified, and spiculated lesion in the upper left lobe.
- No evidence of hilar adenopathy.
- No evidence of soft tissue or bone disease.
- Lungs otherwise reveal hyperexpansion, bullae, and scarring consistent with emphysema.

SPUTUM CYTOLOGY
- Atypical cells suspicious for carcinoma but not diagnostic.

Question 7 What is your interpretation of these findings?

Question 8 What other studies might be indicated?

ADDITIONAL EVALUATION
- She is referred to a pulmonologist.
- CT scan reveals the lesion seen on x-ray, no mediastinal disease.
- Bronchoscopy cannot visualize the lesion, CT-guided fine needle aspiration reveals adenocarcinoma.
- Stage is 1, V/Q scanning and functional status testing indicates operability.
- There is no evidence of another primary tumor.

Question 9   The patient returns for advice prior to surgery, what should she be told?

POSTOPERATIVE FOLLOW-UP

- 3 weeks after left lower lobectomy, the patient returns feeling weak and still having pain at the incision.
- Her dyspnea is gradually improving after getting much worse immediately post-OP.
- She reports that she was told that the operation was a success; there were no complications.
- She is concerned about whether she will need chemotherapy and about her prognosis.

Question 10   What can you tell the patient now?

9

Breast Cancer

DEFINITION

- Neoplastic proliferation of breast cells.
- Classification of breast tumor types include the following:
  - Ductal
    1) Carcinoma in situ (DCIS): 50% of cases will progress to invasive carcinoma.
    2) Infiltrating ductal: most common breast cancer.
    3) Others include medullary, tubular, mucinous, papillary, adenocystic, carcinosarcoma.
  - Lobular
    1) Carcinoma in situ (LCIS).
    2) Infiltrating lobular.
  - Other
    1) Paget disease: oozing and itching of the nipple.
    2) Inflammatory breast cancer: skin edema, redness and warmth.

EPIDEMIOLOGY

- It is the most common cancer affecting women in the United States (185,000 cases in 1999).
- One in every 8 women in the United States develops breast cancer by the age of 85.
- The risk of dying of breast cancer is <4%.
- The peak age is 75 to 79; the major cause of death for women aged 35 to 54.
- Risk factors (50% of women with breast cancer have no risk factors other than age).
  - **Age.**
  - **Family History:** having a first degree relative with breast cancer confers a relative risk of 1.4 to 13.6 (risk rises if relative is young at the time of diagnosis).
  - **Genetics:**
    1) Hereditary (approximately 10% of cases)
       a) Mutation of BRCA1 gene: located on the long arm of chromosome 17; autosomal dominant transmission; 54% risk of breast cancer by age 60, 30% risk of ovarian cancer.
       b) Mutation of BRCA2 gene: located on chromosome 13; 85% lifetime risk for breast cancer; 10% to 20% risk of ovarian cancer; 6% lifetime risk of male breast cancer (100-fold increase in risk over the general population).
       c) Li Fraumeni syndrome: a germline deletion of p53 (p53 is a tumor-suppressor gene that normally induces apoptosis in mutated cells); increase in breast, brain, and adrenal tumors, as well as sarcomas and leukemias.

2) Sporadic (approximately 90% of cases):

   a) Multiple mutations have been identified, including oncogenes Her2/neu (ERBB2), MYC, CPY17, and CCND1, and tumor-suppressor genes p53, RB1, and CDKN2.

   b) Acquired mutations in BRCA1 and BRCA2 are rare in sporadic tumors but there may be some depression in these tumor-suppressor gene products.

- **Reproductive/hormonal:** parity and breast-feeding decrease risk.

  1) Early menarche (<age 12) or late menopause (>age 55)

  2) Nulliparity or late first pregnancy (>age 30).

  3) Termination of pregnancy remains controversial; recent studies suggest no risk.

  4) Level of serum estradiol correlated with breast cancer risk in both pre- and postmenopausal women.

  5) Postmenopausal estrogen replacement: controversy remains over magnitude of risk and the amount, timing, and type of hormones associated with the greatest risk; overall estimated increase in risk is 1.0 to 1.7; risk must be weighed against potential benefits.

  6) Oral contraceptive use before 1975 increases risk; no evidence that more recent use confers risk.

- **Environmental:** incidence of breast cancer cannot be fully explained by genetic and reproductive/ hormonal risks but direct links to environmental toxins have been difficult.

  1) Dietary fats: still controversial; recent data continues to suggest obesity is a risk factor.

  2) Smoking: data suggests that nicotine and N-nitrosamines (carcinogens in cigarette smoke) are concentrated in breast tissue, and that postmenopausal women smokers with a polymorphism of the gene responsible for detoxifying these carcinogens (slow acetylators) have an increased risk for breast cancer.

  3) Alcohol: over 30 to 60 gm/day (2 to 5 drinks) is linked to an increase in breast cancer risk.

  4) Others still being studied include polycyclic aromatic hydrocarbons (fossil fuel pollution), heterocyclic amines (overcooked meat), and ionizing radiation (risk is greatest if exposed before age 19).

- **Proliferative breast disease** (including fibrocysts):

  1) Affects 1.2 million women in the United States.

  2) Benign fibrocysts may be associated with a small increase in risk.

  3) Atypical hyperplasia increases risk of breast cancer 4 fold.

- **Past history of breast cancer** in contralateral breast: 47% of cases will develop carcinoma in situ with 1% per year developing invasive carcinoma.

PATHOPHYSIOLOGY

- The period between menarche and first pregnancy is believed to be the most vulnerable time for mutagenesis of breast cells.

- **Lob 1:**

  - Mammary cancer originates in areas of the breast called Lob 1, which are undifferentiated terminal structures of the mammary gland.

  - Lob 1 contains many undifferentiated cells with high proliferation rates and is particularly sensitive to carcinogens.

  - Pregnancy, especially with breast-feeding, reduces the amount of Lob 1 in the breast. Most of Lob 1 matures to Lob 2 or Lob 3 that are more differentiated and less vulnerable to mutagenesis.

- **BRCA1:**
  - Breast tissue taken from prophylactic mastectomy from patients with mutated BRCA1 gene reveals high amounts of Lob 1, even if the patient was parous.
  - The normal BRCA1 gene product is a growth inhibitor that controls proliferation of breast cells; this gene product is lost when the gene is mutated.
- **p53 gene mutation:**
  - This gene is a transcription regulator, genomic stabilizer, participant in DNA repair, inhibitor of cell cycle progression, and a facilitator of apoptosis of damaged cells.
  - It is a common acquired mutation in breast cancer as well as many other tumors such as lung.

Estrogen receptors (ERs):
  - ERs are cytosol proteins present in the nucleus of normal breast cells and on primary breast tumors or their metastases.
  - Estrogens regulate growth factor production and receptor expression. Estrogen is required for normal breast cell function (withdrawal of estrogen, such as with menopause, results in apoptosis of breast cells) and causes breast maturation and proliferation.
  - In neoplastic cells, ER stimulation results in over-expression of growth factor production and/or receptors resulting in uncontrolled cell proliferation.
  - 60% of primary tumors are considered ER positive. Many tumors also have progesterone receptors (PR). These tumors have slower growth rates, better prognoses, and better responses to hormone manipulation therapy than ER/PR negative tumors.
  - ER negative tumors result from methylation of the DNA (experimentally, blocking of DNA methylation can restore ER receptors) and are capable of autocrine stimulation independent of estrogen, thus are resistant to endocrine therapy and tend to be more aggressive tumors.

- **Other growth factors:**
  - Progesterone receptors are also found on normal cells and 50% of ER positive tumors; these tumors are the most responsive to endocrine therapy.
  - Insulin-like growth factor 1 (IGF_1) is important for normal mammary development but is also a mitogen for cancer cells and promotes anchorage-independent growth. Insulin-like growth factor 2 (IGF_2) regulates IGF_1 activity; receptors for these growth factors are found on ER positive tumors and suggest increased responsiveness to endocrine therapy.
  - Epidermal growth factor (EGF) leads to increased mitosis and resistance to tamoxifen; binds via HER receptors and increases HER2/neu expression (present on 20% to 30% of breast tumors).
  - Others include transforming growth factor β and angiogenesis factors.
- **Cell adhesion molecules:**
  - Tumor cells escape normal cell-basement membrane adhesion molecules in order to invade.
  - One of the most important adhesion molecules in breast tissue is E-cadherin which is down-regulated in breast cancer.
- **Multidrug resistance gene (MDR1):** codes for a glycoprotein "efflux pump" that decreases intracellular concentration of anticancer agents.
- **Matrix metalloproteinases and cathepsins:** breast cancers are high in these extracellular proteinases that modulate cell-basement membrane interactions and can degrade the membrane to allow for invasion and metastasis.

PATIENT PRESENTATION

History

Medical history of breast disease; reproductive history (age of onset of menses, number of pregnancies and age at first pregnancy, age of onset of menopause); history of hormone use; family history of breast cancer; alcohol consumption, smoking history, diet. Risk assessment (consider Gail or Claus model).

Symptoms

Breast and axillary symptoms (mass, pain, nipple discharge or retraction, skin changes, arm swelling); symptoms of metastases (headache, seizure, bone pain, dyspnea); fatigue; weight loss.

Examination

Breast mass (size, location, consistency, fixation to skin); skin changes (erythema, dimpling, edema); nipple changes (retraction, thickening, discharge); nodal status (axillary size, location fixation, supraclavicular nodes).

DIFFERENTIAL DIAGNOSIS

- Fibroadenoma
- Mastitis
- Metastases from another primary tumor

KEYS TO ASSESSMENT

- Screening for breast cancer in the general public.
  - Screening for cancer: monthly self-exam plus yearly clinical exam and mammography.
  - Recommendations for mammography are controversial; it is unclear whether to do screening before age 50 but evidence is mounting that screening beginning at age 40 can reduce mortality in high-risk individuals (more false positive tests in this age group, however).
- Screening of women with an inherited predisposition (BRCA1, BRCA2, Li Fraumeni) for breast cancer.
  - Monthly self-exam beginning at age 18; semiannual clinical exam beginning at age 25.
  - Mammography beginning at age 25 (every other year until age 35, then every year).
  - Ovarian cancer surveillance with yearly transvaginal ultrasound and serum CA-125.
- Assessment once a breast mass is discovered.
  - Careful history of risk factors and family history.
  - Further diagnostics
    1) Mammography: digital mammography is more sensitive (88% to 95%).
    2) Ultrasound: differentiates cystic vs. solid masses, helps to find palpable masses not seen on mammogram (especially in a young woman), and can be used to guide biopsy.
    3) MRI–3D RODEO MRI: highly sensitive but also many false positives; especially useful for finding other foci of cancer in patients with a known primary and for guiding biopsy of small lesions.
    4) Mammoscintigraphy: highly sensitive but does not differentiate malignant from benign and cannot be used to guide biopsy.
    5) Positron emission tomography: still being tested but highly sensitive.

- Tissue diagnosis:
    1) Fine needle aspiration (FNA): 98% accuracy if combined with exam and mammogram.
    2) Core biopsy, excisional biopsy (lumpectomy).
    3) Ductal lavage: provides very early detection in high-risk patients.
- Assessing nodal status:
    1) Sentinel node biopsy: if the sentinel node is negative, then it is highly likely that the rest of the axillary nodes are negative, thus it may eliminate the need for more extensive axillary biopsies; cytokeratin immunohistochemical staining can pick up micrometastases further increasing the sensitivity of this procedure.
    2) Axillary dissection: if sentinel node is positive, full axillary dissection to assess the extent of nodal involvement is indicated.
- Chest x-ray, bone scan if symptomatic for metastases or if alkaline phosphatase is elevated.
- Staging: "TNM" system (*T*umor size, *N*odal status, *M*etastases).

KEYS TO MANAGEMENT

- Prevention of breast cancer:
    - Smoking cessation, decrease alcohol intake.
    - Exercise, decrease fat intake, weight loss.
    - Vitamin E (α-tocopherol): antioxidant; studies are mixed but there is a strong trend toward decreased risk with supplementation, especially in postmenopausal women.
    - Fiber: alters gut microbial enzymes and decreases the amount of estrogens reabsorbed from the gut, also produces phytoestrogens that compete for estrogen receptor binding sites.
    - Selective estrogen receptor modulators (SERMS):
        1) Tamoxifen: approved in 1998 for the primary prevention of breast cancer in high-risk patients; clearly reduces risk but increases the risk of endometrial cancer.
        2) Raloxifene: recent retrospective study found a 75% decrease in risk of invasive breast cancer in women taking raloxifene for osteoporosis for at least 3 years.
    - Prophylactic mastectomy reduces risk of breast cancer by over 90% in high-risk women.
- Surgical:
    - Lumpectomy: used when the tumor is small and there is no obvious axillary involvement; results clearly show survival similar to mastectomy, even if axillary nodes are positive.
    - Modified radical mastectomy: preserves pectoralis muscles with improved cosmesis over radical mastectomy; it is used for stage II to stage III if there is no fixation to muscle.
    - Total mastectomy (simple mastectomy): no axillary dissection; it is used for CIS, prophylactic removal of a contralateral breast, local recurrence after lumpectomy, and palliation of bulky tumor.
    - Radical mastectomy: the breast is removed en bloc, along with all axillary nodes and both pectoralis muscles; is used if the tumor is fixed to the pectoralis muscle or if there is bulky axillary involvement.
- Radiation:
    - Local irradiation after surgery reduces the risk of local recurrence.
    - Recent reports suggest radiation also improves long-term survival in both node positive and node negative cancers.

- Endocrine therapy (hormone manipulation):
  - Used as adjuvant therapy after surgery for both pre- and postmenopausal women with ER or PR positive tumors; used with cytotoxic therapy in node-positive disease.
  - Increases survival and disease-free survival and decreases the risk for disease in the contralateral breast.
  - Tamoxifen: when used in operable ER positive breast cancer; tamoxifen taken for 5 years results in a 50% annual reduction in recurrence rate and a 28% annual decrease in death rate, and can reduce the risk of recurrence in the contralateral breast. Also slows tumor progression in advanced disease. Confers an increased risk of endometrial cancer and thromboembolic disease.
  - Raloxifene probably has equal antitumor effects with less risk of endometrial cancer; studies ongoing.
  - Other hormonal manipulation: luteinizing hormone releasing hormone agonists, ovarian ablation. Progestins, aromatase inhibitors, androgens.
- Chemotherapy:
  - Adjunctive chemotherapy substantially improves long-term, disease free survival in both premenopausal and postmenopausal women up to age 70 with node-positive and node-negative disease.
  - Most patients receive combination chemotherapy containing an anthracycline; taxanes are added for metastatic disease.
  - A high dose of chemotherapy plus supporting granulocyte-colony stimulating factor (G-CSF) and blood stem cells has been found to be an effective and safe outpatient regimen for selected patients.
  - Preoperative chemotherapy can shrink tumors and make lumpectomy a surgical option in some patients with a relatively large primary tumor prior to chemotherapy.
  - High dose of chemotherapy and an autologous bone marrow transplant provide dramatic results in a few patients but is associated with high morbidity and mortality and cannot be recommended for most patients.
- Trastuzumab (Herceptin): Monoclonal antibody to Her2/neu growth factor receptor; for advanced disease, used alone or with chemotherapy it improves response rates and survival time but is associated with significant myocardial toxicity and resultant congestive heart failure.
- Tumor vaccines for tumor-associated antigens are under investigation.
- Bisphosphonates (alendronate) may reduce the risk of skeletal metastases.
- Psychological support: improves survival and slows disease progression

Pathophysiology → Clinical Link

What is going on in the disease process that influences how the patient presents and how he or she should be managed?

What should you do now that you understand the underlying pathophysiology?

Strong genetic component to risk.	The family history is important, and genetic screening should be considered.
Between puberty and pregnancy, the breast contains high amounts of Lob 1. Breast cancer is most likely to arise in Lob 1 tissue.	Nulliparous women are at greater risk; pregnancy, especially with lactation, reduces risk. The interval between puberty and the first pregnancy may be the most vulnerable time for exposure to carcinogens.
Numerous environmental toxins accumulate in breast tissue and are associated with carcinogenesis.	Women should be counseled to exercise and avoid smoking and should consider dietary modification including reduced fat and alcohol intake and increased antioxidant intake. These measures may be most important during the most "vulnerable" time in breast development that occurs between puberty and the first pregnancy.
Mutation of the BRCA1 gene leads to loss of an important growth inhibitor and is associated with high amounts of Lob 1 even in multiparous women.	Patients with BRCA1 gene require careful screening beginning at age 25.
When estrogen receptors are stimulated, they cause the production of growth factors that induce cell division.	Tamoxifen and raloxifene are selective estrogen receptor modulators that block estrogens effect on the breast and can be used in both prevention and treatment. Raloxifene may turn out to be better and safer.
Positive axillary nodes indicate spread of the primary tumor.	Axillary sentinel node biopsy or full axillary dissection is crucial to proper staging for treatment.
When the tumor is small, there is less likelihood of tumor spread.	Early stage tumors should be treated with lumpectomy; most patients will also be treated with adjuvant endocrine, radiation, or chemotherapy.

Suggested Reading

Aebi, S., Gelber, S., Castiglione-Gertsch, M., Gelber, R. D., Collins, J., Thurlimann, B., Rudenstam, C. M., Lindtner, J., Crivellari, D., Cortes-Funes, H., Simoncini, E., Werner, I. D., Coates, A. S., & Goldhirsch, A. (2000). Is chemotherapy alone adequate for young women with oestrogen-receptor-positive breast cancer? *Lancet, 355,* 1869-1874.

Angele, S., & Hall, J. (2000). The ATM gene and breast cancer: Is it really a risk factor? *Mutation Research, 462,* 167-178.

Anonymous. (1997). National Institutes of Health Consensus Development Conference Statement: Breast cancer screening for women ages 40-49, January 21-23, 1997. National Institutes of Health Consensus Development Panel. *Journal of the National Cancer Institute, 89*(14), 1015-1026.

Anonymous. (2000). Adjuvant therapy for breast cancer. *NIH Consensus Statement 2000, 17*(4), 1-23. [Online November 1-3].

Armstrong, K., Eisen, A., & Weber, B. (2000). Assessing the risk of breast cancer. *New England Journal of Medicine, 342,* 564-571.

Bassett, L. W. (2000). Imaging of breast masses. *Radiologic Clinics of North America, 38,* 669-691.

Baynes, R. D., Dansey, R. D., Klein, J. L., Karanes, C., Cassells, L., Abella, E., Wei, W. Z., Galy, A., Du, W., Wood, G., & Peters, W. P. (2000). High-dose chemotherapy and autologous stem cell transplantation for breast cancer. *Cancer Investigation, 18,* 440-455.

Berenson, J. R., & Lipton, A. (1999). Bisphosphonates in the treatment of malignant bone disease. *Annual Review of Medicine, 50,* 237-248.

Black, M. H., & Diamandis, E. P. (2000). The diagnostic and prognostic utility of prostate-specific antigen for diseases of the breast. *Breast Cancer Research & Treatment, 59,* 1-14.

Burke, W., Daly, M., Garber, J., Botkin, J., Kahn, M. J., Lynch, P., McTiernan, A., Offit, K., Perlman, J., Petersen, G., Thomson, E., & Varricchio, C. (1997). Recommendations for follow-up care of individuals with an inherited predisposition to cancer. II. BRCA1 and BRCA2. Cancer Genetics Studies Consortium. *Journal of the American Medical Association, 277*(12), 997-1003.

Cardenosa, G., Quinn, C. A., Chilcote, W. A., Foglietti, M. G., & Barry, M. A. (2000). How new technology is changing mammography and breast cancer management. *Cleveland Clinic Journal of Medicine, 67,* 191-193.

Cheung, K. L., Graves, C. R., & Robertson, J. F. (2000). Tumour marker measurements in the diagnosis and monitoring of breast cancer. *Cancer Treatment Reviews, 26,* 91-102.

Chlebowski, R. T. (2000). Reducing the risk of breast cancer. *New England Journal of Medicine, 343,* 191-198.

Cody, H. S. (1999). Sentinel lymph node mapping in breast cancer. *Oncology, 13*(1), 25-34, discussion 35-36.

Coleman, R. E. (2000). High dose chemotherapy: Rationale and results in breast carcinoma. *Cancer, 88,* 3059-3064.

Crawshaw, A. (2000). Carcinoma of the breast and hormone replacement therapy for osteoporosis. *International Journal of Clinical Practice, 54,* 99-103.

Crown, J., & O'Leary, M. (2000). The taxanes: An update. *Lancet, 355,* 1176-1178.

de Boer, R., Hillen, H. F., Roumen, R. M., Rutten, H. J., van der Sangen, M. J., & Voogd, A. C. (2001). Detection, treatment and outcome of axillary recurrence after axillary clearance for invasive breast cancer. *British Journal of Surgery, 88,* 118-122.

Diel, I. J. (2000). Antitumour effects of bisphosphonates: First evidence and possible mechanisms. *Drugs, 59,* 391-399.

Diel, I. J., Solomayer, E. F., & Bastert, G. (2000). Bisphosphonates and the prevention of metastasis: First evidences from preclinical and clinical studies. *Cancer, 88,* 3080-3088.

Dignam, J. J. (2000). Differences in breast cancer prognosis among African-American and Caucasian women. *Ca: A Cancer Journal for Clinicians, 50,* 50-64.

Dowsett, M. (2000). Use of risk determinants for different breast cancer prevention strategies. *European Journal of Cancer, 36,* 1283-1287.

Eisen, A., Rebbeck, T. R., Wood, W. C., & Weber, B. L. (2000). Prophylactic surgery in women with a hereditary predisposition to breast and ovarian cancer. *Journal of Clinical Oncology, 18,* 1980-1995.

Eisinger, F., Charafe-Jauffret, E., Jacquemier, J., Birnbaum, D., Julian-Reynier, C., & Sobol, H. (2001). Tamoxifen and breast cancer risk in women harboring a BRCA1 germline mutation: Computed efficacy, effectiveness and impact. *International Journal of Oncology, 18,* 5-10.

Feigelson, H. S., McKean-Cowdin, R., Coetzee, G. A., Stram, D. O., Kolonel, L. N., & Henderson, B. E. (2001). Building a multigenic model of breast cancer susceptibility: CYP17 and HSD17B1 are two important candidates. *Cancer Research, 61,* 785-789.

Feldman, A. M., Lorell, B. H., & Reis, S. E. (2000). Trastuzumab in the treatment of metastatic breast cancer: Anticancer therapy versus cardiotoxicity. *Circulation, 102,* 272-274.

Fentiman, I. S. (2000). Future prospects for the prevention and cure of breast cancer. *European Journal of Cancer, 36,* 1085-1088.

Fitzgibbons, P. L., Page, D. L., Weaver, D., Thor, A. D., Allred, D. C., Clark, G. M., Ruby, S. G., O'Malley, F., Simpson, J. F., Connolly, J. L., Hayes, D. F., Edge, S. B., Lichter, A., & Schnitt, S. J. (2000). Prognostic factors in breast cancer. College of American Pathologists Consensus Statement 1999. *Archives of Pathology & Laboratory Medicine, 124,* 966-978.

Fornier, M., Munster, P., & Seidman, A. D. (1999). Update on the management of advanced breast cancer. *Oncology, 13*(5), 647-658.

Freedman, M., San Martin, J., O'Gorman, J., Eckert, S., Lippman, M. E., Lo, S. C., Walls, E. L., & Zeng, J. (2001). Digitized mammography: A clinical trial of postmenopausal women randomly assigned to receive raloxifene, estrogen, or placebo. *Journal of the National Cancer Institute, 93,* 51-56.

Gianni, A. M., & Piccart, M. J. (2000). Optimising chemotherapy dose density and dose intensity. New strategies to improve outcomes in adjuvant therapy for breast cancer. *European Journal of Cancer, 36*(Suppl 1), S1-S3.

Gilewski, T., Seidman, A., Norton, L., & Hudis, C. (2000). An immunotherapeutic approach to treatment of breast cancer: Focus on trastuzumab plus paclitaxel. Breast Cancer Medicine Service. *Cancer Chemotherapy & Pharmacology, 46*(Suppl), S23-S26.

Hansen, R. K., & Bissell, M. J. (2000). Tissue architecture and breast cancer: The role of extracellular matrix and steroid hormones. *Endocrine-Related Cancer, 7,* 95-113.

Henderson, B. E., & Feigelson, H. S. (2000). Hormonal carcinogenesis. *Carcinogenesis, 21,* 427-433.

Higa, G. M. (2000). Altering the estrogenic milieu of breast cancer with a focus on the new aromatase inhibitors. *Pharmacotherapy, 20,* 280-291.

Hortobagyi, G. (2000). Adjuvant therapy for breast cancer. *Annual Review of Medicine, 51,* 377-392.

Hortobagyi, G. N. (2000). Developments in chemotherapy of breast cancer. *Cancer, 88,* 3073-3079:

Hunter, C. P. (2000). Epidemiology, stage at diagnosis, and tumor biology of breast carcinoma in multiracial and multiethnic populations. *Cancer, 88,* 1193-1202.

Jacobs, H. S. (2000). Hormone replacement therapy and breast cancer. *Endocrine-Related Cancer, 7,* 53-61.

Jacobson, J. S., Workman, S. B., & Kronenberg, F. (2000). Research on complementary/ alternative medicine for patients with breast cancer: A review of the biomedical literature. *Journal of Clinical Oncology, 18,* 668-683.

Kaas, R., Hart, A. A., Besnard, A. P., Peterse, J. L., & Rutgers, E. J. (2001). Impact of mammographic interval on stage and survival after the diagnosis of contralateral breast cancer. *British Journal of Surgery, 88,* 123-127.

Kaijser, M., Lichtenstein, P., Granath, F., Erlandsson, G., Cnattingius, S., & Ekbom, A. (2001). In utero exposures and breast cancer: A study of opposite-sexed twins. *Journal of the National Cancer Institute, 93,* 60-62.

Karp, S. E. (2000). Clinical management of BRCA1- and BRCA2-associated breast cancer. *Seminars in Surgical Oncology, 18,* 296-304.

Khayat, D., Antoine, E. C., & Coeffic, D. (2000). Taxol in the management of cancers of the breast and the ovary. *Cancer Investigation, 18,* 242-260.

Kimmick, G. G., & Balducci, L. (2000). Breast cancer and aging. Clinical interactions. *Hematology-Oncology Clinics of North America, 14,* 213-234.

Krag, D. (2000). Sentinel lymph node biopsy for the detection of metastases. *Cancer Journal From Scientific American, 6*(Suppl 2), S121-S124.

Kristensen, V. N., & Borresen-Dale, A. L. (2000). Molecular epidemiology of breast cancer: Genetic variation in steroid hormone metabolism. *Mutation Research, 462,* 323-333.

Liberman, L. (2000). Clinical management issues in percutaneous core breast biopsy. *Radiologic Clinics of North America, 38,* 791-807.

Lien, E. A., & Lonning, P. E. (2000). Selective oestrogen receptor modifiers (SERMs) and breast cancer therapy. *Cancer Treatment Reviews, 26,* 205-227.

Lipton, A. (2000). Bisphosphonates and breast carcinoma: Present and future. *Cancer, 88,* 3033-3037.

Lipworth, L., Bailey, L. R., & Trichopoulos, D. (2000). History of breast-feeding in relation to breast cancer risk: A review of the epidemiologic literature. *Journal of the National Cancer Institute, 92,* 302-312.

Marbella, A. M., & Layde, P. M. (2001). Racial trends in age-specific breast cancer mortality rates in US women. *American Journal of Public Health, 91,* 118-121.

Menard, S., Tagliabue, E., Campiglio, M., & Pupa, S. M. (2000). Role of HER2 gene overexpression in breast carcinoma. *Journal of Cellular Physiology, 182,* 150-162.

Minton, S. E. (2000). Chemoprevention of breast cancer in the older patient. *Hematology-Oncology Clinics of North America, 14,* 113-130.

Morrow, M., & Jordan, V. C. (2000). Tamoxifen for the prevention of breast cancer in the high-risk woman. *Annals of Surgical Oncology, 7,* 67-71.

Nass, S. J., & Davidson, N. E. (1999). The biology of breast cancer. *Hematology-Oncology Clinics of North America, 13*(2), 311-332.

Nicholson, R. I., & Gee, J. M. (2000). Oestrogen and growth factor cross-talk and endocrine insensitivity and acquired resistance in breast cancer. *British Journal of Cancer, 82,* 501-513.

Nicolini, A., & Carpi, A. (2000). Postoperative follow-up of breast cancer patients: Overview and progress in the use of tumor markers. *Tumour Biology, 21,* 235-248.

Orel, S. G. (2000). MR imaging of the breast. *Radiologic Clinics of North America, 38,* 899-913.

Page, D. (2001). Re: Short-term breast cancer prediction by random periareolar fine-needle aspiration cytology and the Gail risk model. *Journal of the National Cancer Institute, 93,* 68.

Paterson, A. H. (2000). The potential role of bisphosphonates as adjuvant therapy in the prevention of bone metastases. *Cancer, 88,* 3038-3046.

Pathak, D. R., Osuch, J. R., & He, J. (2000). Breast carcinoma etiology: Current knowledge and new insights into the effects of reproductive and hormonal risk factors in black and white populations. *Cancer, 88,* 1230-1238.

Peters, J. A., & Rubinstein, W. S. (2000). Genetics and the multidisciplinary breast center. *Surgical Oncology Clinics of North America, 9,* 367-396.

Pike, M. C., & Spicer, D. V. (2000). Hormonal contraception and chemoprevention of female cancers. *Endocrine-Related Cancer, 7,* 73-83.

Pisano, E. D., & Parham, C. A. (2000). Digital mammography, sestamibi breast scintigraphy, and positron emission tomography breast imaging. *Radiologic Clinics of North America, 38,* 861-869.

Powers, A., Cox, C., & Reintgen, D. S. (2000). Breast cancer screening in childhood cancer survivors. *Medical & Pediatric Oncology, 34,* 210-212.

Pritchard, K. I. (2000). Current and future directions in medical therapy for breast carcinoma: Endocrine treatment. *Cancer, 88,* 3065-3072.

Pritchard, K. I. (2000). Endocrine therapy for breast cancer. *Oncology (Huntington), 14,* 483-492.

Rabinowitz, B. (2000). Psychologic issues, practitioners' interventions, and the relationship of both to an interdisciplinary breast center team. *Surgical Oncology Clinics of North America, 9,* 347-365.

Recht, A. (2000). Locally advanced breast cancer and postmastectomy radiotherapy. *Surgical Oncology Clinics of North America, 9,* 603-620.

Rodenhuis, S., Huitema, A. D., van Dam, F. S., de Vries, E. G., & Beijnen, J. H. (2000). High-dose chemotherapy with peripheral blood progenitor cell transplantation in the adjuvant treatment of breast cancer. *Cancer Journal From Scientific American, 6*(Suppl 2), S125-S130.

Rodriguez, C., Calle, E. E., Patel, A. V., Tatham, L. M., Jacobs, E. J., & Thun, M. J. (2001). Effect of body mass on the association between estrogen replacement therapy and mortality among elderly US women. *American Journal of Epidemiology, 153,* 145-152.

Roe, E. B., Chiu, K. M., & Arnaud, C. D. (2000). Selective estrogen receptor modulators and postmenopausal health. *Advances in Internal Medicine, 45,* 259-278.

Russo, I. H., & Russo, J. (2000). Hormonal approach to breast cancer prevention. *Journal of Cellular Biochemistry—Supplement 34,* 1-6.

Sakorafas, G. H., & Tsiotou, A. G. (2000). Ductal carcinoma in situ (DCIS) of the breast: Evolving perspectives. *Cancer Treatment Reviews, 26,* 103-125.

Sakorafas, G. H., & Tsiotou, A. G. (2000). Sentinel lymph node biopsy in breast cancer. *American Surgeon, 66,* 667-674.

Sapunar, F., & Smith, I. E. (2000). Neoadjuvant chemotherapy for breast cancer. *Annals of Medicine, 32,* 43-50.

Schwartz, G. F., Solin, L. J., Olivotto, I. A., Ernster, V. L., & Pressman, P. I. (2000). Consensus conference on the treatment of in situ ductal carcinoma of the breast, April 22-25, 1999. *Cancer, 88,* 946-954.

Shuster, T. D., Girshovich, L., Whitney, T. M., & Hughes, K. S. (2000). Multidisciplinary care for patients with breast cancer. *Surgical Clinics of North America, 80,* 505-533.

Silverstein, M. J. (2000). Ductal carcinoma in situ of the breast. *Annual Review of Medicine, 51,* 17-32.

Simpson, J. F., & Page, D. L. (2000). The p53 tumor suppressor gene in ductal carcinoma in situ of the breast [comment]. *American Journal of Pathology, 156,* 5-6.

Speirs, V., & Kerin, M. J. (2000). Prognostic significance of oestrogen receptor beta in breast cancer. *British Journal of Surgery, 87,* 405-409.

Stebbing, J., Copson, E., & O'Reilly, S. (2000). Herceptin (trastuzamab) in advanced breast cancer. *Cancer Treatment Reviews, 26,* 287-290.

Stockler, M., Wilcken, N. R., Ghersi, D., & Simes, R. J. (2000). Systematic reviews of chemotherapy and endocrine therapy in metastatic breast cancer. *Cancer Treatment Reviews, 26,* 151-168.

Tabar, L., Dean, P. B., Duffy, S. W., & Chen, H. H. (2000). A new era in the diagnosis of breast cancer. *Surgical Oncology Clinics of North America, 9,* 233-277.

Tonin, P. N. (2000). Genes implicated in hereditary breast cancer syndromes. *Seminars in Surgical Oncology, 18,* 281-286.

Vaziri, S. A., Krumroy, L. M., Rostai, M., & Casey, G. (2001). Frequency of BRCA1 and BRCA2 mutations in a clinic-based series of breast and ovarian cancer families. *Human Mutation, 17,* 74.

Vogel, V. G. (2000). Breast cancer prevention: A review of current evidence. *Ca: A Cancer Journal for Clinicians, 50,* 156-170.

Weiss, N. S. (2001). Re: Tumor characteristics and clinical outcome of elderly women with breast cancer. *Journal of the National Cancer Institute, 93,* 65-66.

Welcsh, P. L., Owens, K. N., & King, M. C. (2000). Insights into the functions of BRCA1 and BRCA2. *Trends in Genetics, 16,* 69-74.

Winchester, D. P., Jeske, J. M., & Goldschmidt, R. A. (2000). The diagnosis and management of ductal carcinoma in-situ of the breast. *Ca: A Cancer Journal for Clinicians, 50,* 184-200.

Wohlfahrt, J., & Melbye, M. (2001). Age at any birth is associated with breast cancer risk. *Epidemiology, 12,* 68-73.

Wolff, A. C., & Davidson, N. E. (2000). Primary systemic therapy in operable breast cancer. *Journal of Clinical Oncology, 18,* 1558-1569.

Case Study*

Breast Cancer

INITIAL HISTORY
- 44-year-old white premenopausal woman.
- Presents for annual GYN examination.
- States her breasts are "cystic."
- Concerned about a "lump" in her left breast.
- History of 7 to 8 year use of birth control pills.
- Denies pain, nipple discharge, or skin changes of her breasts.

Question 1   What is your differential diagnosis based on the information you now have?

Question 2   What other questions would like to ask this patient?

ADDITIONAL HISTORY
- The patient does practice breast self-exam, but not routinely.
- She never had a mammogram.
- She noticed the lump approximately 8 weeks ago.
- Maternal grandmother was diagnosed with breast cancer at age 78.
- No previous breast biopsies.
- One child, age 10; has never breast fed.
- No significant health history, no medications, exercises 3 times a week.
- Menarche age 12, first child at age 34.

_____

*Kathleen R. Haden contributed this case study.

Question 3   What are the major risk factors of breast cancer?

Question 4   What are the controversial risk factors associated with breast cancer?

PHYSICAL EXAMINATION
- Well appearing 44-year-old white female in no acute distress.
- Afebrile, vital signs stable.
- Weight stable at 125 lbs.
- Height 5' 4"

HEENT
- Head exam normal.
- Neck supple, no JVD.
- No palpable cervical, supraclavicular, infraclavicular or axillary adenopathy.
- Thyroid nonpalpable.

Breast Exam
- Symmetrical breasts.
- No dimpling, puckering, or nipple discharge.
- Normal skin appearance.
- Diffuse small mobile cystic nodules palpable in the upper outer quadrants of both breasts.
- One is approximately 1 cm, firm, nonmobile nodule palpable in the left upper outer quadrant of the left breast.

Chest, Cardiac, Abdomen, Gynecologic
- Exam unremarkable.

Question 5   What do you think of her exam findings?

Question 6   What would you do at this point?

Question 7   What would you tell the patient about her examination and the scheduled testing?

ADDITIONAL FINDINGS

- Mammogram reveals an approximately 2 cm noncystic dominant mass with irregular borders within the left upper outer quadrant of the left breast.
- During her exam, the radiologist informs you about the findings and the patient agrees to undergo a core biopsy of the lesion.
- Results reveal an infiltrating ductal carcinoma.

Question 8   What do you do now?

ADDITIONAL INFORMATION

- All laboratory tests and chest x-ray are normal.
- Breast surgeon educates patient about two surgical options including:
  - Lumpectomy with axillary dissection followed by local irradiation.
  - Mastectomy with axillary lymph node dissection with or without reconstruction surgery.

PATIENT ALSO MET WITH RADIATION ONCOLOGIST TO DISCUSS THE POTENTIAL SIDE EFFECTS OF RADIATION THERAPY

- Acute changes, such as skin changes (erythema and desquamation), lymphedema of the breast, and fatigue.
- Chronic problems, such as rib fracture, breast retraction, scarring of lumpectomy incision, and the potential of pneumonitis.

Question 9 On what basis is breast conservation therapy (lumpectomy) based?

MORE INFORMATION

- The patient elects breast conservation therapy (lumpectomy) and axillary dissection with RT.
- The pathology reveals a 1.8 cm infiltrating ductal carcinoma.
- Graded III/III
  - None of the 12 lymph nodes are positive.
  - All surgical margins are clear.
  - Estrogen receptors/progesterone receptors are negative.
- Stage IA

Question 10 Would you refer her to a medical oncologist at this time?

Question 11 What therapy would be recommended?

Question 12 What side effects would be discussed with the patient?

ADDITIONAL INFORMATION

- Patient elects CMF chemotherapy for 6 months, followed by 6 weeks of radiation treatment since she had breast-conserving therapy.
- Following therapy, the patient will be followed every 3 to 4 months for the first 2 years, then every 6 months until 5 years, and then annually.
- Only routine yearly chest x-ray, routine chemistries, and mammography are ordered for follow-up unless clinical suspicion for recurrence.

Question 13 Where are the most common sites of breast cancer recurrence that would be important to ask during routine review of system history taken during follow-up visits?

10

Cutaneous Malignant Melanoma

DEFINITION

- Intraepidermal proliferation of malignant melanocytes with or without extension into the subcutaneous layers.
- Melanoma types include the following:
  - Superficial spreading melanoma
  - Acral lentiginous melanoma
  - Lentigo maligna
  - Nodular melanoma

EPIDEMIOLOGY

- It is the 7th most common cancer in the United States.
- Incidence has increased dramatically over the past 2 decades (approximately 4% per year); estimated lifetime risk 1:75; incidence increases with age.
- Worldwide, Australia has the highest incidence; in the United States, California has the highest incidence.
- Overall mortality rate for melanoma in the U.S. is 2.2 per 100,000; accounts for the vast majority of deaths from cutaneous malignancies.
- Risk factors:
  - Sun exposure: intermittent intense sun exposures (especially repeated sunburns as children) have the highest risk (blistering sunburns between the ages or 15 to 20 increase risk 2.2 fold); occupational exposure; tanning beds have also been implicated.
  - Pigment traits: blue eyes, fair complexion, red hair, freckling, sunburns easily.
  - Nevi: the total number of benign melanocytic nevi has been related to up to a 10-fold increased melanoma risk; dysplastic nevi are the precursor lesion to melanoma; the dysplastic nevus syndrome is an inherited entity associated with 25 to 75, such nevi per individual and a high risk for melanoma.
  - Family history: one relative = 2 times the risk; 2 relatives = 14 times the risk.
  - Genetics: melanoma susceptibility loci have been identified on chromosomes 9 (p16 or CDKN2A), 12 (CDK4), 1, and 6; melanoma tumor suppressor genes mutations have been identified on chromosome 11; acquired gene abnormalities include melanoma differentiation associated gene (mda-7), and loss of p53 activity.
  - Immunosuppression: risk is increased by 4- to 8-fold.

PATHOPHYSIOLOGY

- Ultraviolet radiation can act as an initiator, a promoter, a cocarcinogen, and an immunosuppressive agent.

- Melanin functions to absorb ultraviolet protons, skin that is low in melanin is more vulnerable to ultraviolet damage; melanomas tend to occur in areas that are not usually tanned but have been severely burned intermittently (ex. trunk on men, legs on women).

- UVA and UVB radiation are absorbed by the deoxyribonucleic acid (DNA) resulting in DNA mutations, proliferation of melanocytes, increased deposition of melanin in keratinocytes, and skin thickening.

- Melanocytes have high levels of the anti-apoptotic protein Bcl-2, thus mutations result in diminished apoptosis and damaged melanocytes can continue to divide with little or no DNA repair.

- Mutated melanocytes produce high levels of basic fibrinogen growth factor (bFGF) which stimulates autonomous melanocyte proliferation; an increased activity of bFGF is associated with a p53 mutation.

- Numerous other autocrine and paracrine growth factors further stimulate melanoma cell proliferation, including interleukins 1,8, and 10, platelet derived growth factor, epidermal growth factors, vasculare endothelial growth factors, and angiogenesis factors. Tumor necrosis factor and interleukins 2 and 6 inhibit melanocyte division.

- Mutation of CDK4 locus results in inactivation of inhibitors of melanocyte division.

- Melanoma cells frequently express specific tumor antigens, such as the MAGE antigens.

- Disordered cellular "cross-talk" by cadherins, connexins and adhesion receptors result in abnormalities in cell growth and differentiation, apoptosis, and migration.

- Intraepidermal proliferation of malignant melanocytes (radial growth phase) are followed by malignant cell nests and single cells spreading outward and down through the dermis and into the subcutaneous fat.

- The intraepidermal phase is not associated with metastasis; once growth is vertical (nodular with penetration through the dermis), then metastasis is likely.

- 30% of melanomas arise from dysplastic nevi that occur in about 10% of the Caucasian population; there is stepwise progression from a symmetrical, uniformly pigmented macule to an increasingly asymmetrical, variegated, elevated lesion with atypia, and patchy lymphocyte invasion.

PATIENT PRESENTATION

History

Fair skinned with a history of frequent sunburns as a child; multiple nevi; outdoor occupation; residence in sunny location; family history; immunosuppression.

Symptoms

Enlarging pigmented lesion commonly on the trunk in men and on the legs in women; also occurs on the neck, head or arms, genitalia, mucus membranes, occasionally on palms, soles, or nail plate; may present with dyspnea, diarrhea, or neurologic symptoms from pulmonary, gastrointestinal or central nervous system involvement.

Examination (palpate for satellite nodules and lymph nodes)

- **Superficial spreading:** lesions occur on the back or the legs with irregular, asymmetric borders and color variegation; size is generally >6 mm to 8 mm.

- **Acral lentiginous:** occurs on soles, palms, and beneath the nail plate with irregular pigmentation and large size (≥3 cm); pigmentation of the proximal or lateral nail folds (Hutchinson sign) is diagnostic of subungual melanoma.

- **Lentigo maligna:** often occurs in the elderly with lesions on head, neck, and arms occurring in a previously benign lesion (often present for numerous years); tan on brown patch with hypopigmented areas and nodular areas.

- **Nodular melanoma:** located on the back and the trunk with rapid growth and the presence of a raised dark nodule with frequent bleeding and ulceration.

DIFFERENTIAL DIAGNOSIS

- Seborrheic keratoses
- Common acquired melanocytic nevi
- Traumatized benign nevi (bleeding mole)
- Blue nevus
- Spitz nevus
- Congenital melanocytic nevi
- Dysplastic nevi

KEYS TO ASSESSMENT

- Visually recognize suspicious nevi.
  - Recent change, location in unusual areas (palms, soles, under breasts).
  - Asymmetry, irregular border; variegated coloring from brown to black with areas of white (regression at the periphery); size greater than 6 mm; nodularity; bleeding or crusting.
- Full thickness punch biopsy for large lesions; excisional biopsy with 1 mm to 2 mm margin for small or medium lesions.
- Determination of prognostic indicators include the following:
  - Anatomic level of invasion (Clark): 5 levels of invasion based on anatomic landmarks (e.g., I is intraepidermal only, V is infiltration of the subcutaneous fat).
  - Linear depth of invasion (Breslow): millimeters from the top to the deepest tumor cell.
  - Histiogenic type (superficial spreading, acral lentiginous).
  - Evidence of regression or ulceration.
- Lymphoscintigraphy to identify lymphatic basins draining the primary melanoma followed by sentinel node biopsy: sensitivity is high (especially with special stains of the node specimen) and if positive, complete regional lymph node dissection (LND) is indicated in most patients.
- Polymerase chain reaction (PCR) detection of melanoma markers detect nodal micrometastases (can also use PCR to detect circulating melanoma cells in the blood).
- Tumor/Nodes/Metastasis (TNM) staging according to the1997 American Joint Committee on Cancer TNM Staging System for Malignant Melanoma of the Skin.
- Chest x-ray; liver function tests, complete blood count.
- Chest, head, or abdominal computerized tomography (CT) or magnetic resonance imaging (MRI) are indicated only from evaluation of symptoms that may be related to metastases.
- Positron emission tomography can be used to evaluate for recurrent melanoma, its use in primary diagnosis is not yet determined.

KEYS TO MANAGEMENT

Prevention

- Avoidance of excessive sunlight, especially prior to age 20, is the most effective prevention.
- Sunscreens may be helpful but studies are not conclusive.

- Thorough Skin Self-Exam (TSSE) is recommended and in one study reduced melanoma mortality by 63%.
- Regular primary care or dermatological screening results in lesions being diagnosed at thinner (earlier) stages.

Surgical management

- Wide excision of primary lesion (1 to 4 cm margins depending on the thickness of the lesion).
- Sentinel node biopsy after lymphatic mapping: if negative, the procedure is terminated; if positive, then complete lymph node dissection is performed.
- Complications include postoperative lymphedema.
- Local recurrences are widely excised.
- Resection of distant metastases is indicated if there is a small number of lesions (<4) and a disease-free interval after primary resection of 1 to 2 years: subcutaneous, pulmonary, and gastrointestinal.
- Stereotactic radiosurgery for palliation of brain metastases.

Adjuvant therapy

- Interferon alpha-2b is used as adjuvant therapy in patients at high risk for recurrence. It increases 5-year survival in patients with positive nodes, but has a high toxicity. Use in patients with negative nodes is controversial and has not been definitively shown to change outcomes.
- Interferons are also used for metastatic disease, alone or in combination with other chemotherapy agents.
- Interleukin-2, given alone or in combination with lymphokine-activated killer cells, has provided response rates of 15% to 25% but with high toxicity.
- Nonspecific immunotherapy with bacille Calmette-Guerin (BCG) via intralesional injection controls local disease but does not improve the ultimate outcome.
- Tumor vaccines made from tumor cells or antigens cause induction of cytotoxic T cells and antibodies with some clinical response.
- Passive immunotherapy with human antimelanoma monoclonal antibodies has shown partial remissions.
- Adaptive cellular therapy, in which tumor infiltrating leukocytes are extracted from the primary tumor, activated with interleukin-2, and re-infused, show response rates of 20% to 35%.
- Isolated limb perfusion with melphalan, with or without tumor necrosis factor or interferon for limb recurrence or intransit melanoma or as an adjunct to primary excision, improves survival and decreases the need for major amputation.
- Chemotherapy for metastatic disease consists of single agent or combinations of dacarbazine, nitroso-ureas, or taxanes and interleukin-2, or interferon alpha; toxicity is high and response rates are variable.
- Radiation is used as primary therapy for inoperable tumors, as adjuvant therapy for mucosal and uveal melanomas, and as palliation for unresectable loco-regional disease and brain metastases.

Pathophysiology →	**Clinical Link**
What is going on in the disease process that influences how the patient presents and how he or she should be managed?	*What should you do now that you understand the underlying pathophysiology?*
UVA and UVB radiation, especially when associated with recurrent childhood sunburns, cause changes in melanocyte DNA and increase melanoma risk.	Protection from excessive sun exposure, especially in children, is essential for the prevention of melanoma.
Melanin functions to absorb UV radiation and is protective of the skin.	Malignant melanomas tend to arise in areas that are not normally tanned but which have been burned intermittently.
Many melanomas arise from dysplastic nevi, especially in inherited dysplastic nevus syndrome.	Patients with multiple nevi require frequent examinations to screen for malignancy.
Melanocytes possess high levels of anti-apoptotic proteins and lack the ability for effective DNA repair.	Damaged melanocytes can be long-lived and proliferate even when there is significant DNA mutation with the possibility of tumor progression years after initial exposure to ultraviolet radiation.
There are four melanoma types, each with somewhat different likely locations and appearances.	Patients must be examined carefully for suspicious lesions.
Malignant lesions initially spread within the epidermis and have little risk of metastasis. Once intradermal invasion occurs with formation of a nodular lesion, there is significant risk for distant spread.	Careful biopsy to evaluate for Clark level and depth of invasion (Breslow) is essential to staging and prognostic evaluation.
Melanoma spread first through the lymphatics, and outcomes can be improved with lymph node removal if positive nodes are found on biopsy.	Lymphoscintigraphy and sentinel node biopsy are used to determining the appropriate extent of surgical removal.
Melanoma cells are relatively responsive to immunologic intervention.	Interferons, interleukins, monoclonal antibodies, tumor vaccines, and passive immunotherapy are all being used as adjunctive treatment for malignant melanoma.

Selected Reading

Anonymous. (1999). Ultraviolet light: A hazard to children. American Academy of Pediatrics. Committee on Environmental Health. *Pediatrics, 104*(2 Pt 1), 328-333.

Arienti, F., Belli, F., Napolitano, F., Sule-Suso, J., Mazzocchi, A., Gallino, G. F., Cattelan, A., Santantonio, C., Rivoltini, L., Melani, C., Colombo, M. P., Cascinelli, N., Maio, M., Parmiani, G., & Santantonio, C. (1999). Vaccination of melanoma patients with interleukin 4 gene-transduced allogeneic melanoma cells. *Human Gene Therapy, 10*(18), 2907-2916.

Ascierto, P. A., & Palmieri, G. (1999). Adjuvant therapy of cutaneous melanoma. *Lancet, 353*(9149), 328.

Autier, P., Dore, J. F., Negrier, S., Lienard, D., Panizzon, R., Lejeune, F. J., Guggisberg, D., & Eggermont, A. M. (1999). Sunscreen use and duration of sun exposure: A double-blind, randomized trial. *Journal of the National Cancer Institute, 91*(15), 1304-1309.

Black, J. (1999). Malignant melanoma: An update on treatments. *Plastic Surgical Nursing, 19*(3), 143-147.

Buettner, P. G., & Garbe, C. (2000). Agreement between self-assessment of melanocytic nevi by patients and dermatologic examination. *American Journal of Epidemiology, 151*(1), 72-77.

Bullock, G. J., Green, J. L., & Baron, P. L. (1999). Impact of p16 expression on surgical management of malignant melanoma and pancreatic carcinoma. *American Journal of Surgery, 177* (1), 15-18.

Burton, R. C. (2000). Malignant melanoma in the year 2000. *Ca: A Cancer Journal for Clinicians, 50*(4), 209-213.

Carson, J. J., Gold, L. H., Barton, A. B., & Biss, R. T. (1998). Fatality and interferon alpha for malignant melanoma. *Lancet, 352*(9138), 1443-1444.

Crosby, T., Fish, R., Coles, B., & Mason, M. D. (2000). Systemic treatments for metastatic cutaneous melanoma. *Cochrane Database of Systematic Reviews* (2), *[computer file]*, CD001215

Curiel-Lewandrowski, C., & Demierre, M. F. (2000). Advances in specific immunotherapy of malignant melanoma. *Journal of the American Academy of Dermatology, 43*(2 Pt 1), 167-185.

Dummer, R., Hauschild, A., Henseler, T., & Burg, G. (1998). Combined interferon-alpha and interleukin-2 as adjuvant treatment for melanoma. *Lancet, 352*(9131), 908-909.

Dunn, C. L., & Zitelli, J. A. (2000). Standards of care for patients with malignant melanoma. *Journal of the American Academy of Dermatology, 43*(1 Pt 1), 155-158.

Dunton, C. J., & Berd, D. (1999). Vulvar melanoma, biologically different from other cutaneous melanomas. *Lancet, 354*(9195), 2013-2014.

Edman, R. L., & Klaus, S. N. (2000). Is routine screening for melanoma a benign practice? *Journal of the American Medical Association, 284*(7), 883-886.

Epstein, D. S., Lange, J. R., Gruber, S. B., Mofid, M., & Koch, S. E. (1999). Is physician detection associated with thinner melanomas? *Journal of the American Medical Association, 281*(7), 640-643.

Finkel, E. (1998). Sorting the hype from the facts in melanoma. *Lancet, 351*(9119), 1866.

Fisher, S. R. (1999). Considerations in the surgical treatment of malignant melanoma. *Archives of Otolaryngology—Head & Neck Surgery, 125*(1), 116-117.

Fletcher, W. S., Pommier, R. F., Lum, S., & Wilmarth, T. J. (1998). Surgical treatment of metastatic melanoma. *American Journal of Surgery, 175*(5), 413-417.

Fraser, M., Marentay, P., & Bertha, R. (2000). A collaborative approach to isolated limb perfusion. *AORN Journal, 70*(4), 642-647.

Gadd, M. A., Cosimi, A. B., Yu, J., Duncan, L. M., Yu, L., Flotte, T. J., Souba, W. W., Ott, M. J., Wong, L. S., Sober, A. J., Mihm, M. C., Haluska, F. G., & Tanabe, K. K. (1999). Outcome of patients with melanoma and histologically negative sentinel lymph nodes. *Archives of Surgery, 134*(4), 381-387.

Gogel, B. M., Kuhn, J. A., Ferry, K. M., Fisher, T. L., Preskitt, J. T., O'Brien, J. C., Lieberman, Z. H., Stephens, J. S., & Krag, D. N. (1998). Sentinel lymph node biopsy for melanoma. *American Journal of Surgery, 176*(6), 544-547.

Goldberg, E. K., Glendening, J. M., Karanjawala, Z., Sridhar, A., Walker, G. J., Hayward, N. K., Rice, A. J., Kurera, D., Tebha, Y., & Fountain, J. W. (2000). Localization of multiple melanoma tumor-suppressor genes on chromosome 11 by use of homozygosity mapping-of-deletions. *American Journal of Human Genetics, 67*(2), 417-431.

Goldstein, A. M., Struewing, J. P., Chidambaram, A., Fraser, M. C., & Tucker, M. A. (2000). Genotype-phenotype relationships in U.S. melanoma-prone families with CDKN2A and CDK4 mutations. *Journal of the National Cancer Institute, 92*(12), 1006-1010.

Hadzantonis, M., & O'Neill, H. (1999). Review: Dendritic cell immunotherapy for melanoma. *Cancer Biotherapy & Radiopharmaceuticals, 14*(1), 11-22.

Healy, E., Flannagan, N., Ray, A., Todd, C., Jackson, I. J., Matthews, J. N., Birch-Machin, M. A., & Rees, J. L. (2000). Melanocortin-1-receptor gene and sun sensitivity in individuals without red hair. *Lancet, 355*(9209), 1072-1073.

Juergensen, A., Holzapfel, U., Hein, R., Stolz, W., Buettner, R., & Bosserhoff, A. (2001). Comparison of two prognostic markers for malignant melanoma: MIA and S100 beta. *Tumour Biology, 22,* 54-58.

Kirkwood, J. M., Ibrahim, J. G., Sondak, V. K., Richards, J., Flaherty, L. E., Ernstoff, M. S., Smith, T. J., Rao, U., Steele, M., & Blum, R. H. (2000). High- and low-dose interferon alfa-2b in high-risk melanoma: First analysis of intergroup trial E1690/S9111/C9190. *Journal of Clinical Oncology, 18*(12), 2444-2458.

Kraehn, G. M., Utikal, J., Udart, M., Greulich, K. M., Bezold, G., Kaskel, P., Leiter, U., & Peter, R. U. (2001). Extra c-myc oncogene copies in high risk cutaneous malignant melanoma and melanoma metastases. *British Journal of Cancer, 84,* 72-79.

Lamberg, L. (2000). New and emerging dermatologic therapies presented at conference. *Journal of the American Medical Association, 283*(18), 2377-2378.

Lazar-Molnar, E., Hegyesi, H., Toth, S., & Falus, A. (2000). Autocrine and paracrine regulation by cytokines and growth factors in melanoma. *Cytokine, 12*(6), 547-554.

Lee, J. E., Mansfield, P. F., & Ross, M. I. (1998). Cutaneous melanoma metastases. *New England Journal of Medicine, 338*(13), 922-923.

Li, G., & Herlyn, M. (2000). Dynamics of intercellular communication during melanoma development. *Molecular Medicine Today, 6*(4), 163-169.

Lin, E. Y., Piepkorn, M., Garcia, R., Byrd, D., Tsou, R., & Isik, F. F. (1999). Angiogenesis and vascular growth factor receptor expression in malignant melanoma. *Plastic & Reconstructive Surgery, 104*(6), 1666-1674.

Lucas, S., De Plaen, E., & Boon, T. (2000). MAGE-B5, MAGE-B6, MAGE-C2, and MAGE-C3: New members of the MAGE family with tumor-specific expression. *International Journal of Cancer, 87*(1), 55-60.

Middleton, M. R., Grob, J. J., Aaronson, N., Fierlbeck, G., Tilgen, W., Seiter, S., Gore, M., Aamdal, S., Cebon, J., Coates, A., Dreno, B., Henz, M., Schadendorf, D., Kapp, A., Weiss, J., Fraass, U., Statkevich, P., Muller, M., & Thatcher, N. (2000). Randomized phase III study of temozolomide versus dacarbazine in the treatment of patients with advanced metastatic malignant melanoma. *Journal of Clinical Oncology, 18*(1), 158-166.

Monzon, J., Liu, L., Brill, H., Goldstein, A. M., Tucker, M. A., From, L., McLaughlin, J., Hogg, D., & Lassam, N. J. (1998). CDKN2A mutations in multiple primary melanomas. *New England Journal of Medicine, 338*(13), 879-887.

Nauman, C. (2000) Interferon for melanoma: Another application of immunopharmacology. *Journal of the American Medical Association, 279*(16), 1263-29.

Ng, A. K., Jones, W. O., & Shaw, J. H. (2001). Analysis of local recurrence and optimizing excision margins for cutaneous melanoma. *British Journal of Surgery, 88,* 137-142.

Nichols, L., & Hanzlick, R. (2000). Case of the month: What killed the patient—The disease or the experimental treatment? *Archives of Internal Medicine, 160*(15), 2253-2254.

Nielsen, M. B., & Marincola, F. M. (2000). Melanoma vaccines: The paradox of T cell activation without clinical response. *Cancer Chemotherapy & Pharmacology, 46*(Suppl), S62-S66.

NIH Consensus Panel on Early Melanoma. (1992). Diagnosis and treatment of early melanoma. *Journal of the American Medical Association, 268,* 1314-1319.

Platz, A., Ringborg, U., & Hansson, J. (2000). Hereditary cutaneous melanoma. *Seminars in Cancer Biology, 10*(4), 319-326.

Pu, L. L., Cruse, C. W., Wells, K. E., Cantor, A., Glass, L. F., Messina, J. L., & Reintgen, D. S. (1999). Lymphatic mapping and sentinel lymph node biopsy in patients with melanoma of the lower extremity. *Plastic & Reconstructive Surgery, 104*(4), 964-969.

Schrader, A. J. (2000). Combined chemoimmunotherapy in metastatic melanoma—Is there a need for the double? *Anti-Cancer Drugs, 11*(3), 143-148.

Shivers, S. C., Wang, X., Li, W., Joseph, E., Messina, J., Glass, L. F., DeConti, R., Cruse, C. W., Berman, C., Fenske, N. A., Lyman, G. H., & Reintgen, D. S. (1998). Molecular staging of malignant melanoma: Correlation with clinical outcome. *Journal of the American Medical Association, 280*(16), 1410-1415.

Stadelmann, W. K., McMasters, K., Digenis, A. G., & Reintgen, D. S. (2000). Cutaneous melanoma of the head and neck: Advances in evaluation and treatment. *Plastic & Reconstructive Surgery, 105*(6), 2105-2126.

Stam-Posthuma, J. J., van Duinen, C., Scheffer, E., Vink, J., & Bergman, W. (2001). Multiple primary melanomas. *Journal of the American Academy of Dermatology, 44,* 22-27.

Stratton, S. P., Dorr, R. T., & Alberts, D. S. (2000). The state-of-the-art in chemoprevention of skin cancer. *European Journal of Cancer, 36*(10), 1292-1297.

Swerlick, R. A., & Solomon, A.R. (1998). Clinical diagnosis of moles vs melanoma. *Journal of the American Medical Association, 280*(10), 881.

Valmori, D., Dutoit, V., Rubio-Godoy, V., Chambaz, C., Lienard, D., Guillaume, P., Romero, P., Cerottini, J. C., & Rimoldi, D. (2001). Frequent cytolytic T-cell responses to peptide MAGE-A10(254-262) in melanoma. *Cancer Research, 61*(2), 509-512.

Virgo, K. S., Chan, D., Handler, B. S., Johnson, D. Y., Goshima, K., & Johnson, F. E. (2000). Current practice of patient follow-up after potentially curative resection of cutaneous melanoma. *Plastic & Reconstructive Surgery, 106*(3), 590-597.

Vollmer, R. T., & Seigler, H. F. (2001). Using a continuous transformation of the Breslow thickness for prognosis in cutaneous melanoma. *American Journal of Clinical Pathology, 115,* 205-212.

Wagner, J. D., Corbett, L., Park, H. M., Davidson, D., Coleman, J. J., Havlik, R. J., & Hayes, J. T. (2000). Sentinel lymph node biopsy for melanoma: Experience with 234 consecutive procedures. *Plastic & Reconstructive Surgery, 105*(6), 1956-1966.

Wagner, J. D., Gordon, M. S., Chuang, T. Y., & Coleman, J. J., III. (2000). Current therapy of cutaneous melanoma. *Plastic & Reconstructive Surgery, 105*(5), 1774-1799.

Weinstock, M. A. (2000). Early detection of melanoma. *Journal of the American Medical Association, 284*(7), 886-889.

Westerdahl, J., Ingvar, C., Masback, A., & Olsson, H. (2000). Sunscreen use and malignant melanoma. *International Journal of Cancer, 87*(1), 145-150.

Whiteman, D., & Green, A. (1999). The pathogenesis of melanoma induced by ultraviolet radiation. *New England Journal of Medicine, 341*(10), 766-767.

Case Study*
Melanoma

INITIAL HISTORY
- 39-year-old white, red-haired, green-eyed male with light, freckled skin.
- History of numerous nevi since childhood.
- Now with a larger dark, irregular-shaped skin lesion on his midback.
- Physical education teacher.
- Positive family history of dysplastic nevus syndrome.

Question 1   What of this patient's history are considered risk factors for melanoma, and what are other warning signs?

Question 2   Is there a relationship between dysplastic nevus syndrome and melanoma?

Question 3   What would be the relationship between sunlight and melanoma for this patient?

_____

*Patrice Y. Neese contributed this case study.**

PHYSICAL EXAMINATION

HEENT, Neck, Lungs, Cardiac, Abdomen, Neurological
- Conjunctival and fundoscopic exam without lesions.
- No supraclavicular or cervical adenopathy.
- Clear to auscultation and percussion, no axillary adenopathy.
- Regular rate and rhythm (RRR) without murmurs.
- Soft, nontender, no liver enlargement.
- Strength and reflex +2 and equal bilaterally.

Integument
- Numerous nevi and freckles
- 5 mm, irregularly-shaped, darker lesion, midback
- Moderate sun damage to face, neck, chest, and back

Question 4   What are the pertinent positive and negative findings of this patient's physical exam?

Question 5   Does melanoma always appear on the skin?

Question 6   What are the most common sites of metastases?

Question 7   What type of biopsy should be done for this patient?

BIOPSY RESULTS
- Clark level IV
- Breslow 2.2 mm
- Superficial spreading melanoma

Question 8 What does this tell you about his prognosis?

Question 9 What is the significance of this histologic subgroup of melanoma?

Question 10 What tests should be ordered for staging?

MANAGEMENT
- Patient proceeds with wide local excision and sentinel lymph node biopsy.

Question 11 What is the role of sentinel lymph node mapping and biopsy in melanoma for this patient?

RESULTS OF SURGERY
- Lymphoscintigraphy results: one hot spot identified in right axilla.
- Lymph node biopsy negative.
- Scar and inflammatory changes in remainder of wide local excision.

Question 12 Should adjuvant therapy be offered to this patient?

Question 13 What is the pertinent patient education the practitioner should convey?

Question 14 What is the appropriate follow-up for this patient?

11

Type 2 Diabetes Mellitus*

DEFINITION

- In 1997, the Expert Committee on the Diagnosis and Classification of Diabetes Mellitus in the United States recommended replacing the term noninsulin-dependent diabetes mellitus (NIDDM) with type 2 diabetes, although both terms are still used throughout the world literature.

- As defined by the National Diabetes Data Group and the World Health Organization, type 2 diabetes is carbohydrate intolerance characterized by insulin resistance, relative (rather than absolute) insulin deficiency, excessive hepatic glucose production and hyperglycemia. Because complete insulin deficiency seldom occurs, ketoacidosis is unusual in this form of diabetes.

EPIDEMIOLOGY

- It is the most common endocrine disease and the most common form of diabetes.

- Prevalence in the United States is 6% to 7% in persons 45 to 65 years old and 10% to 12% in persons over 65 years old; approximately 16 million people in the United States have been diagnosed with diabetes, of whom 90% have type 2 diabetes.

- There is an emerging epidemic of type 2 diabetes in youth that parallels the rise of obesity and sedentary lifestyle in this age group.

- It has been estimated that because of the lengthy latent onset, the average time from onset of type 2 diabetes to diagnosis is 7 to 12 years; many patients already have long-term complications at diagnosis.

- It is the 7th leading cause of death in the United States, causing 17% of all deaths in persons over 25 years old; it is responsible for 300,000 deaths annually.

- It is the leading cause of blindness, end-stage renal disease, and lower extremity amputations.

- It increases risk of coronary disease and stroke 2 to 5 times.

PATHOPHYSIOLOGY

- Genetics: Carbohydrate tolerance is controlled by a myriad of genetic influences. Diabetes type 2, therefore, is a polygenic disorder with multiple metabolic factors that interact with exogenous influences to produce the phenotype. Genetic concordance for diabetes type 2 in identical twins approaches 90%.

- Insulin resistance
  - The major mechanisms of insulin resistance in skeletal muscle include impairments in glycogen synthase activation, metabolic regulatory dysfunction, receptor down-regulation, and glucose transporter abnormalities.
  - This results in reduced insulin-mediated cellular glucose uptake.

---

*Eugene C. Corbett, Jr., Lucy R. Paskus and Valentina L. Brashers contributed this chapter.

- The liver also becomes resistant to insulin, which would ordinarily respond to hyperglycemia with a decrease in glucose production. In diabetes type 2, hepatic glucose production continues despite hyperglycemia, leading to inappropriately raised basal hepatic glucose output.

- Obesity, particularly abdominal obesity, is directly correlated with increasing degrees of insulin resistance.

- Beta-cell dysfunction:

  - Beta-cell dysfunction results in the inability of the pancreatic islet cells to produce sufficient insulin to compensate for insulin resistance and to provide adequately for post ingestion insulin secretion.

  - It is theorized that hyperglycemia may render the beta-cells increasingly unresponsive to glucose due to glucose toxicity.

  - Insulin secretion normally occurs in two phases. The first phase occurs within minutes of glucose loading and represents release of the insulin stored in the beta-cells; the second phase represents the release of newly synthesized insulin over a period of hours post ingestion. In type 2 diabetes the first phase of insulin release is progressively impaired.

  - Beta-cell function (including early phase insulin secretion) and insulin resistance improve with weight loss and increased physical activity.

PATIENT PRESENTATION

History

A positive family history of diabetes mellitus is the rule. Look for associated cardiovascular risk factors (hypertension, dyslipidemia, smoking). Assess level of physical activity, development of obesity, personal history of impaired glucose tolerance or gestational diabetes. Assess nutritional pattern including total caloric intake and carbohydrate ingestion pattern.

Symptoms

Frequently asymptomatic in early stages, a patient may have significant hyperglycemia without loss of sense of well-being. Classical symptoms of hyperglycemia include chronic fatigue, polyuria, polydipsia, nocturia and delayed wound healing. Weight gain or loss can occur. Yeast infections of the skin and vagina are common. Early presentation can include symptoms of diabetic complications such as visual blurring or loss (retinopathy). Decreased sensory perception and paresthesia especially of the feet (diabetic neuropathy) is common.

Examination

Truncal obesity with increased waist to hip ratio, sensory or vibration sense impairment (neuropathy) of the feet, yeast skin rashes or ulcers; decrease in visual acuity; hypertension, loss of peripheral pulses, hyperpigmented lesions especially of lower extremity, abnormalities of retinal exam.

DIFFERENTIAL DIAGNOSIS

- Type 1 diabetes (insulin-dependent diabetes mellitus).

- Latent autoimmune diabetes in adults (rare).

- Gestational diabetes mellitus.

- Secondary diabetes mellitus: pancreatic disorder (hemochromatosis, chronic pancreatitis, pancreatectomy), hormonal disorder (Cushing syndrome, acromegaly), medication induced (steroids, thiazides).

- There are several other rare clinical and genetic syndromes associated with diabetes.

KEYS TO ASSESSMENT

- Screening for diabetes.
    - All patients, particularly those who:
        1) Are obese (>120% ideal body weight) or gaining significant weight.
        2) Have relatives with diabetes.
        3) Are members of a high-risk ethnic population (African American, Hispanic, Native American, Pacific Islander).
        4) Have a history of gestational diabetes.
        5) Are hypertensive and/or have dyslipidemia (HDL <35, triglyceride >250).
        6) Have diabetic symptoms of any kind including unexplained fatigue.
        7) Have recurrent infections especially of the skin, urinary tract and vagina.
- Establishing the diagnosis.
    - The Expert Committee on the Diagnosis and Classification of Diabetes Mellitus in the United States in 1997 stated that diabetes is diagnosed by any one of three criteria:
        1) Fasting plasma glucose (FPG) $\geq$7 mmol/L (126 mg/dL).
        2) Any casual plasma glucose concentration $\geq$11.1 mmol/L (200 mg/dl).
        3) A 2-hour plasma glucose level of $\geq$11.1 mmol/L during an oral glucose tolerance test (OGTT).
    - **Glycosylated hemoglobin** (HbA1c) is a measure of the percent of hemoglobin molecules that have a glucose molecule bonded onto their structure. This percent reflects the average level of blood sugar over the lifetime of the red blood cell. Therefore it is an indication of overall glycemic control over the preceding 2 to 3 month period. Generally, a glycosylated hemoglobin above 7% is considered an abnormal blood sugar average consistent with the diagnosis of diabetes.
    - **C-peptide** is the inactive fragment which is cleaved from proinsulin, resulting in the active insulin molecule. Measurement of c-peptide helps to establish the insulin making capacity of beta cells, thus, offering a test which helps to distinguish type 1 from type 2 diabetes. Individuals with type 2 diabetes generally have normal or elevated levels of c-peptide.
- Look for associated complications.
    - Proteinuria/albuminuria as well as glycosuria in urine analysis; a 24-hour urinary collection for creatinine clearance and total protein and albumin evaluates for the presence of diabetic nephropathy.
    - On blood examination, evaluate renal function (BUN, creatinine), cholesterol, and triglyceride levels.

KEYS TO MANAGEMENT

- Prevention:
    - An underlying singular cause for diabetes type 2 remains unclear. Because of this, approaches to the prevention of the disease are based upon the control of known factors which have been identified to reverse insulin resistance and prevent obesity.
        1) Maintenance of body weight within 120% of ideal body weight, particularly when family history is positive for the disease.
        2) Maintain exercise program throughout one's lifetime.

- The second most important preventive strategy pertains to the early detection and therefore prevention of the complications of type 2 diabetes. Strict glycemic control has been demonstrated to be preventive for all of the following:
    1) Retinopathy and lens cataract: annual ophthalmologic examination.
    2) Nephropathy: annual assessment for degree of albuminuria and use of angiotensin converting enzyme inhibitor drugs.
    3) Nephropathy: meticulous hypertension prevention and control.
    4) Neuropathy: monitoring for evidence of early sensory impairment particularly of the feet.
  - In addition to the above, careful monitoring for comorbid cardiovascular risk factors is essential.
    1) Avoidance of cigarette smoke.
    2) Optimal management of cholesterol and triglyceride levels.
    3) Observation of peripheral pulses for signs of peripheral vascular impairment.

- **Therapeutic goals** include optimizing blood glucose control, reducing body weight, increasing physical activity, normalizing lipid disturbances, and reducing hypertension. Identifying organ-system complications as early as possible so that they may be treated is also key. Improving the patient's sense of well-being and self-care attitude and habit are important for ensuring the healthiest outcomes long term.

- **Goals for glycemic control** include fasting and preprandial serum glucose of less than 126 mg/dL, postprandial glucose less than 160, and a glycosylated hemoglobin of less than 7.

- **Self-monitoring of blood glucose** is most desirable in patients with type 2 diabetes, sufficient to ensure optimal glycemic control.

- **Exercise:** within limits guided by cardiovascular ability, patients should begin an individualized exercise regime emphasizing aerobic exercise at least 3 days per week for 30 minutes. They should begin gradually and build up as exercise capacity increases. Exercise reduces insulin resistance.

- **The diabetic diet** aims to normalize blood glucose and lipid levels, as well as to obtain and maintain optimal body weight and balance caloric intake with caloric expenditure.
  - Current dietary recommendations advocate:
    1) Carbohydrates should be complex and rich in fiber and make up 55% to 60% of the total energy intake.
    2) Total fat should be reduced to 30% to 35% of total energy intake; animal fats should be replaced with monounsaturated or polyunsaturated fats.
    3) Protein should be reduced to 10% of total caloric intake.
    4) Cholesterol intake should be limited to 300 mg per day.
    5) Alcohol consumption should be limited to the equivalent of 4 oz. of wine per day.
  - Recent studies have reported a more favorable lipid, glucose, and insulin profile following the ingestion of a diet that predominates in monounsaturated fats.

- **Oral hypoglycemics and insulin:**
  - When glycemic control is not sufficiently achieved with dietary and exercise interventions, oral hypoglycemic agents are warranted. Home glucose monitoring is essential when striving for glycemic control and the avoidance of hypoglycemia.

- There are five categories of oral hypoglycemics:
  1) **Sulfonylureas** (tolbutamide, acetohexamide, chlorpropamide, glyburide, glipizide, glimepiride)
     a) They primarily stimulate insulin release from beta cells during the pharmacologic life of the drug (4 to 24 hours).
     b) They are often successful when used alone.
     c) Side effects include weight gain and hypoglycemia.
     d) Drug interactions: sulfonamides, salicylates, probenecid and beta-blockers may enhance hypoglycemia.
     e) They are contraindicated in insulin deficiency (diabetes type 1), pregnancy, and lactation. The perioperative patient is best managed with insulin.
  2) **Biguanides** (metformin)
     a) They lower blood glucose by decreasing intestinal glucose absorption, enhancing insulin sensitivity and peripheral glucose uptake, and inhibiting hepatic glucose production.
     b) They do not cause hypoglycemia.
     c) Other benefits include decreased total cholesterol, triglyceride, and LDL levels.
     d) Due to the occasional side effects of reduced appetite and weight loss, this drug is preferred in the treatment of the obese patient.
     e) Side-effects include minor gastrointestinal (GI) effects that can be controlled by lowering dosage. A rare serious consequence is lactic acidosis; this usually occurs when a contraindication such as renal insufficiency has been overlooked.
     f) They are contraindicated in renal impairment, pregnancy, and insulin deficiency, and should be used with caution in patients with liver, heart, or lung disease; cimetidine increases metformin serum levels.
  3) **Benzoic acid derivatives** (meglitinide, repaglinide)
     a) Are structurally distinct from sulfonylureas but similar in their insulin secretion stimulation mechanism.
     b) Are designed to increase mealtime insulin secretion and should be taken at mealtime.
  4) **Alpha-glucosidase inhibitors** (acarbose, voglibose, miglitol)
     a) They act by interfering with enzymes in the intestine which break down complex sugars. They slow the rate of polysaccharide digestion, resulting in some limitation in the absorption of glucose from ingested carbohydrate. They have been shown to improve postprandial blood glucose levels and lower glycosylated hemoglobin.
     b) They do not cause hypoglycemia.
     c) Side effects are similar to those of lactose intolerance because of the effect of undigested sugars upon colonic bacteria (diarrhea, abd pain, flatus, abd distention).
  5) **Thiazolidinediones** (rosiglitazone, pioglitazone)
     a) They enhance hepatic sensitivity and reduce insulin resistance.
     b) Side effects are minimal and include fluid retention and occasional reversible increases in liver function enzymes. Because of concerns for hepatic impairment, the latter is an indication for discontinuation of the drug.

- **Insulin:**
  - Exogenous insulin substitutes for the beta-cell defect by reducing glucose levels, suppressing hepatic glucose production, and increasing glucose uptake into cells.
  - Insulin treatment is initiated after insufficient metabolic control is obtained with maximal doses of oral hypoglycemic agents; large doses (200 to 300 units daily) may be required to overcome the insulin resistance.
  - Side-effects of insulin administration include weight gain, hypoglycemia, and hyperinsulinemia.
  - Insulin may be useful during acute medical or surgical events when more careful management of blood glucose is needed.

- **For general management,** treatment is initiated with one of the oral hypoglycemic agents (metformin, sulfonylurea, benzoic acid derivative). If ineffective, 2 or 3 drug therapy using other classes of oral agents is indicated. Because of cost factors, thiazolidinediones are more selectively used although they can be effective as monotherapy.

- **Combinations** of oral agents and selected insulin regimens have been shown to have benefit in diabetes type 2.

- **Monitoring and management of diabetic complications:**
  - Microvascular disease, including retinopathy, nephropathy, and neuropathy, may all be delayed or prevented by tight glycemic control (HbA1c averaging 7% or less) and aggressive treatment of hypertension when present.
    1) Retinopathy includes microaneurysms and vitreous and retinal hemorrhage and proliferative retinopathy. Yearly eye examinations are recommended. Laser photocoagulation may be beneficial in the early stages of disease.
    2) Nephropathy results in early urinary albumin excretion in excess of 30 mg in 24 hours due to glomerular injury. The use of angiotensin converting enzyme inhibitors has been shown to delay the progress of diabetic renal disease in both normotensive and hypertensive patients, and delay the decline in glomerular filtration rate.
    3) Neuropathy, both sensory and motor, is best avoided and treated with tight glycemic control. It is the primary factor in the pathogenesis of diabetic foot ulcers. Practicing consistent foot observation and care, and avoiding physical injury decreases the risk of foot ulcers and potential infection and amputation.
  - Poor glucose control results in increased bacterial and fungal infections, itching, and eventually more severe variations in diabetic skin disease.
    1) Diabetic foot infections account for nearly half of all nontraumatic lower-extremity amputations in the United States. Patients should examine their feet daily and wear appropriate footwear. Foot examination with particular attention to vascular and neurologic function and nail integrity should be done regularly.
  - Atherosclerosis is accelerated in the diabetic individual. Careful attention to other cardiovascular risk factors including smoking, hypertension, lipid abnormalities and sedentary lifestyle is mandatory. Observation for evidence of developing cardiac, cerebral and peripheral vascular disease is important for the purpose of early detection and treatment. The silent nature of vascular disease in its early stages is complicated in the diabetic because of the occurrence of autonomic sensory neuropathy, which diminishes the ability to perceive organ dysfunction.

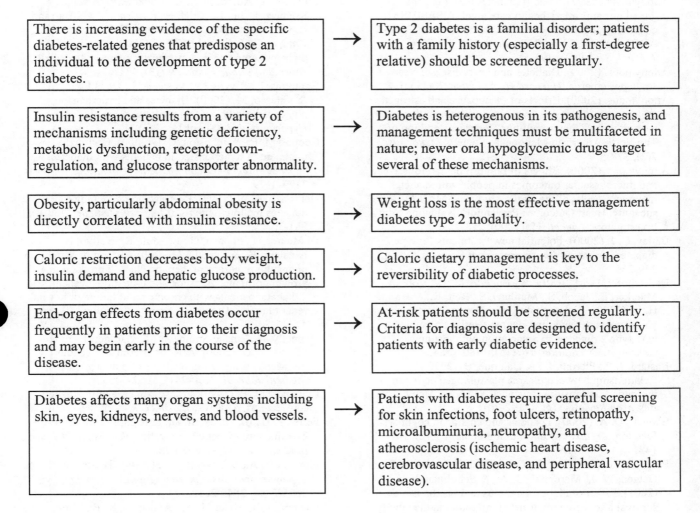

Pathophysiology → ## Clinical Link

What is going on in the disease process that influences how the patient presents and how he or she should be managed?

What should you do now that you understand the underlying pathophysiology?

Pathophysiology	Clinical Link
There is increasing evidence of the specific diabetes-related genes that predispose an individual to the development of type 2 diabetes.	Type 2 diabetes is a familial disorder; patients with a family history (especially a first-degree relative) should be screened regularly.
Insulin resistance results from a variety of mechanisms including genetic deficiency, metabolic dysfunction, receptor down-regulation, and glucose transporter abnormality.	Diabetes is heterogenous in its pathogenesis, and management techniques must be multifaceted in nature; newer oral hypoglycemic drugs target several of these mechanisms.
Obesity, particularly abdominal obesity is directly correlated with insulin resistance.	Weight loss is the most effective management diabetes type 2 modality.
Caloric restriction decreases body weight, insulin demand and hepatic glucose production.	Caloric dietary management is key to the reversibility of diabetic processes.
End-organ effects from diabetes occur frequently in patients prior to their diagnosis and may begin early in the course of the disease.	At-risk patients should be screened regularly. Criteria for diagnosis are designed to identify patients with early diabetic evidence.
Diabetes affects many organ systems including skin, eyes, kidneys, nerves, and blood vessels.	Patients with diabetes require careful screening for skin infections, foot ulcers, retinopathy, microalbuminuria, neuropathy, and atherosclerosis (ischemic heart disease, cerebrovascular disease, and peripheral vascular disease).

Suggested Reading

Ahren, B. (2000). Autonomic regulation of islet hormone secretion—Implications for health and disease. *Diabetologia, 43*(4), 393-410.

Anonymous. (1997). Type II diabetes mellitus clinical guidelines at primary health care level. A SEMDSA consensus document, 1997, in association with DESSA, ADSA [review, 13 refs]. *South African Medical Journal, 87*(4 Pt 3), 493-512.

Anonymous. (2000). Diabetes and heart disease: New strategies emerge. *Harvard Heart Letter, 10*(11), 1-4.

Anonymous. (2000). Effects of menopause and estrogen replacement therapy or hormone replacement therapy in women with diabetes mellitus: Consensus opinion of The North American Menopause Society. *Menopause, 7*(2), 87-95.

Anonymous. (2000). Effects of ramipril on cardiovascular and microvascular outcomes in people with diabetes mellitus: Results of the HOPE study and MICRO-HOPE substudy. Heart Outcomes Prevention Evaluation Study Investigators. *Lancet, 355*(2000), 253-259.

Bailey, C. J. (2000). Potential new treatments for type 2 diabetes. *Trends in Pharmacological Sciences, 21*(7), 259-265.

Balletshofer, B. M., Rittig, K., Enderle, M. D., Volk, A., Maerker, E., Jacob, S., Matthaei, S., Rett, K., & Haring, H. U. (2000). Endothelial dysfunction is detectable in young normotensive first-degree relatives of subjects with type 2 diabetes in association with insulin resistance. *Circulation, 101*(15), 1780-1784.

Bastard, J. P., Pieroni, L., & Hainque, B. (2000). Relationship between plasma plasminogen activator inhibitor 1 and insulin resistance. *Diabetes/Metabolism Research Reviews, 16*(3), 192-201.

Bennett, D. A. (2000). Diabetes and change in cognitive function. *Archives of Internal Medicine, 160*(2), 141-143.

Berger, A. K., Breall, J. A., Gersh, B. J., Johnson, A. E., Oetgen, W. J., Marciniak, T. A., & Schulman, K. A. (2001). Effect of diabetes mellitus and insulin use on survival after acute myocardial infarction in the elderly (the Cooperative Cardiovascular Project). *American Journal of Cardiology, 87*, 272-277.

Borg, W. P., & Sherwin, R. S. (2000). Classification of diabetes mellitus. *Advances in Internal Medicine, 45*, 279-295.

Brown, D. L., & Brillon, D. (1999). New directions in type 2 diabetes mellitus: An update of current oral antidiabetic therapy. *Journal of the National Medical Association, 91*(7), 389-395.

Burak, W., & Grzeszczak, W. (1999). Diagnosis of cardiac autonomic neuropathy in diabetic patients. *Diabetes Care, 22*(8), 1387-1388.

Ceriello, A. (2000). The post-prandial state and cardiovascular disease: Relevance to diabetes mellitus. *Diabetes/Metabolism Research Reviews, 16*(2), 125-132.

Chantrel, F., Moulin, B., & Hannedouche, T. (2000). Blood pressure, diabetes and diabetic nephropathy. *Diabetes & Metabolism, 26*(Suppl 4), 37-44.

Chin, M. H., Auerbach, S. B., Cook, S., Harrison, J. F., Koppert, J., Jin, L., Thiel, F., Karrison, T. G., Harrand, A. G., Schaefer, C. T., Takashima, H. T., Egbert, N., Chiu, S. C., & McNabb, W. L. (2000). Quality of diabetes care in community health centers. *American Journal of Public Health, 90* (3), 431-434.

Contreras, F., Rivera, M., Vasquez, J., De la Parte, M. A., & Velasco, M. (2000). Diabetes and hypertension physiopathology and therapeutics. *Journal of Human Hypertension, 14*(Suppl 1), S26-S31.

Cooper, M. E., & Johnston, C. I. (2000). Optimizing treatment of hypertension in patients with diabetes. *Journal of the American Medical Association, 283*(24), 3177-3179.

DeFronzo, R. A. (1999). Pharmacologic therapy for type 2 diabetes mellitus. *Annals of Internal Medicine, 131*(4), 281-303.

Di Mauro, M., Papalia, G., Le Moli, R., Nativo, B., Nicoletti, F., & Lunetta, M. (2001). Effect of octreotide on insulin requirement, hepatic glucose production, growth hormone, glucagon and c-peptide levels in type 2 diabetic patients with chronic renal failure or normal renal function. *Diabetes Research & Clinical Practice, 51*, 45-50.

Donnelly, R., Emslie-Smith, A. M., Gardner, I. D., & Morris, A. D. (2000). ABC of arterial and venous disease: Vascular complications of diabetes. *British Medical Journal, 320*(7241), 1062-1066.

Edmonds, M. E. (1999). Progress in care of the diabetic foot. *Lancet, 354*(9175), 270-272.

Ferris, F. L., III, Davis, M. D., & Aiello, L. M. (1999). Treatment of diabetic retinopathy. *New England Journal of Medicine, 341*(9), 667-678.

Florence, J. A., & Yeager, B. F. (1999). Treatment of type 2 diabetes mellitus. *American Family Physician, 59*(10), 2835-2844, 2849-2850.

Folsom, A. R., Kushi, L. H., Anderson, K. E., Mink, P. J., Olson, J. E., Hong, C. P., Sellers, T. A., Lazovich, D., & Prineas, R. J. (2000). Associations of general and abdominal obesity with multiple health outcomes in older women: The Iowa Women's Health Study. *Archives of Internal Medicine, 160*(14), 2117-2128.

Friedrich, M. J. (2000). Enhancing diabetes care in a low-income, high-risk population. *Journal of the American Medical Association, 283*(4), 467-468.

Fuller, J., Stevens, L. K., Chaturvedi, N., & Holloway, J. F. (2000). Antihypertensive therapy for preventing cardiovascular complications in people with diabetes mellitus. *Cochrane Database of Systematic Reviews [computer file]*, CD002188.

Gale, E. A. (2001). Two cheers for inhaled insulin. *Lancet, 357*, 324-325.

Gaster, B., & Hirsch, I. B. (1998). The effects of improved glycemic control on complications in type 2 diabetes. *Archives of Internal Medicine, 158*(2), 134-140.

Geffken, G., & Winter, W. E. (2001). Hardware and software in diabetes mellitus: Performance characteristics of hand-held glucose testing devices and the application of glycemic testing to patients' daily diabetes management. *Clinical Chemistry, 47,* 11-12.

Gibbons, G. R., & Newton, W. (2000). Noninvasive glucose monitoring. *Journal of Family Practice, 49*(2), 110-111.

Goldberg, R. B. (2000). Cardiovascular disease in diabetic patients. *Medical Clinics of North America, 84*(1), 81-93.

Griffin, S., & Kinmonth, A. L. (2000). Diabetes care: The effectiveness of systems for routine surveillance for people with diabetes. *Cochrane Database of Systematic Reviews [computer file],* CD000541.

Harrower, A. D. (2000). Comparative tolerability of sulphonylureas in diabetes mellitus. *Drug Safety, 22*(4), 313-320.

Heales, S. J. (2001). Catalase deficiency, diabetes, and mitochondrial function. *Lancet, 357,* 314.

Herman, W. H. (1999). Clinical evidence: Glycaemic control in diabetes. *British Medical Journal, 319*(7202), 104-106.

Hirayama, H., Sugano, M., Abe, N., Yonemoch, H., & Makino, N. (2001). Troglitazone, an antidiabetic drug, improves left ventricular mass and diastolic function in normotensive diabetic patients. *International Journal of Cardiology, 77,* 75-79.

Jovanovic, L., & Gondos, B. (1999). Type 2 diabetes: The epidemic of the new millennium. *Annals of Clinical & Laboratory Science, 29*(1), 33-42.

Kilpatrick, E. S. (2000). Glycated haemoglobin in the year 2000. *Journal of Clinical Pathology, 53*(5), 335-339.

Kolhlroser, J., Mathai, J., Reichheld, J., Banner, B. F., & Bonkovsky, H. L. (2000). Hepatotoxicity due to troglitazone: Report of two cases and review of adverse events reported to the United States Food and Drug Administration. *American Journal of Gastroenterology, 95*(1), 272-276.

Kopelman, P. G., & Hitman, G. A. (1998). Diabetes. Exploding type II. *Lancet, 352*(Suppl 4), SIV5.

Krein, S. L., Hayward, R. A., Pogach, L., & BootsMiller, B. J. (2000). Department of Veterans Affairs' quality enhancement research initiative for diabetes mellitus. *Medical Care, 38*(6 Suppl 1), I38-I48.

Lovell, H. G. (2000). Angiotensin converting enzyme inhibitors in normotensive diabetic patients with microalbuminuria. *Cochrane Database of Systematic Reviews [computer file],* CD002183.

Mak, K. H., & Topol, E. J. (2000). Emerging concepts in the management of acute myocardial infarction in patients with diabetes mellitus. *Journal of the American College of Cardiology, 35*(3), 563-568.

Mangan, D., Selwitz, R. H., & Genco, R. (2000). Infections associated with diabetes mellitus. *New England Journal of Medicine, 342*(12), 896.

Marshall, S. M., & Barth, J. H. (2000). Standardization of HbA1c measurements—A consensus statement. *Diabetic Medicine, 17*(1), 5-6.

McGuire, D. K. (2000). Influence of proteinuria on long-term outcome among patients with diabetes: The evidence continues to accumulate. *American Heart Journal, 139*(6), 934-935.

Morello, C. M., Leckband, S. G., Stoner, C. P., Moorhouse, D. F., & Sahagian, G. A. (1999). Randomized double-blind study comparing the efficacy of gabapentin with amitriptyline on diabetic peripheral neuropathy pain. *Archives of Internal Medicine, 159*(16), 1931-1937.

Paron, N. G., & Lambert, P. W. (2000). Cutaneous manifestations of diabetes mellitus. *Primary Care Clinics in Office Practice, 27*(2), 371-383.

Parulkar, A. A., Pendergrass, M. L., Granda-Ayala, R., Lee, T. R., & Fonseca, V. A. (2001). Nonhypoglycemic effects of thiazolidinediones. *Annals of Internal Medicine, 134,* 61-71.

Philis-Tsimikas, A., & Walker, C. (2001). Improved care for diabetes in underserved populations. *Journal of Ambulatory Care Management, 24,* 39-43.

Pickup, J. (2000). Sensitive glucose sensing in diabetes. *Lancet, 355*(9202), 426-427.

Pi-Sunyer, F. X. (2000). Overnutrition and undernutrition as modifiers of metabolic processes in disease states. *American Journal of Clinical Nutrition, 72*(2 Suppl), 533S-537S.

Plouin, P. F. (2000). The importance of diabetes as a cardiovascular risk factor. *International Journal of Clinical Practice Supplement, 110,* 3-8.

Price, P., & Harding, K. (2000). The impact of foot complications on health-related quality of life in patients with diabetes. *Journal of Cutaneous Medicine & Surgery, 4*(1), 45-50.

Quintao, E. C., Medina, W. L., & Passarelli, M. (2000). Reverse cholesterol transport in diabetes mellitus. *Diabetes/Metabolism Research Reviews, 16*(4), 237-250.

Raj, D. S., Choudhury, D., Welbourne, T. C., & Levi, M. (2000). Advanced glycation end products: A nephrologist's perspective. *American Journal of Kidney Diseases, 35*(3), 365-380.

Ramlo-Halstead, B. A., & Edelman, S. V. (1999). The natural history of type 2 diabetes. Implications for clinical practice. *Primary Care Clinics in Office Practice, 26*(4), 771-789.

Rockwood, K., Awalt, E., MacKnight, C., & McDowell, I. (2000). Incidence and outcomes of diabetes mellitus in elderly people: Report from the Canadian Study of Health and Aging. *Canadian Medical Association Journal, 162*(6), 769-772.

Rosenbloom, A. L., Joe, J. R., Young, R. S., & Winter, W. E. (1999). Emerging epidemic of type 2 diabetes in youth. *Diabetes Care, 22*(2), 345-354.

Scheen, A. J., & Lefebvre, P. J. (1999). Troglitazone: Antihyperglycemic activity and potential role in the treatment of type 2 diabetes. *Diabetes Care, 22*(9), 1568-1577.

Schoonjans, K., & Auwerx, J. (2000). Thiazolidinediones: An update. *Lancet, 355*(9208), 1008-1010.

Schrezenmeir, J., & Jagla, A. (2000). Milk and diabetes. *Journal of the American College of Nutrition, 19*(2 Suppl), 176S-190S.

Seidell, J. C. (2000). Obesity, insulin resistance and diabetes—A worldwide epidemic. *British Journal of Nutrition, 83*(Suppl 1), S5-S8.

Shulman, G. I. (2000). Cellular mechanisms of insulin resistance. *Journal of Clinical Investigation, 106*(2), 171-176.

Smith, S. A., & Poland, G. A. (2000). Use of influenza and pneumococcal vaccines in people with diabetes. *Diabetes Care, 23*(1), 95-108.

Sonksen, P., & Sonksen, J. (2000). Insulin: Understanding its action in health and disease. *British Journal of Anaesthesia, 85*(1), 69-79.

Steppan, C. M., Bailey, S. T., Bhat, S., Brown, E. J., Banerjee, R. R., Wright, C. M., Patel, H. R., Ahima, R. S., & Lazar, M. A. (2001). The hormone resistin links obesity to diabetes. *Nature, 409*, 307-312.

Streja, D. A., & Rabkin, S. W. (1999). Factors associated with implementation of preventive care measures in patients with diabetes mellitus. *Archives of Internal Medicine, 159*(3), 294-302.

Sumpio, B. E. (2000). Foot ulcers. *New England Journal of Medicine, 343*(11), 787-793.

Vaag, A. (1999). On the pathophysiology of late onset non-insulin dependent diabetes mellitus. Current controversies and new insights. *Danish Medical Bulletin, 46*(3), 197-234.

Vajo, Z., & Duckworth, W. C. (2000). Genetically engineered insulin analogs: Diabetes in the new millenium. *Pharmacological Reviews, 52*(1), 1-9.

Valdmanis, V., Smith, D. W., & Page, M. R. (2001). Productivity and economic burden associated with diabetes. *American Journal of Public Health, 91,* 129-130.

Vessby, B. (2000). Dietary fat and insulin action in humans. *British Journal of Nutrition, 83*(Suppl 1), S91-S96.

Warren-Boulton, E., Greenberg, R., Lising, M., & Galliva, J. (1999). An update on primary care management of type 2 diabetes. *Nurse Practitioner, 24*(12), 14-6, 19-20, 23-24 passim; quiz 32-33.

White, W. B., Prisant, L. M., & Wright, J. T., Jr. (2000). Management of patients with hypertension and diabetes mellitus: Advances in the evidence for intensive treatment. *American Journal of Medicine, 108*(3), 238-245.

Wright, J. (2000). Total parenteral nutrition and enteral nutrition in diabetes [review, 48 refs]. *Current Opinion in Clinical Nutrition & Metabolic Care, 3*(1), 5-10.

Young, T. K., & Mustard, C. A. (2001). Undiagnosed diabetes: Does it matter? *CMAJ: Canadian Medical Association Journal, 164,* 24-28.

Case Study

Type 2 Diabetes Mellitus

INITIAL HISTORY

- 52-year-old African American female.
- Diagnosed with type 2 diabetes 6 years ago but did not follow-up with recommendations for care.
- Now complaining of weakness in her right foot and an itching rash in her groin area.

Question 1   What questions would you like to ask her about her symptoms?

ADDITIONAL HISTORY

- She says her foot has been weak for about a month and is difficult to dorsiflex; it also feels numb.
- She denies any other weakness, numbness, difficulty speaking or walking, change in vision, syncope, or seizures.
- She has had some increased thirst and gets up more often at night to urinate.
- She says she has had the rash on and off for many years. It is worst when the weather is warm. She gets some relief from salt baths.
- She denies any chest pain, shortness of breath, edema, change in bowel habit, or skin ulcers.

Question 2   What other questions would you like to ask her about her diabetes?

DIABETES HISTORY

- She remembers being told her blood sugar was "around 200" when she was first diagnosed. She had gone for a work physical and felt fine at the time and saw no need for expensive drugs.

- Her mother and her sister have diabetes; both of them were diagnosed in their 40s and are on both pills and shots.
- She has been completely asymptomatic, except for the rash, until the foot weakness.
- She has gained 18 pounds over the past year and eats a diet high in fats and refined sugars.
- She works as a banking executive and gets little exercise.

Question 3 What would you like to ask about her past medical history?

PHYSICAL EXAMINATION

- Obese female in no acute distress.
- T = 37°F orally; P = 80 and regular; RR = 15 and unlabored; BP = 162/98 right arm sitting; Wgt 84 kg.

Skin

- Erythematous moist rash in both inguinal areas and in the axillae.
- No petechia or ecchymoses.
- Many hyperpigmented spots on the anterior shins.

HEENT, Neck

- Pupils equal and round, fundi with mild vascular narrowing.
- Nares and tympanic membranes clear.
- Pharynx clear.
- Neck without bruits or thyromegaly.

Lungs, Cardiac

- Lungs clear to auscultation and percussion.
- Cardiac exam with distant heart tones, a regular rate and rhythm without murmurs or gallops.

Abdomen, Extremities

- Abdomen moderately obese with bowel sounds heard in all four quadrants; no abdominal bruits, tenderness, masses, or organomegaly.
- Extremities without edema; pulses diminished but palpable in both feet.

Neurological
- Alert and oriented.
- Cranial nerves II-XII intact (including good visual acuity).
- Strength 5/5 throughout except 2/5 on dorsiflexion of the right foot.
- Sensory to light touch, diminished on anterior soles of both feet.
- Deep tendon reflexes 1+ and symmetrical throughout.
- Gait normal except for right foot drop, negative Romberg.

Question 4   What are the pertinent positives and negatives on exam?

Question 5   What laboratory tests would you order now?

LABORATORY RESULTS

- Serum electrolytes, including BUN and creatinine, calcium, and magnesium all within normal limits.
- Random glucose = 253 mg/dL.
- HbA1c = 9.1%.
- Urine dipstick positive for glucose, negative for protein; microscopic without significant cellular or infectious findings.
- Wet prep of smear from skin rash consistent with fungal spores and mycelia.
- ECG with evidence of early left ventricular hypertrophy (LVH) by voltage.

BLOOD PRESSURE AND FOLLOW-UP LABORATORY RESULTS THE FOLLOWING WEEK

- BP = 150/100 both arms sitting.
- Fasting glucose = 168 mg/dL.
- Fasting total cholesterol = 246 mg/dL with HDL = 28 mg/dL and triglucerides = 458 mg/dL.
- 24-hour urine for protein = 100 mg/24 hrs.
- Electromyography consistent with peripheral neuropathy of right foot.

Question 6   How would you interpret these laboratory findings?

Question 7   What would you recommend at this time?

12

Anemia

DEFINITION

- A decrease in red blood cells (RBC): often reported as a decrease in hematocrit (HCT) or a decrease in hemoglobin concentration (Hgb). The World Health Organization defines anemia as a Hgb concentration of less than 13 g/dL in men, less than 12 g/dL in women and in children aged 6 to 14 years, and less than 11 g/dL in children 6 months to 6 years old.
- Results in decreased oxygen carrying capacity of the blood.
- Selected causes of anemia:
  - Insufficient production
    1) Microcytic anemia (iron deficiency, anemia of chronic disease [ACD])
    2) Macrocytic anemia (vitamin B_{12} or folate deficiency, alcoholism)
    3) Marrow disease (leukemia, aplastic anemia, other myelodysplastic diseases)
    4) Renal disease with decreased erythropoietin
  - Increased destruction
    1) Immune hemolytic anemia
    2) Inherited hemolytic anemia
       a) Hereditary spherocytosis
       b) Sickle cell disease
       c) Thalassemias

EPIDEMIOLOGY

- Iron deficiency occurs in an estimated 30% of the world's population.
- In the U.S., 9% of toddlers aged 1 to 2 years and 9% to 11% of adolescent girls and women of childbearing age are iron deficient; less than 1% of older male children and men are iron deficient.
- Vitamin B12 deficiency affects 10% to 15% of the U.S. population over the age of 60 years.
- Pernicious anemia occurs in an estimated 3% of the white U.S. population over age 60 years.
- Immune hemolytic anemias are common in hospitalized patients and results from many medications.
- Hereditary spherocytosis is the most common inherited anemia in people of northern European descent.
- Sickle cell trait occurs in about 8% of African Americans, with disease present in 0.15%.
- Thalassemia affects 3% to 10% of persons from Asia, Africa, and the Mediterranean.

PATHOPHYSIOLOGY

Insufficient production (decreased reticulocytes)

- Microcytic anemia

- Iron deficiency anemia:

    1) Normally, approximately 1 mg of iron is absorbed and lost per day; an imbalance between intake, requirements, and loss of iron leads to iron deficiency.

    2) Dietary iron deficiency is common in states of increased iron requirements such as infancy and pregnancy; inadequate iron absorption can occur after partial gastrectomy, atrophic gastritis (as with *H. pylori*) and in diseases of the intestine (celiac disease).

    3) Increased iron loss occurs in menstruation (up to 20 mg with each period) and with chronic blood loss (e.g., peptic ulcer disease, colon cancer, repetitive phlebotomy).

    4) Iron deficiency leads to decreased ferritin (in response to iron-regulatory protein 1 gene) and decreased bone marrow iron stores with resultant abnormal RBC production.

    5) RBCs are small (microcytic; decreased mean corpuscular volume [MCV]) and pale (hypochromic; decreased mean corpuscular hemoglobin concentration [MCHC]).

- Anemia of chronic disease (ACD) is the most common anemia in hospitalized patients.

    1) Anemia is associated with underlying inflammatory and neoplastic conditions.

    2) Mechanisms of the anemia are not well understood but include impaired erythropoiesis, relative erythropoietin deficiency, decreased utilization of iron, abnormal hemoglobin synthesis and decreased RBC survival.

    3) Because ferritin is an acute phase protein, it is frequently normal or elevated in ACD.

- Macrocytic anemia

    - Alcoholism is the most common cause of macrocytic anemia, followed by certain drugs, vitamin B_{12} and folate deficiency, liver disease, and hypothyroidism.

    - Alcohol interferes with RBC maturation and is also associated with vitamin B_{12} and folate deficiency, thus is a common cause of macrocytic anemia (high MCV).

    - In B_{12} and folate deficiency, RBCs have abnormal deoxyribonucleic acid (DNA) synthesis in their precursor marrow stem cells (megaloblastic) with inadequate and abnormal RBC production. Hypersegmented neutrophils as well as macrocytes can be seen on smear.

    - Some patients are unable to absorb vitamin B_{12} due to autoimmune destruction of intrinsic factor, which is made in the stomach and is necessary for normal B_{12} absorption in the ileum (pernicious anemia). Patients with atrophic gastritis (as with *H. pylori*) and postgastrectomy patients also are at risk for B_{12} malabsorption.

- Marrow disease

    - Abnormalities of the marrow lead to decreased RBC production and include:

        1) Displacement of erythropoietic stem cells by leukemic or metastatic tumor cells.

        2) Aplasia of the marrow (aplastic anemia).

        3) Abnormal differentiation of the hematopoietic stem cells seen in myelodysplastic syndromes.

- Renal disease

    - Patients with chronic renal disease have inadequate erythropoietin and diminished RBC production.

    - Treatment with recombinant erythropoietin is highly effective but can result in a state of relative iron deficiency requiring iron supplementation.

Increased Destruction (increased reticulocytes)

- Immune hemolytic anemia

    - Binding of antibodies and/or complement to RBC.

- May be mediated by IgG antibody that reacts with RBC at body temperature (warm antibody) or by IgM that reacts with RBC at colder temperatures (cold antibody).
- 50% are idiopathic; secondary causes include:
    1) Neoplasia (chronic leukemia, lymphoma)
    2) Collagen vascular disorders (systemic lupus erythematosus, rheumatoid arthritis)
    3) Drugs (α-methyldopa, penicillin)
    4) Infections (mycoplasma, infectious mononucleosis)
- RBCs may be lysed or are removed from the circulation by the spleen. Polychromasia (due to increased reticulocytes) and fragmented cells (schistocytes) are seen on blood smear.

- Inherited hemolytic anemia
    - Hereditary spherocytosis:
        1) Autosomal dominant inheritance; common in northern Europeans.
        2) Defect in the proteins of the red cell cytoskeleton results in spherocytes that have reduced membrane surface area compared with cell volume.
        3) RBCs are fragile and are removed by the spleen.

- Sickle cell anemia
    - Substitution of an amino acid (Hgb S) results in intracellular polymerization of the hemoglobin molecule in response to deoxygenation, low temperature, and acidosis. In sickle trait, 40% of the total hemoglobin is Hgb S and anemia is mild. There are other hemoglobin mutations that can cause sickling including Hgb C.
    - Sickled cells adhere to the endothelium and cause microvascular obstruction (vasoocclusive disease) with organ infarcts.
    - The acute chest syndrome is a common complication resulting from vasoocclusion of pulmonary vessels with pulmonary infiltrates, infarcts, effusions, and hypoxemia.
    - Sickled cells are removed by the spleen, which can result in sickle cell crisis with severe pain and profound anemia.
    - Complications include susceptibility to infection and sepsis (especially to *S. pneumoniae* due to splenic dysfunction), delayed growth and development, lung and kidney dysfunction, stroke, skin ulcers, bone necrosis, pulmonary failure, retinal hemorrhage, and narcotic addiction.

- Thalassemias
    - Hereditary defects in hemoglobin synthesis: α-thalassemia results from decreased production of alpha globin and β-thalassemia is from abnormal beta globin synthesis resulting in ineffective erythropoiesis.
    - Accumulation and precipitation of abnormal hemoglobin tetramers results in erythroblast and RBC apoptosis and splenic destruction.
    - Hemolysis results in significant iron overload with multiorgan damage, especially to the liver.
    - Several forms of each thalassemia (including carrier, trait, and disease states) result in varying degrees of microcytic hypochromic anemia with hemolysis.

PATIENT PRESENTATION

History

Pregnancy; menorrhagia; unusual diet (e.g., strict vegetarian); alcohol abuse; chronic underlying illness; gastric surgery; drugs; family history; history of pain crises or sepsis.

Symptoms

Mild cases are often asymptomatic; fatigue; dyspnea on exertion; weakness; palpitations; edema; symptoms of underlying disease; more severe cases may present with congestive heart failure, transient ischemic attacks, syncope, or angina.

- Iron deficiency is associated with menometrorrhagia or other blood loss (melena, hematochezia, hematemesis, hemoptysis, hematuria); patients may complain of pica for starch, ice, or clay.
- Sickle cell disease is characterized by pain crises, skin ulcers, and organ infarcts that may be manifested by acute pain, neurologic deficits, or symptoms of other specific organ dysfunction. The acute chest syndrome is characterized by fever, pleuritic chest pain, and cough.

Examination

Pallor and/or jaundice (from hemolysis); tachycardia; systolic murmurs; edema; splenomegaly; severe anemia may be manifested with evidence of congestive heart failure; signs of alcohol abuse; signs of specific underlying illnesses.

- Iron deficiency is associated with glossitis, angular cheilitis, and brittle nails.
- Sickle cell disease is associated with evidence of organ infarction including focal neurologic deficits, skin ulcers, evidence of infection or kidney disease, and pulmonary congestion with infiltrates and hypoxemia (acute chest syndrome).

KEYS TO ASSESSMENT

- Mild anemia may be asymptomatic and should be suspected in infants, women of menstruation age, and pregnant women.
- Alcohol abuse can be associated with direct marrow toxicity, vitamin deficiency, and upper gastrointestinal (GI) blood loss and is a common cause of a mixed microcytic and macrocytic anemia.
- A family history of anemia is common, especially in certain racial and ethnic groups.
- A logical progression of investigative studies should be undertaken (Fig. 12-1 [top of next page]).
- Specific tests:
  - Iron deficiency: serum iron, iron binding capacity, and marrow iron stores; serum ferritin, transferrin receptor assay and reticulocyte hemoglobin concentration (differentiate iron deficiency anemia from anemia of chronic disease).
  - Macrocytic anemia: serum and RBC folate, serum B_{12}, and Schilling test (B_{12} absorption), bone marrow biopsy for megaloblasts; liver function and thyroid function tests if not megaloblastic or vitamin deficient.
  - Immune hemolysis: measurement of specific warm and cold antibodies; Coombs test.
  - Hereditary hemolytic anemias: hemoglobin electrophoresis and genetic profiles.

KEYS TO MANAGEMENT

- Treating any underlying systemic disease is vital. Discontinuation of alcohol intake should be recommended for most patients.

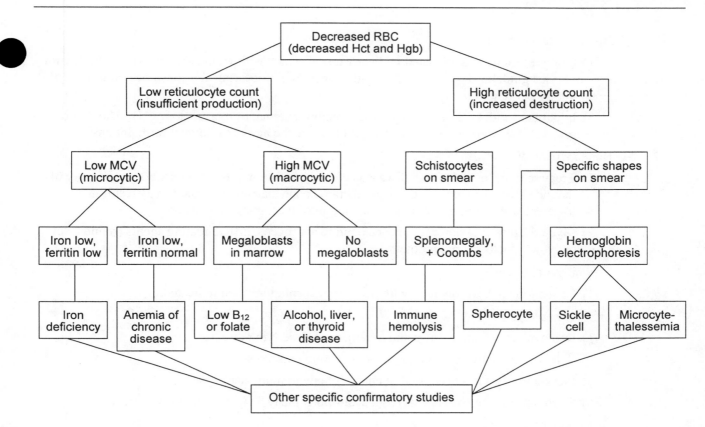

Fig. 12-1 Logical Progression for Assessment of Anemia

- Transfusion should be limited to those patients with severe anemia and symptoms such as chest pain, dyspnea at rest, congestive heart failure, or neurologic complaints.

- Unexplained iron deficiency in adult males and postmenopausal women must be evaluated thoroughly, including a complete GI work-up.

- Recent articles suggest that up to 12% of premenopausal women with iron deficiency have GI lesions (not all of their iron loss is via menstruation). Upper and lower endoscopy in premenopausal patients is indicated if there are any GI complaints or guaiac positive stools.

- Specific therapies.

  - Iron deficiency

    1) Oral iron (60 mg three times a day): GI side effects, such as dyspepsia and constipation, are common; normalization of Hct usually occurs in 6 to 8 weeks.

    2) Malabsorption or iron losses exceeding the maximal oral replacement are indications for parenteral iron replacement with iron dextran; toxicity is high including anaphylaxis and patients should receive a test dose with epinephrine at the bedside.

    3) In patients with *H. pylori*-associated atrophic gastritis, treatment with appropriate antibiotic combinations may reverse the iron deficiency (see Chapter 15).

  - Anemia of chronic disease (ACD)

    1) Successful treatment of the underlying disease will result in normalization of the HCT.

    2) Erythropoietin therapy has been used in rheumatoid arthritis and is being tested in other causes of ACD.

- B_{12} and folate deficiency
    1) Oral replacement is indicated in dietary insufficiency without malabsorption. Public Health Service guidelines recommend that all women of childbearing age consume a minimum of 400μg per day of folate.
    2) In patients with B12 malabsorption (pernicious anemia, postgastrectomy), B_{12} should be given monthly via intramuscular injection or via the newer sublingual formulations.
- Bone marrow disease
    1) Treatment of the underlying disease is the only way to improve anemia, however, many of the indicated treatments (e.g., chemotherapy, bone marrow transplant) may result in a transient worsening of the RBC count and may necessitate transfusion.
    2) Myelodysplastic syndromes may respond to androgens, differentiating agents (retinoic acid), or growth factors (erythropoietin).
- Chronic renal disease
    1) Recombinant erythropoietin with iron supplementation when indicated.
- Immune hemolysis
    1) Removal of causative drugs and treatment of underlying disease.
    2) Splenectomy may be necessary in some chronic diseases.
    3) Plasmapheresis has been used in cold antibody immune hemolysis.
    4) Steroids and cytotoxic agents (e.g., cyclosporin) may be indicated in severe cases.
- Hereditary spherocytosis
    1) Splenectomy.
    2) Vaccination to reduce the risk of infection after splenectomy.
- Sickle cell disease
    1) Pain crises: oxygen, hydration, pain control (patient-controlled analgesia has been effective in emergency room and clinic settings).
    2) Severe anemia (aplastic crisis) is treated with oxygen and transfusion.
    3) Chronic therapy with hydroxyurea or 5-azacitidine (increase Hgb F) decreases symptoms and extends time between transfusions.
    4) Clotrimazole and magnesium help retain RBC water content by reducing potassium and water efflux; early trials have documented decreased sickling when these are used.
    5) Bone marrow transplant has been successful in selected extreme cases.
    6) Monitor and treat the many potential complications; patient education is crucial.
    7) Neonatal screening is available; regular transfusions in children may decrease the risk of stroke but remains controversial.
    8) Daily penicillin for patients age 3 months to 5 years; pneumococcal vaccine.
- Thalassemia
    1) Many patients require no treatment.
    2) Plasmapheresis with transfusions followed by iron chelation therapy is indicated in severe anemia.
    3) Bone marrow transplant has been successful in selected extreme cases.
    4) If thalassemia is diagnosed in utero; successful cord blood transplantation has been reported.

Pathophysiology	→	Clinical Link
What is going on in the disease process that influences how the patient presents and how he or she should be managed?		*What should you do now that you understand the underlying pathophysiology?*

Iron deficiency can result from increased requirement for iron, decreased intake of iron, or increased loss of iron.

→ Patients at risk for iron deficiency anemia include infants, women of menstrual age, pregnant women, those with atrophic gastritis, postgastrectomy patients, and patients with chronic blood loss.

Normally, iron is recycled in the body after RBC destruction and is reused to make new RBCs such that only 1 gm of iron is lost and needs to be replaced per day.

→ Men and postmenstrual women who become iron deficient should be evaluated for sites of blood loss, especially from the GI tract (ulcers, cancers). Iron deficient premenopausal women with GI complaints should also be evaluated.

Macrocytosis can result form direct toxicity from alcohol, or from abnormal RBC maturation due to B_{12} and/or folate deficiency, which are common in alcoholism. Vitamin deficiency results in megaloblastic changes in the marrow.

→ A patient with macrocytic anemia should be questioned about alcohol use and have B_{12} and folate levels measured in the blood.

Intrinsic factor is produced in the stomach and is necessary for adequate B_{12} absorption in the ileum. Some patients have autoimmune antibodies to intrinsic factor (pernicious anemia); other patients have atrophic gastritis or are postgastrectomy and have low levels of intrinsic factor.

→ Patients with pernicious anemia can be diagnosed by measuring intrinsic factor antibodies. Patients who cannot absorb B_{12} will have an abnormal Schilling Test. Treatment for these patients requires intramuscular injection or sublingual administration of B_{12}.

Immune hemolytic anemias are associated with a variety of underlying conditions and the intake of certain drugs; patients will demonstrate autoimmune antibodies to their own RBCs.

→ Patients with lymphoma, chronic leukemia, rheumatoid arthritis, systemic lupus erythematosus, mycoplasma, or Epstein Barr virus infections, or who are on penicillin or α-methyldopa who develop anemia should be evaluated with a Coombs test for autoantibodies.

Inherited hemolytic anemias can result in significant clinical disease and require specific therapy.

→ A thorough family history is important in evaluating childhood anemia with testing to identify specific etiologies.

Suggested Reading

Annibale, B., Marignani, M., Monarca, B., Antonelli, G., Marcheggiano, A., Martino, G., Mandelli, F., Caprilli, R., & Delle, F. G. (1999). Reversal of iron deficiency anemia after *Helicobacter pylori* eradication in patients with asymptomatic gastritis. *Annals of Internal Medicine, 131*(9), 668-672.

Ashley-Koch, A., Yang, Q., & Olney, R. S. (2000). Sickle hemoglobin (HbS) allele and sickle cell disease: A HuGE review. *American Journal of Epidemiology, 151*(9), 839-845.

Bain, B. J. (1999). Pathogenesis and pathophysiology of anemia in HIV infection. *Current Opinion in Hematology, 6*(2), 89-93.

Beard, J. L. (2000). Effectiveness and strategies of iron supplementation during pregnancy. *American Journal of Clinical Nutrition, 71*(5 Suppl), 1288S-1294S.

Beutler, E., & Luzzatto, L. (1999). Hemolytic anemia. *Seminars in Hematology, 36*(4 Suppl 7), 38-47.

Bini, E. J., Micale, P. L., & Weinshel, E. H. (1998). Evaluation of the gastrointestinal tract in premenopausal women with iron deficiency anemia. *American Journal of Medicine, 105*(4), 281-286.

Blot, I., Diallo, D., & Tchernia, G. (1999). Iron deficiency in pregnancy: Effects on the newborn. *Current Opinion in Hematology, 6*(2), 65-70.

Bogen, D. L., Duggan, A. K., Dover, G. J., & Wilson, M. H. (2000). Screening for iron deficiency anemia by dietary history in a high-risk population. *Pediatrics, 105*(6), 1254-1259.

Domen, R. E. (1998). An overview of immune hemolytic anemias. *Cleveland Clinic Journal of Medicine, 65*(2), 89-99.

Farrell, R. J., & LaMont, J. T. (1998). Rational approach to iron-deficiency anaemia in premenopausal women. *Lancet, 352*(9145), 1953-1954.

Fernando, O. V., & Grimsley, E. W. (1998). Prevalence of folate deficiency and macrocytosis in patients with and without alcohol-related illness. *Southern Medical Journal, 91*(8), 721-725.

Fishman, S. M., Christian, P., & West, K. P. (2000). The role of vitamins in the prevention and control of anaemia. *Public Health Nutrition, 3*(2), 125-150.

Freeman, A. G. (1999). Sublingual cobalamin for pernicious anaemia. *Lancet, 354*(9195), 2080.

Gladwin, M. T., & Rodgers, G. P. (2000). Pathogenesis and treatment of acute chest syndrome of sickle-cell anaemia. *Lancet, 355*(9214), 1476-1478.

Gorman, K. (1999). Sickle cell disease. Do you doubt your patient's pain? *American Journal of Nursing, 99*(3), 38-43.

Hashimoto, C. (1998). Autoimmune hemolytic anemia. *Clinical Reviews in Allergy & Immunology, 16*(3), 285-295.

Hoffbrand, A. V., & Herbert, V. (1999). Nutritional anemias. *Seminars in Hematology, 36*(4 Suppl 7), 13-23.

Iolascon, A., Miragliad, G., Perrotta, S., Alloisio, N., Morle, L., & Delaunay, J. (1998). Hereditary spherocytosis: From clinical to molecular defects. *Haematologica, 83*(3), 240-257.

Joosten, E., Ghesquiere, B., Linthoudt, H., Krekelberghs, F., Dejaeger, E., Boonen, S., Flamaing, J., Pelemans, W., Hiele, M., & Gevers, A. M. (1999). Upper and lower gastrointestinal evaluation of elderly inpatients who are iron deficient. *American Journal of Medicine, 107*(1), 24-29.

Kaltwasser, J. P., & Gottschalk, R. (1999). Erythropoietin and iron. *Kidney International—Supplement, 69*, S49-S56.

Khattab, T., Fryer, C., Felimban, S., Yousef, A., & Noufal, M. (2001). Unusual complication of sickle cell crisis. *Journal of Pediatric Hematology/Oncology, 23*, 71-72.

Krishnamurti, L., Blazar, B. R., & Wagner, J. E. (2001). Bone marrow transplantation without myeloablation for sickle cell disease. *New England Journal of Medicine, 344*, 68.

Little, D. R. (1999). Ambulatory management of common forms of anemia. *American Family Physician, 59*(6), 1598-1604.

Mahomed, K. (2000). Iron supplementation in pregnancy. *Cochrane Database of Systematic Reviews (2) [computer file]*, CD000117

Marignani, M., Delle, F. G., Mecarocci, S., Bordi, C., Angeletti, S., D'Ambra, G., Aprile, M. R., Corleto, V. D., Monarca, B., & Annibale, B. (1999). High prevalence of atrophic body gastritis in patients with unexplained microcytic and macrocytic anemia: A prospective screening study. *American Journal of Gastroenterology, 94*(3), 766-772.

Mawji, Z., & Mishriki, Y. Y. (2001). An unusual vertebral radiographic finding. "H-type" vertebral deformity due to sickle cell disease. *Postgraduate Medicine, 109*, 133-135.

Means, R. T., Jr. (1999). Advances in the anemia of chronic disease. *International Journal of Hematology, 70*(1), 7-12.

Mitchell, R. (1999). Sickle cell anemia. *American Journal of Nursing, 99*(5), 36-37.

Nissenson, A. R., & Strobos, J. (1999). Iron deficiency in patients with renal failure. *Kidney International—Supplement, 69*, S18-S21.

Olivieri, N. F. (1999). The beta-thalassemias. *New England Journal of Medicine, 341*(2), 99-109.

Platt, O. S. (2000). Sickle cell anemia as an inflammatory disease. *Journal of Clinical Investigation, 106*(3), 337-338.

Provan, D. (1999). Mechanisms and management of iron deficiency anaemia. *British Journal of Haematology, 105*(Suppl 1), 19-26.

Provan, D., & Weatherall, D. (2000). Red cells II: Acquired anaemias and polycythaemia. *Lancet, 355*(9211), 1260-1268.

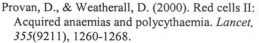

Rund, D., & Rachmilewitz, E. (2000). New trends in the treatment of beta-thalassemia. *Critical Reviews in Oncology-Hematology, 33*(2), 105-118.

Sackey, K. (1999). Hemolytic anemia: Part 1. *Pediatrics in Review, 20*(5), 152-158.

Sackey, K. (1999). Hemolytic anemia: Part 2. *Pediatrics in Review, 20*(6), 204-208.

Saibara, T., Okumiya, T., & Eguchi, T. (1999). Unrecognised iron deficiency in critical illness. *Lancet, 353*(9155), 842-843.

Savage, D. G., Ogundipe, A., Allen, R. H., Stabler, S. P., & Lindenbaum, J. (2000). Etiology and diagnostic evaluation of macrocytosis. *American Journal of the Medical Sciences, 319*(6), 343-352.

Sifakis, S., & Pharmakides, G. (2000). Anemia in pregnancy. *Annals of the New York Academy of Sciences, 900*, 125-136.

Steinberg, M. H. (1999). Management of sickle cell disease. *New England Journal of Medicine, 340* (13), 1021-1030.

Stopeck, A. (2000). Links between *Helicobacter pylori* infection, cobalamin deficiency, and pernicious anemia. *Archives of Internal Medicine, 160*(9), 1229-1230.

Vichinsky, E. P., Neumayr, L. D., Earles, A. N., Williams, R., Lennette, E. T., Dean, D., Nickerson, B., Orringer, E., McKie, V., Bellevue, R., Daeschner, C., & Manci, E. A. (2000). Causes and outcomes of the acute chest syndrome in sickle cell disease. National Acute Chest Syndrome Study Group. *New England Journal of Medicine, 342*(25), 1855-1865.

Weatherall, D. J., & Provan, A. B. (2000). Red cells I: Inherited anaemias. *Lancet, 355*(9210), 1169-1175.

Case Study

Anemia

INITIAL HISTORY

- 47-year-old male presents with the gradual onset of dyspnea on exertion and fatigue.
- Also complains of frequent dyspepsia with nausea and occasional epigastric pain.
- Has a history of alcohol abuse.

Question 1   What questions would you like to ask this patient about his symptoms?

ADDITIONAL HISTORY

- He says he has not had his usual energy levels for several months; the dyspnea has become much worse in the past few weeks.
- He denies chest pain, orthopnea, edema, cough, wheezing, or recent infections.
- He states he has had occasional episodes of hematemesis after drinking heavily, and subsequently had several days of dark stools.
- He drinks up to a 2 six-packs of beer a day for the past 8 years since losing his job.
- Nothing seems to make his breathing any better, but antacids help his epigastric discomfort and dyspepsia.

Question 2   What questions would you like to ask about his past medical history?

PAST MEDICAL HISTORY
- He denies any history of cardiac or pulmonary disease.
- He has been diagnosed with a duodenal ulcer in the past and was on "three drugs at once" for a while 2 years ago, but stopped them due to expense.
- His only surgery was a childhood tonsillectomy.
- He does not smoke.
- He is on no medications except over-the-counter antacids.
- He has no known allergies.

PHYSICAL EXAMINATION
- Thin, pale, white male looking older than stated age in no acute distress.
- T = 37 orally; P = 95 and regular; RR = 16 and unlabored; BP = 128/72 sitting, right arm

Skin, HEENT, Neck
- Skin pale without rash; no spider angiomata.
- Sclera pale; no icterus.
- PERRL, fundi without lesions.
- Pharynx clear without postnasal drainage.
- No thyromegaly or adenopathy.
- No bruits.

Lungs, Cardiac
- Good lung expansion; lungs clear to auscultation and percussion.
- PMI at the 5th ICS at the midclavicular line.
- RRR with a II/VI systolic ejection murmur at the left sternal border.
- No gallops, heaves, or thrills.

Abdomen, Rectal
- Abdomen nondistended; bowel sounds present.
- Liver 8 cm at the midclavicular line.
- Moderate epigastric tenderness without rebound or guarding.
- Prostate not enlarged and nontender.
- Stool guaiac positive.

Extremities, Neurological
- No joint deformity or muscle tenderness.
- No edema.
- Alert and oriented x3.
- Strength 5/5 throughout and sensation intact.
- Gait normal.
- DTR 2+ and symmetrical throughout.

Question 3   What are the pertinent positives and negatives on examination?

Question 4   What is your differential diagnosis at this time?

Question 5   What laboratory studies should be obtained at this time?

LABORATORY RESULTS

- WBC = normal with a normal differential; platelets normal.
- HCT = 29%; MCV = normal; MCHC = slightly decreased; RDW = markedly increased; reticulocyte count <2%.
- Smear with mixed microcytic/hypochromic and macrocytic/normochromic red blood cells; WBC and platelets appear normal.
- PT/PTT, liver function tests, electrolytes, and amylase normal.
- Upper endoscopy with 2 cm duodenal ulcer with evidence of recent but no acute hemorrhage.

Question 6   What might the hematologic findings indicate and what should be done to further evaluate them?

ADDITIONAL LABORATORY RESULTS

- Serum iron, total iron binding capacity, saturation, and ferritin all reduced.
- Bone marrow biopsy with megaloblastic changes and low iron stores.
- Serum folate and red cell folate low; B_{12} normal.

Question 7 Based on these findings, what are the diagnoses for this patient?

Question 8 How should this patient be managed?

13

Bleeding Disorders

DEFINITION

- Bleeding disorders can be divided into platelet disorders or coagulation disorders.
- They include many possible etiologies; a few common selected ones include the following:

Platelet disorders	**Coagulation disorders**
Thrombocytopenia	Hemophilia
Platelet dysfunction	von Willebrand syndrome
	Liver dysfunction
	Disseminated intravascular coagulation (DIC)

PATHOPHYSIOLOGY

- Fig. 13-1.

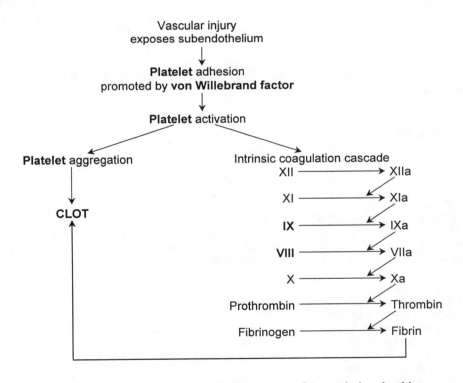

Fig. 13-1 The Clotting Cascade Components frequently involved in bleeding disorders are indicated by bold type (see Boxes 13-1 and 13-2).

- Bleeding disorders result from a defect in one or more of the steps in clot formation.
- Defects can be due to inadequate quantities of platelets and/or clotting factors, or to the abnormal function of these elements.
- Defects in clotting can be inherited or acquired.

PATIENT PRESENTATION

- In general, platelet disorders present with petechiae. Bleeding usually stops easily with local pressure and does not recur once the pressure is removed, unless the platelet count is very low.
- In general, coagulation factor disorders present with ecchymoses and deep tissue hemorrhages (hematomas, hemarthroses). Bleeding is slow to stop with local pressure and tends to recur when pressure is removed.

History

History of easy bruising; history of bleeding after surgery or dental work; family history of bleeding disorder; history of alcohol abuse; history of medication use; history of one of the many diseases listed in Boxes 13-1 and 13-2.

Symptoms

"Rashes" (petechiae); bruises (purpura and ecchymoses); mucosal membrane bleeding; gum bleeding with tooth brushing; epistaxis; deep soft tissue hematomas; bleeding into joints; sustained bleeding after injury or surgery; menorrhagia; hematuria; symptoms of liver disease or other underlying systemic illness as in Boxes 13-1 and 13-2.

Examination

Petechiae; purpura and ecchymoses; hematomas; heme positive stools; hemarthroses; evidence of liver disease or other underlying systemic illness as in Boxes 13-1 and 13-2.

DIFFERENTIAL DIAGNOSIS

- Boxes 13-1 and 13-2.

Box 13-1 Selected Platelet Problems

THROMBOCYTOPENIA
  A. Must be differentiated from pseudothrombocytopenia (spuriously low platelet count obtained from an automated complete blood count [CBC] counter) and dilutional thrombocytopenia caused by a transfusion greater than 10 to 12 units of red blood cells (RBC)
  B. "True" thrombocytopenia can be divided into three major causes
    1. Diminished production
      a. Congenital
      b. Acute viral infections (cytomegalovirus [CMV], rubella, Epstein-Barr virus [EBV])
      c. Vitamin B_{12}, folate, or iron deficiency
      d. Aplastic anemia
      e. Malignant marrow replacement (e.g., leukemia, metastases)
      f. Drugs (chemotherapeutic agents, estrogens, thiazide diuretics)
      g. Toxins (ethanol, cocaine)
    2. Altered distribution
      a. Hypersplenism (cirrhosis, heart failure, portal vein obstruction).
    3. Increased destruction
      a. Primary autoimmune (immune thrombocytopenic purpura [ITP], HIV-related)
      b. Secondary autoimmune (systemic lupus erythematosus, malignancy, drug-induced [heparin, gold, quinidine, furosemide, anticonvulsants, penicillin, sulfonylurea, cimetidine], and infection-induced)
      c. Disseminated intravascular coagulation
      d. Thrombotic thrombocytopenic purpura
      e. Extracorporeal circulation

Continued.

Box 13-1 continued

PLATELET DYSFUNCTION
- A. Can be divided into three main categories
    1. Hereditary
        a. Defects in platelet adhesion (Bernard-Soulier syndrome)
        b. Defects in platelet aggregation (Glanzmann's thrombasthenia)
    2. Acquired
        a. Uremia
        b. Myeloproliferative syndromes (leukemia, multiple myeloma)
        c. Autoimmune diseases (collagen vascular disease, platelet antibodies)
        d. Disseminated intravascular coagulation
        e. Liver disease
    3. Drug-induced
        a. Nonsteroidal antiinflammatory drugs
        b. Aspirin
        c. Antibiotics
        d. Psychiatric drugs
        e. Cardiovascular drugs
        f. Anesthetics
        g. Antihistamines

Box 13-2 Selected Coagulation Disorders

HEMOPHILIA
- A. Inherited coagulation factor deficiency, sex-linked recessive primarily affecting males
- B. 30% of cases are due to new mutations with no family history
    1. Hemophilia A: factor VIII deficiency
    2. Hemophilia B: factor IX deficiency
    3. Several more rare hereditary factor deficiencies

von WILLEBRAND SYNDROME
- A. von Willebrand factor is necessary for proper adhesion between platelets and vascular subendothelial structures, and between adjacent platelets
- B. A carrier for factor VIII; without von Willebrand factor, factor VIII has a very short half life
    1. Inherited
        a. It is the most common inherited bleeding disorder in humans
        b. It is autosomal dominant with variable penetrance
        c. There are three types
            1) Type I (moderate decrease in von Willebrand factor and factor VIII)
            2) Type II (functional abnormality in von Willebrand factor)
            3) Type III (severe decrease in von Willebrand factor and factor VIII)
    2. Acquired
        a. Antibodies to von Willebrand factor
        b. Is associated with many disease states and some drugs: lymphoproliferative disease (leukemia, lymphoma); autoimmune disease (collagen vascular); solid tumors (Wilms tumor); hyperthyroidism; valvular heart disease; dextrans; and valproate

LIVER DYSFUNCTION
- A. The liver synthesizes most of the factors of the clotting system except for von Willebrand factor
- B. Also responsible for the clearance of activated clotting or fibrinolytic factors
- C. Vitamin K is important in hepatic synthesis of functioning clotting factors
- D. Liver disease causes coagulopathy
    1. Impaired factor synthesis
    2. Abnormally functioning clotting factors
    3. Increased consumption of coagulation factors
    4. Disturbed clearance of circulating components of the coagulation system

DISSEMINATED INTRAVASCULAR COAGULATION
- A. Disseminated intravascular coagulation is associated with infection, trauma, shock, anoxia, burns, transfusion reactions, and obstetric emergencies
- B. Results in diffuse clotting with depletion of clotting factors, increased clot lysis and production of fibrin degradation products, and subsequent bleeding
- C. Fibrin degradation products are anticoagulants and exacerbate the bleeding disorder.

KEYS TO ASSESSMENT

- The approach to the patient with bleeding disorders should be systematic and include a logical selection of laboratory evaluations.

- Alcohol can cause thrombocytopenia, platelet dysfunction, and coagulation disorders and should be suspected in any bleeding patient.

- After a careful history, family history, and physical exam, obtaining basic laboratories in the majority of patients should include the following:

  - CBC with platelet count and careful examination of the peripheral blood smear.

  - Hematocrit (HCT) and hemoglobin (HGB) with RBC indices (mean corpuscular volume [MCV], mean corpuscular hemoglobin concentration [MCHC]).

  - Chemistries, including blood urea nitrogen (BUN) and creatinine (Cr); liver function tests.

  - Prothrombin time (PT) and activated partial thromboplastin time (aPTT).

  - Fibrinogen and fibrin degradation products.

- **If thrombocytopenia is found:**

  - A blood smear should be obtained.

    1) If the smear is normal and PT/PTT are normal, suspect autoimmune or drug-induced thrombocytopenia.

    2) If the smear is normal and the PT/PTT are abnormal, suspect liver dysfunction and evaluate for acute or chronic hepatic disease, and alcohol abuse.

    3) If the smear is abnormal and hemolysis is present, suspect disseminated intravascular coagulation or autoimmune destruction.

    4) If the smear is abnormal and the white blood cell (WBC) and RBC number or appearance is abnormal, suspect bone marrow disease and obtain bone marrow biopsy for diseases such as aplastic anemia, metastases, or leukemia.

- **If platelet disorder is suspected, but platelet count is normal, suspect platelet dysfunction:**

  - Template bleeding time in adults or petechiometer test in children confirms platelet dysfunction.

  - Review medication history carefully, check BUN and Cr.

  - Other specific tests of platelet function include aggregation to adenosine, epinephrine, collagen arachidonate, and thrombin; and the prothrombin consumption test.

- **Platelets are normal in number and function but PT and/or PTT are abnormal:**

  - If both PT and PTT are abnormal, suspect liver disease.

  - If only the PT is abnormal, suspect warfarin use.

  - If only PTT is abnormal, suspect inherited disease or heparin treatment; look again for a family history and measure von Willebrand antigen and factor VIII and IX levels.

KEYS TO MANAGEMENT

- The control of hemorrhage and the stabilization of the patient are of primary importance in acute bleeding.

- All patients should discontinue alcohol intake and nonessential medications especially nonsteroidal antiinflammatory drugs.

- The choice of therapy is based on the underlying causes as follows:

- **Thrombocytopenia**

    1) Treat underlying marrow disease; replace nutritional deficit; discontinue causative medication if possible; avoid toxins.

    2) Hematopoietic growth factors (IL-3, IL-6, IL-11).

    3) Platelet transfusion: for platelet count ≤10,000/μL; recheck counts at 1 hour and again at 12 to 20 hours after transfusion with a goal of 50,000/μL; single-donor platelets are preferred.

    4) Antifibrinolytic therapy with aminocaproic acid can be effective for patients with chronic mucosal bleeding but who do not require frequent platelet transfusions.

    5) Treat underlying disease as appropriate.

- **Platelet dysfunction**

    1) Hereditary defects are treated with platelet concentrates.

    2) Acquired defects require discontinuation of associated drugs, dialysis for uremia, correction of severe anemia, or treatment of the underlying systemic illness.

- **Hemophilia**

    1) Replacement with recombinant factor VIII or concentrated factor IX for acute hemorrhage.

    2) Recombinant factor VII for patients unresponsive to conventional factor replacement.

    3) 1-deamino-(8-D-arginine)-vasopressin (DDAVP) will increase factor VIII in mild cases of Hemophilia A.

    4) Antifibrinolytic agents.

    5) Liver transplant is effective but not easily available.

    6) Gene therapy is promising.

- **von Willebrand syndrome**

    1) The goal is to raise the factor VIII and von Willebrand factor up to 50% of normal levels.

    2) DDAVP indirectly releases von Willebrand factor from endothelial cell storage sites; it is useful for type I and type II; side effects include facial flushing and headache.

    3) Plasma-derived products are used in patients who have type III or who do not respond to DDAVP; They contain factor VIII concentrates with von Willebrand factor multimers.

    4) Fibrinolytic inhibitors and estrogens have been used as adjunctive therapy in some patients.

- **Liver dysfunction**

    1) Discontinuation of alcohol and drugs with hepatic toxicity.

    2) Fresh frozen plasma for acute bleeding.

    3) Vitamin K replacement when indicated.

    4) Antifibrinolytic therapy during hepatic surgery.

- **Disseminated intravascular coagulation (DIC)**

    1) Reverse underlying pathophysiologic condition.

    2) Support circulation, oxygenation and ventilation, and fluid and electrolyte balance.

    3) Avoid transfusion of blood products unless life-threatening exsanguination occurs.

    4) Heparin or antithrombin III infusion and plasmapheresis have been used in extreme cases with mixed success.

Pathophysiology → Clinical Link

What is going on in the disease process that influences how the patient presents and how he or she should be managed?

What should you do now that you understand the underlying pathophysiology?

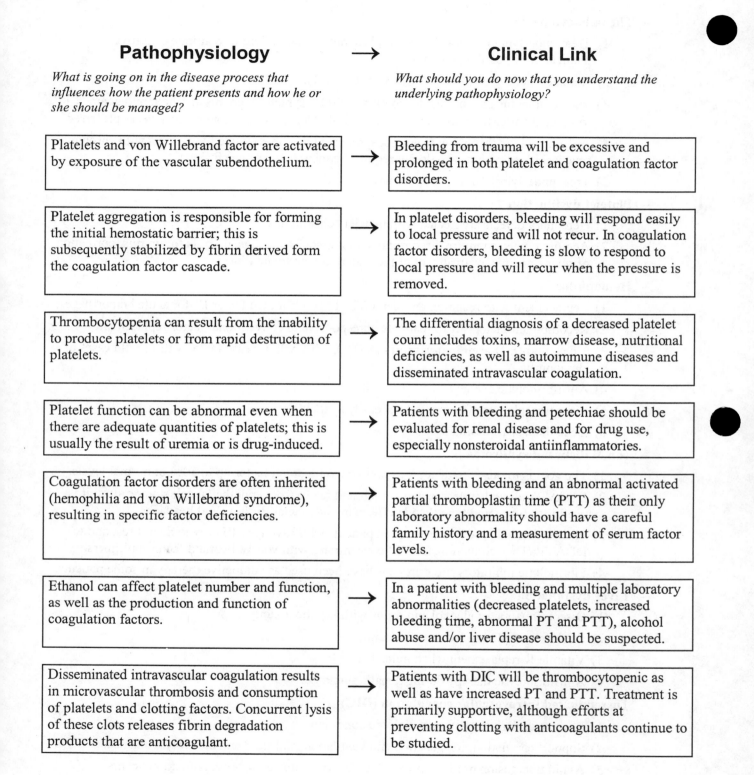

Pathophysiology	Clinical Link
Platelets and von Willebrand factor are activated by exposure of the vascular subendothelium.	Bleeding from trauma will be excessive and prolonged in both platelet and coagulation factor disorders.
Platelet aggregation is responsible for forming the initial hemostatic barrier; this is subsequently stabilized by fibrin derived form the coagulation factor cascade.	In platelet disorders, bleeding will respond easily to local pressure and will not recur. In coagulation factor disorders, bleeding is slow to respond to local pressure and will recur when the pressure is removed.
Thrombocytopenia can result from the inability to produce platelets or from rapid destruction of platelets.	The differential diagnosis of a decreased platelet count includes toxins, marrow disease, nutritional deficiencies, as well as autoimmune diseases and disseminated intravascular coagulation.
Platelet function can be abnormal even when there are adequate quantities of platelets; this is usually the result of uremia or is drug-induced.	Patients with bleeding and petechiae should be evaluated for renal disease and for drug use, especially nonsteroidal antiinflammatories.
Coagulation factor disorders are often inherited (hemophilia and von Willebrand syndrome), resulting in specific factor deficiencies.	Patients with bleeding and an abnormal activated partial thromboplastin time (PTT) as their only laboratory abnormality should have a careful family history and a measurement of serum factor levels.
Ethanol can affect platelet number and function, as well as the production and function of coagulation factors.	In a patient with bleeding and multiple laboratory abnormalities (decreased platelets, increased bleeding time, abnormal PT and PTT), alcohol abuse and/or liver disease should be suspected.
Disseminated intravascular coagulation results in microvascular thrombosis and consumption of platelets and clotting factors. Concurrent lysis of these clots releases fibrin degradation products that are anticoagulant.	Patients with DIC will be thrombocytopenic as well as have increased PT and PTT. Treatment is primarily supportive, although efforts at preventing clotting with anticoagulants continue to be studied.

Suggested Reading

Barrow, R. T., Healey, J. F., Jacquemin, M. G., Saint-Remy, J. M., & Lollar, P. (2001). Antigenicity of putative phospholipid membrane-binding residues in factor VIII. *Blood, 97,* 169-174.

Bick, R. L., Arun, B., & Frenkel, E. P. (1999). Disseminated intravascular coagulation. Clinical and pathophysiological mechanisms and manifestations. *Haemostasis, 29*(2-3), 111-134.

Buchanan, G. R. (1999). Quantitative and qualitative platelet disorders. *Clinics in Laboratory Medicine, 19*(1), 71-86.

Carter, S. (1954). Overview of common obstetric bleeding disorders. *Nurse Practitioner, 24*(3), 50-51.

Casonato, A., Pontara, E., Sartorello, F., Bertomoro, A., Durante, C., & Girolami, A. (2001). Type 2M von Willebrand disease variant characterized by abnormal von Willebrand factor multimerization. *Journal of Laboratory & Clinical Medicine, 137,* 70-76.

Cattaneo, M., & Gachet, C. (1999). ADP receptors and clinical bleeding disorders. *Arteriosclerosis, Thrombosis & Vascular Biology, 19*(10), 2281-2285.

Cho, Y. S., Kim, K. W., & Yang, S. N. (2001). Disseminated intravascular coagulation after a surgery for a mandibular fracture. *Journal of Oral & Maxillofacial Surgery, 59,* 98-102.

Cobos, E., Cruz, J. C., & Day, M. (2000). Etiology and management of coagulation abnormalities in the pain management patient. *Current Review of Pain, 4*(5), 413-419.

Dahlback, B. (2000). Blood coagulation. *Lancet, 355*(9215), 1627-1632.

de Jonge, E., Levi, M., Stoutenbeek, C. P., & van Deventer, S. J. (1998). Current drug treatment strategies for disseminated intravascular coagulation. *Drugs, 55*(6), 767-777.

DiMichele, D., & Neufeld, E. J. (1998). Hemophilia. A new approach to an old disease. *Hematology—Oncology Clinics of North America, 12*(6), 1315-1344.

Drews, R. E., & Weinberger, S. E. (2000). Thrombocytopenic disorders in critically ill patients. *American Journal of Respiratory Critical Care Medicine, 162*(2 Pt 1), 347-351.

Esmon, C. T., Fukudome, K., Mather, T., Bode, W., Regan, L. M., Stearns-Kurosawa, D. J., & Kurosawa, S. (1999). Inflammation, sepsis, and coagulation. *Haematologica, 84*(3), 254-259.

Fausett, B., & Silver, R. M. (1999). Congenital disorders of platelet function. *Clinical Obstetrics & Gynecology, 42*(2), 390-405.

Favaloro, E. J. (1999). Laboratory assessment as a critical component of the appropriate diagnosis and subclassification of von Willebrand's disease. *Blood Reviews, 13*(4), 185-204.

Federici, A. B. (1998). Diagnosis of von Willebrand disease. *Haemophilia, 4*(4), 654-660.

Federici, A. B., & Mannucci, P. M. (1998). Optimizing therapy with factor VIII/von Willebrand factor concentrates in von Willebrand disease. *Haemophilia, 4*(Suppl 3), 7-10.

Ginsburg, D. (1999). Molecular genetics of von Willebrand disease. *Thrombosis & Haemostasis, 82*(2), 585-591.

Gobel, B. H. (1999). Disseminated intravascular coagulation. *Seminars in Oncology Nursing, 15*(3), 174-182.

Hawkins, R. (2000). Disseminated intravascular coagulation. *Clinical Journal of Oncology Nursing, 3*(3), 127.

Hedner, U. (2000). NovoSeven as a universal haemostatic agent. *Blood Coagulation & Fibrinolysis, 11*(Suppl 1), S107-S111.

Hord, J. D. (2000). Anemia and coagulation disorders in adolescents. *Adolescent Medicine, 10*(3), 359-367.

Hortelano, G., & Chang, P. L. (2000). Gene therapy for hemophilia. *Artificial Cells, Blood Substitutes, & Immobilization Biotechnology, 28*(1), 1-24.

Kadir, R. A. (1999). Women and inherited bleeding disorders: Pregnancy and delivery. *Seminars in Hematology, 36*(3 Suppl 4), 28-35.

Lee, C. (1999). Recombinant clotting factors in the treatment of hemophilia. *Thrombosis & Haemostasis, 82*(2), 516-524.

Levi, M., de Jonge, E., van der, P. T., & ten Cate, H. (2000). Novel approaches to the management of disseminated intravascular coagulation. *Critical Care Medicine, 28*(9 Suppl), S20-S24.

Levi, M., & ten Cate, H. (1999). Disseminated intravascular coagulation. *New England Journal of Medicine, 341*(8), 586-592.

Lillicrap, D. (1999). Molecular diagnosis of inherited bleeding disorders and thrombophilia. *Seminars in Hematology, 36*(4), 340-351.

Ljung, R. C. (1999). Prenatal diagnosis of haemophilia. *Haemophilia, 5*(2), 84-87.

Ljung, R. C. (1999). Prophylactic infusion regimens in the management of hemophilia. *Thrombosis & Haemostasis, 82*(2), 525-530.

Lockwood, C. J. (1999). Heritable coagulopathies in pregnancy. *Obstetrical & Gynecological Survey, 54*(12), 754-765.

Ludlam, C. A. (1998). Treatment of haemophilia. *British Journal of Haematology, 101*(Suppl 1), 13-14.

Madan, M., & Berkowitz, S. D. (1999). Understanding thrombocytopenia and antigenicity with glycoprotein IIb-IIIa inhibitors. *American Heart Journal, 138*(4 Pt 2), 317-326.

Mannucci, P. M. (1998). Treatment of von Willebrand disease. *International Journal of Clinical & Laboratory Research, 28*(4), 211-214.

Mannucci, P. M., & Tuddenbam, E. G. (1999). The hemophilias: Progress and problems. *Seminars in Hematology, 36*(4 Suppl 7), 104-117.

Matsuo, T., Kobayashi, H., Kario, K., & Suzuki, S. (2000). Fibrin D-dimer in thrombogenic disorders. *Seminars in Thrombosis & Hemostasis, 26*(1), 101-107.

Mehta, A. B., & McIntyre, N. (1998). Haematological disorders in liver disease. *Forum, 8*(1), 8-25.

Mittelman, M., & Zeidman, A. (2000). Platelet function in the myelodysplastic syndromes. *International Journal of Hematology, 71*(2), 95-98.

Mohlke, K. L., Nichols, W. C., & Ginsburg, D. (1999). The molecular basis of von Willebrand disease. *International Journal of Clinical & Laboratory Research, 29*(1), 1-7.

Montgomery, R. R., & Gill, J. C. (2000). Interactions between von Willebrand factor and factor VIII: Where did they first meet? *Journal of Pediatric Hematology/ Oncology, 22*(3), 269-275.

Nurden, A. T. (1999). Inherited abnormalities of platelets. *Thrombosis & Haemostasis, 82*(2), 468-480.

Phillips, M. D., & Santhouse, A. (1998). von Willebrand disease: Recent advances in pathophysiology and treatment. *American Journal of the Medical Sciences, 316*(2), 77-86.

Rao, A. K., & Gabbeta, J. (2000). Congenital disorders of platelet signal transduction. *Arteriosclerosis, Thrombosis & Vascular Biology, 20*(2), 285-289.

Rapaport, S. I. (2000). Coagulation problems in liver disease. *Blood Coagulation & Fibrinolysis, 11*(Suppl 1), S69-S74.

Reiss, R. F. (2000). Hemostatic defects in massive transfusion: Rapid diagnosis and management. *American Journal of Critical Care, 9*(3), 158-165.

Rodgers, G. M. (1999). Overview of platelet physiology and laboratory evaluation of platelet function. *Clinical Obstetrics & Gynecology, 42*(2), 349-359.

Schetz, M. R. (1998). Coagulation disorders in acute renal failure. *Kidney International—Supplement, 66*, S96-S101.

Storey, R. F., & Heptinstall, S. (1999). Laboratory investigation of platelet function. *Clinical & Laboratory Haematology, 21*(5), 317-329.

Teitel, J. M. (1999). Recombinant factor VIIa versus aPCCs in haemophiliacs with inhibitors: Treatment and cost considerations. *Haemophilia, 5*(Suppl 3), 43-49.

Triplett, D. A. (2000). Coagulation and bleeding disorders: Review and update. *Clinical Chemistry, 46*(8 Pt 2), 1260-1269.

Vermeer, C., & Schurgers, L. J. (2000). A comprehensive review of vitamin K and vitamin K antagonists. *Hematology—Oncology Clinics of North America, 14*(2), 339-353.

Veyradier, A., Fressinaud, E., & Meyer, D. (1998). Laboratory diagnosis of von Willebrand disease. *International Journal of Clinical & Laboratory Research, 28*(4), 201-210.

Vischer, U. M., & de Moerloose, P. (1999). von Willebrand factor: From cell biology to the clinical management of von Willebrand's disease. *Critical Reviews in Oncology-Hematology, 30*(2), 93-109.

Vlot, A. J., Koppelman, S. J., Bouma, B. N., & Sixma, J. J. (1998). Factor VIII and von Willebrand factor. *Thrombosis & Haemostasis, 79*(3), 456-465.

Case Study*

Bleeding Disorders

INITIAL HISTORY

- Mr. H. is a 58-year-old male who has just been transferred in stable condition at 2:15 p.m. from the operating room to the intensive care unit (ICU) after undergoing an uncomplicated but lengthy (5 hours) right lung decortication procedure.
- His estimated blood loss during the procedure was 550 cc, and he received approximately 2500 cc of IV fluid during the operation.
- The initial drainage amount from his right pleural chest tube on arrival to the ICU is 120 cc.

Question 1   What essential information do you want to be sure to receive in report from the anesthesiologist and surgeon?

ADDITIONAL HISTORY

- Mr. H. has a previous medical history significant for a right lower lobectomy for a benign tumor resection, complicated by right empyema.
- He has a 40 pack/year smoking history (quit 3 years ago).
- He is otherwise in good health.
- Mr. H.'s home medications include only PRN albuterol inhaler use.
- He has no medication allergies.
- His surgery progressed with moderate difficulty as the visceral pleura was badly scarred.

HIS INITIAL PHYSICAL EXAMINATION ON ARRIVAL TO THE ICU FROM THE OPERATING ROOM

- Rectal T is 35.8° C; P = 90 and regular.
- No spontaneous respirations on ventilator at intermittent mandatory ventilation (IMV) 10 breaths/minute.
- BP via right radial arterial line 112/60, correlates with cuff.

Skin

- Grossly intact, pale, cool, dry.
- Three second capillary refill throughout.
- Good turgor.
- Right thoracotomy surgical dressing intact with scant bloody drainage present.

---

*Kathryn B. Reid contributed this case study.

Pulmonary

- #8.0 oral endotracheal tube, 23 cm @ lips.
- Fully ventilated with FIO_2 = 1.00, IMV = 10, positive end-expiratory pressure (PEEP) = 5; O_2 sat = 100%.
- No spontaneous respirations present.
- Bilateral breath sounds present, slightly diminished in the bases.
- Right lateral pleural chest tube at 20 cm H_2O suction via chest drainage system with 120 cc bloody drainage present, no air leak.

Cardiovascular

- S_1 S_2 clear; no murmurs or gallops present.
- Pulses full throughout.

Gastrointestinal

- Left nasogastric tube to low constant suction, minimal drainage.
- Hypoactive bowel sounds.

Genitourinary

- Urinary catheter draining clear yellow urine.
- Specific gravity 1.010.

Neurological

- Remains anesthetized and sedated, unable to communicate.
- Glasgow coma scale = 2T; PERRL = 2 mm.

ADDITIONAL ASSESSMENTS

- Endotracheal suction reveals scant, thin white secretions.
- Initial arterial blood gas: pH = 7.45; $PaCO_2$ = 36; PaO_2 = 433.
- Electrocardiogram monitor lead II shows normal sinus rhythm, no ectopy, rate = 92.

VASCULAR ACCESS

- Right subclavian triple lumen catheter: proximal port with D_5W @ KVO, middle heparin locked, distal with central venous pressure (CVP) monitor and flush per protocol, CVP = 6 mmHg.
- Bilateral upper extremity IV is with normal saline infusing at KVO from operating room.

POSTOPERATIVE COURSE

- Mr. H. is stable and receives the routine postoperative care and monitoring. He is placed on an FIO_2 of 50% to begin normalizing his arterial blood gases after transport.
- At 2:45 p.m. (after 30 minutes), you note that his chest tube output is an additional 175 cc.

Question 2   What will you evaluate related to his blood loss at this time?

RAPID ASSESSMENT AND LABORATORY RESULTS

- No evidence of hypovolemia.
- Postoperative chest radiograph reveals proper endotracheal tube and chest tube placement, bilateral lung expansion, and no evidence of hemothorax.
- Initial postoperative laboratory results:
  - Hemoglobin = 6.8 mg/dl; hematocrit = 20%.
  - Platelets = 85,000/mm^3.
  - PT/PTT are normal.
  - His electrolytes are within normal limits, except for potassium of 3.4 mEq/l and an ionized calcium of 3.8 mg/dl.

Question 3   What do these values represent?

Question 4   What is your primary concern related to this patient' chest tube drainage?

Question 5   What actions should be taken at this time to attempt to reduce his postoperative hemorrhage?

CONTINUED POSTOPERATIVE COURSE

- At 3:00 p.m., he has an additional 200 cc of chest tube drainage (postoperative total = 495 cc).
- In addition to the normal postoperative volume resuscitation, the patient receives a rapid transfusion of 2 units packed red blood cells, 2 units fresh frozen plasma, 1 unit single donor platelets, and 1 ampule of calcium chloride intravenously.

ADDITIONAL POSTOPERATIVE DEVELOPMENTS

- At 4:00 p.m., his chest drainage equals 275 cc (770 cc total). His hematological studies at this time are:
  - Hemoglobin = 7.0 mg/dl; HCT = 21%
  - PLTs = 65,000/mm^3
  - PT = 15 sec; PTT = 42 sec
- Mr. H. receives an additional 1 unit packed red blood cells and 2 units fresh frozen plasma.

Question 6   What is your assessment of the situation at this time?

Question 7   What other laboratory information will guide your decision-making at this time?

CONTINUED POSTOPERATIVE COURSE

- At 4:30 p.m., Mr. H.'s chest tube drainage is 220 ccs (postoperative total = 990 ccs). Due to his continued excessive bleeding, he is emergently returned to the operating room for re-exploration.
- While Mr. H. is in the operating room undergoing re-exploration, his blood work returns as follows:
  - Hemoglobin = 6.2 mg/dl; HCT = 19%
  - PLTs = 48,000/mm^3
  - PTT = 47 sec; PT = 19 sec
  - Fibrinogen = 120 mg/dl
  - Fibrinogen degradation products = 150 mcg/ml
  - D-dimer = 220 ng/ml
  - Ca^{++} = 3.9 mg/dl

CHAPTER 13 Bleeding Disorders **191**

Question 8   What does this lab work indicate?

Question 9   What are the possible causes for Mr. H.'s bleeding problem?

Question 10   Based on this information, what other information do you want to acquire?

Question 11   What are the recommended therapeutic approaches in the management of Mr. H.'s DIC-like coagulopathy?

Copyright © 2002 Mosby, Inc. All rights reserved.

AFTER RETURNING FROM THE OPERATING ROOM
- Mr. H. returns from the operating room at 5:15 p.m., after his re-exploration procedure.
- The surgeon reports that no single source of bleeding could be identified and that there was heavy generalized diffuse oozing of blood from the chest wall. The surgeon's diagnosis of the bleeding problem is DIC and orders that all blood products be placed on hold.
- Care of Mr. H.'s bleeding problem is supportive in nature with administration of crystalloid fluids as needed to maintain adequate volume status.

CONTINUED POSTOPERATIVE CARE
- Over the next 6 hours, Mr. H.'s chest tube drainage improves from 210 cc per hour to 45 cc per hour.
- He does not demonstrate other evidence of a transfusion reaction.
- His hematocrit reaches a low of 17, and on the first postoperative day he is gently transfused 2 units of packed red blood cells without complication to bring his hematocrit over 30.
- He is placed on an iron supplement and he is instructed in dietary measures that will help improve his postoperative anemia.

14

Urinary Tract Infection*

DEFINITION

- Urinary tract infection (UTI) is an inflammation of the urinary tract epithelium in response to a bacterial pathogen that is usually associated with pyuria and bacteriuria.
- Cystitis is an infection of the bladder producing characteristic symptoms including dysuria, lower abdominal or suprapubic discomfort, and frequency of urination.
- Bacteriuria is the presence of bacteria in the urine; this condition may or may not be associated with UTI symptoms.
- Pyelonephritis is an infection of the upper urinary tracts, including the renal pelvis and renal parenchyma, also called afebrile UTI or upper tract UTI.
- Acute pyelonephritis is a clinical syndrome of chills, fever and flank pain accompanied by bacteriuria and involving the upper urinary tracts.
- Chronic pyelonephritis is a term used to describe a scarred or damaged kidney owing to previous episodes of pyelonephritis that is diagnosed on radiographic or other imaging study. It may or may not be associated with a current urinary tract infection.
- Urosepsis is a systemic extension of febrile UTI; urine and blood cultures are positive for a common pathogen that can progress to septic shock and death unless successfully treated.
- Isolated urinary tract infection is an initial infection or an infection that is remote in time from previous episodes.
- Recurrent urinary tract infection is a new infection following successful resolution of previous episode(s).
- Persistent urinary infection is lasting bacteriuria caused by inappropriate or incomplete therapy, or arising from bacterial persistence within some focus within the urine, such as a calculus or a foreign object.
- Nosocomial urinary infection is a hospital-acquired UTI.
- Domiciliary UTI occurs in persons who reside in the community at the time of infection.
- Complicated urinary tract infection is associated with hematuria, fever, or an infection in the patient with an indwelling catheter, obstruction, urinary calculus, or anatomic abnormality of the urinary system.

EPIDEMIOLOGY

- 4% to 6% of young adult women have bacteriuria at any given time; the majority are asymptomatic.
- Incidence of symptomatic urinary tract infections among young adult women are approximately 0.2 per month.
- Prevalence of asymptomatic bacteriuria in elderly community-dwelling women is 20%.

---

*Mikel Gray authored this chapter.

193

- Patients with an initial UTI are at risk for subsequent infections; for example, 61% of elderly women treated for a UTI will seek treatment for one or more recurrent infections within a decade.

- Prevalence of asymptomatic bacteriuria in women with diabetes mellitus is 26%, including a prevalence of 21% in women with type 1 diabetes mellitus and 29% with type 2 diabetes mellitus.

- Patients with HIV have a higher incidence of UTI when compared to controls.

- Prevalence increases to approximately 20% to community-dwelling elderly women (>65 years of age).

- Prevalence of young adult men is <1%; it increases to approximately 10% of community-dwelling elderly men.

- Prevalence of bacteriuria among functionally-impaired elderly women and men is 24%, compared to 12% of nonfunctionally-impaired women and men.

- The incidence of antimicrobial resistant UTI continues to grow.

PATHOPHYSIOLOGY

- Route of infection: ascending urethral course is most common.

- The pathogen typically arises from the intestinal bacterial reservoir; it may arise from vaginal flora or cutaneous source.

- *Escherichia coli* is the most common pathogen among domiciliary UTI but Enterococci is more common among persons with HIV infection.

- Pyelonephritis occurs when bacteria ascends from lower to upper urinary tract via the ureter.

- UTI via a hematogenous route is uncommon; it occasionally occurs with septicemia from *Staphylococcus aureus* from oral infections or from *Candida* fungemia; lymphogenous infection rarely occurs from severe bowel infection or retroperitoneal abscess, particularly when obstruction is present.

Source	Common Pathogen
Community-acquired	Intestinal flora *Escherichia coli* (accounts for 85% of all infections) *Proteus* *Klebsiella* *Enterococcus fecalis* *Staphylococcus saprophytics* Cutaneous/vaginal flora *Staphylococcus epidermidis* *Candida albicans*
Nosocomial infections	*Escherichia coli* (accounts for 50% of all infections) *Klebsiella* *Enterobacter* *Citrobacter* *Pseudomonas aeruginosa* *Providencia* *Enterococcus fecalis* *Staphylococcus epidermidis*

- Virulence of pathogen is directly related to its ability to adhere to epithelial cells.

- Adherence is related to host epithelial cell receptivity, a genotypic predisposition that primarily affects women.

- Women with a history of recurring UTI are more likely to be nonsecretors of specific Lewis blood group antigens leading to increased reservoirs of *E. coli* in vaginal epithelium and greater susceptibility to bacterial adherence.

- Additional risk factors increasing the risk of recurring UTI in young women include use of a diaphragm and spermicide during intercourse, and use of a nonlubricated condom.
- Use of antibiotics within 15 to days increases the risk or a subsequent UTI in young women.
- Risk factors for recurring UTI in postmenopausal women include incomplete bladder emptying, cystocele, urinary incontinence, history of UTI prior to menopause, and nonsecretor status.
- Urine osmolality, urea concentration, and pH influence bacterial reproduction; a dilute urine or a concentrated urine with a low pH are bacteriostatic.
- Glucosuria associated with diabetes may increase bacterial reproduction and urinary tract infection risk.
- The average urinary pH of a pregnant woman tends to favor bacterial reproduction more than the average urinary pH of a nonpregnant woman.
- Pregnancy exacerbates the risk of progression of asymptomatic bacteriuria to clinically relevant UTI and it increases the risk of preterm delivery.
- Pyelonephritis leads to immunoglobulin synthesis and antibodies in the urine; cystitis produces little or no detectable serologic response.
- Obstruction and vesicoureteral reflux increase the risk of febrile urinary infection.
- Constipation increases the perianal and vaginal bacterial reservoir and has been associated with urinary tract infections in children.
- Voiding dysfunction (particularly detrusor sphincter dyssynergia) increases risk of cystitis and febrile urinary tract infection.

PATIENT PRESENTATION

History

Previous urinary tract infection; history of "gastroenteritis" as child; congenital defect of urinary system; urinary retention; recent onset of sexual activity (women).

Symptoms

Lower abdominal discomfort or nausea in child; dysuria, urinary frequency, lower abdominal, or suprapubic discomfort in young adult; lower abdominal discomfort or urinary incontinence in elderly adult; symptoms of cystitis and flank pain with chills and sweating, nausea, and vomiting with pyelonephritis; urine may or may not be odorous or cloudy.

Examination

Suprapubic discomfort or no physical findings with cystitis, costovertebral angle tenderness, fever, dehydration with pyelonephritis.

DIFFERENTIAL DIAGNOSIS

- Vaginitis
- Urethritis
- Interstitial cystitis
- Pelvic pain
- Prostatitis
- Gastroenteritis (particularly in children with pyelonephritis)
- Urinary calculus
- Urinary system tumor (may be confused with hemorrhagic cystitis)

KEYS TO ASSESSMENT

- Urine specimen collection: clean catch urine adequate for community-dwelling patients; catheterized specimen for patients with complicated infection, persistent bacteriuria, immobile patient, individual with urinary or fecal incontinence requiring incontinent brief.

- Centrifuge urine for 5 minutes at 2000 rpm prior to dipstick urinalysis and microscopic examination.

- Urine culture and sensitivity if:
  - Patient with first febrile infection, recurrent afebrile infection (more than 1 per year), complicated urinary tract infection, history of urinary system conditions including congenital defect, urinary calculi.
  - The dipstick urinalysis shows nitrates and leukocytes.
  - Bacteriuria and pyuria are seen on microscopic examination.

- An ultrasound and voiding cystourethrogram for an infant or child with first febrile urinary tract infection or recurrent cystitis.

- Imaging study in otherwise healthy adult with first febrile UTI, persistent bacteriuria, or suspicion of foreign body or obstruction.

KEYS TO MANAGEMENT

- Prevention
  - Avoid dehydration: recommended daily allowance (RDA) for fluids in the active adult is approximately 30 ml/kg/day.
  - Avoid constipation (encourage fluids, dietary fiber, and recreational exercise).
  - Manage urinary retention, urinary incontinence or bladder outlet obstruction.
  - Consider repair of cystocele in the postmenopausal woman with incomplete bladder emptying and recurring UTI.
  - Teach women about proper hygiene after toileting and urination after intercourse.
  - Treat infections early, particularly in patients with compromised immune function or those with urinary retention, or voiding dysfunction.
  - Remove indwelling catheter and treat patients with voiding dysfunction with an alternative management program such as bladder retraining, pharmacotherapy for urinary incontinence, intermittent catheterization and/or scheduled voiding.

- Acute urinary tract infection
  - Empiric treatment is adequate for first time infection in otherwise healthy, young women; begin empiric treatment before the culture and sensitivity results for complicated or febrile urinary tract infection.
  - Antipyretics and hospitalization with intravenous fluids is necessary if pyelonephritis is associated with significant nausea and vomiting or urosepsis.
  - Select an antibiotic according to the culture and sensitivity report (when indicated), frequency of administration, risk of associated vaginitis, cost to the patient, and risk of promoting bacterial resistance (Table 14-1).

Table 14-1 Common Antibiotic Choices for UTI

Antibiotic	Typical Dosage and Administration Schedule	Implications
Trimethoprim-Sulfamethoxazole (TMP-SMX)	1 double strength tablet PO BID	- BID dosage promotes compliance - Relatively inexpensive - Risk of secondary vaginitis
Nitrofurantoin (Macrodantin or Macrobid)	Macrodantin given as 50 to 100 mg PO QID; Macrobid given as 1 capsule PO BID	- BID dosage promotes compliance - More expensive than TMP-SMX - Risk of vaginitis negligible - May be used for enterococcus infection, may be effective when managing vancomycin resistant enterococcus in certain patients
Ampicillin	500 mg QID	- QID dosage may reduce compliance - Relatively inexpensive - Risk of secondary vaginitis
Amoxicillin	500 mg PO TID	- TID dosage may reduce compliance - Relatively inexpensive compared to TMP-SMX, other penicillins
Cephalexin	500 mg PO QID	- QID dosage may reduce compliance - Relatively expensive when compared to penicillins, TMX-SMZ - Risk of secondary vaginitis
Levofloxacin	500 mg PO QID	- QD dosage promotes compliance - Relatively expensive - Risk of secondary vaginitis - Reserved for complicated infections
Ciprofloxacin	500 mg PO BID	- BID dosage promotes compliance - Relatively expensive - Risk of secondary vaginitis - Reserved for complicated infections
Norfloxacin	400 mg PO BID	- BID dosage promotes compliance - Relatively expensive - Risk of secondary vaginitis - Reserved for complicated infections

- Emphasize compliance with antibiotic course; treat uncomplicated infection for 3 days, complicated infection for 7 days, and febrile UTI for 14 days.
- Supplement antibiotic treatment with urinary analgesic (Pyridium is available as over-the-counter medication) or a combination agent, such as Urised.
- Begin prophylactic treatment using an antifungal cream for woman with a history of vaginitis when receiving antibiotic therapy, unless nitrofurantoin is administered.
- Encourage adequate fluid intake; avoid bladder irritants.
- Prevention of recurrent infection
  - Obtain a culture and sensitivity with persistent symptoms.
  - Obtain an imaging study (ultrasound, kidneys/ureter/bladder [KUB], intravenous pyelogram) when hematuria persists, when hematuria is found in isolation of a UTI, or refer the patient to a urologist.
  - Refer to urologist if infection with *Proteus, Klebsiella* or *Pseudomonas* species or obtain imaging study to rule out urinary calculi.
  - Rule out prostatitis in men.
  - Refer to urologist when an explanation of persistent bacteriuria is not identified.
  - Obtain upper urinary tract imaging (ultrasonography) with febrile urinary tract infection.
  - Consider low-dose, suppressive therapy for recurrent, febrile infections.

- Consider self-start, intermittent therapy (where the patient is taught to obtain a culture with a dip-slide device followed by empiric treatment).
- Consider postintercourse suppressive antibiotic therapy when the relation between intercourse and UTI is established.

Pathophysiology → Clinical Link

What is going on in the disease process that influences how the patient presents and how he or she should be managed?

What should you do now that you understand the underlying pathophysiology?

Bacterial adherence is influenced by genotypic epithelial cell receptivity.	There is a risk for recurrent urinary tract infections, particularly among otherwise healthy adult women.
Ascending urethral course is the most common route of bacterial invasion.	Risk of recurrent infection is increased with sexual intercourse; teach the patient to urinate immediately following intercourse and to have proper hygiene following urination. Consider postcoital suppression antibiotic therapy.
Dilute urine is bacteriostatic.	Adequate fluid intake.
Gastrointestinal flora account for the majority of pathogens in the community-dwelling population.	Maintain proper hygiene following urination and avoid constipation, which increases intestinal bacterial reservoir.
Risk of pyelonephritis is greater in patients with voiding dysfunction, foreign object in urinary system (including indwelling catheter), vesicoureteral reflux, and diabetics.	Identify and manage risk factors. Treat UTI promptly in the patient at-risk; treat complicated infection for 7 days and febrile UTI for 14 days.
Enterococcus is predominant pathogen in patients with HIV infection.	Nitrofurantoin is often effective in the treatment of an enterococcus UTI, and it may be effective in cases of vancomycin resistant enterococcus *provided the infection is limited to the lower urinary tract.*
The incidence and prevalence of UTI with antimicrobial resistant pathogens continues to rise.	Suppressive or prophylactic treatment of UTI increases the risk of infection with antimicrobial resistant pathogens. Fluoroquinolones and related agents should be reserved for complicated infections.
Pregnancy increases the risk of asymptomatic bacteriuria progressing to cystitis and the risk of preterm delivery.	Consult the obstetrician concerning treatment of asymptomatic bacteriuria in a pregnant woman.

Suggested Reading

Barry, H. C., Ebell, M. H., & Hickner, J. (1997). Evaluation of suspected urinary tract infection in ambulatory women: A cost utility analysis of office-based strategies. *Journal of Family Practice, 44*, 49-60.

Bartkowski, D. P. (2001). Recognizing UTIs in infants and children. Early treatment prevents permanent damage. *Postgraduate Medicine, 109*, 171-172.

Bjornson, D. C., Rovers, J. P., Burian, J. A., & Hall, N. L. (1997). Pharmacoepidemiology of urinary tract infection in Iowa medicaid patients in long-term care facilities. *Annals of Pharmacotherapy, 31*, 837-841.

Childs, S. J., & Egan, R. J. (1996). Bacteriuria and urinary infections in the elderly. *Urologic Clinics of North American, 23*, 45-54.

Cockerill, F. R., & Edson, R. S. (1991). Trimethoprim-sulfamethoxazole. *Mayo Clinic Proceedings, 66*, 1249-1251.

Connolly, A., & Throp, J.M. 1999). Urinary tract infections in pregnancy. *Urologic Clinics of North America, 26*, 779-87.

Dellagrammaticas, H. D., Iacovidou, N., Papadimitriou, M., Daskalaki, A., & Papadoyannis, M. (2001). Mild dilatation of renal pelvis in term neonates with urinary tract infection. *Biology of the Neonate, 79,* 1-4.

Eron, L. J. & Passos, S. (2001). Early discharge of infected patients through appropriate antibiotic use. *Archives of Internal Medicine, 161,* 61-65.

Foxman, B., Marsh, J., Gillespie, B., Rubin, M., Koopman, J. S., & Spear, S. (1997). Condom use and first time urinary tract infection. *Epidemiology, 8,* 612-614.

Goettsch, W., van Pelt, W., Kagelkerke, N., Hendrix, M.G., Buiting, A.G., Sabbe, L. J. et al. (2000). Increasing resistance to fluoroquinolones in *Escherichia coli* from urinary tract infections in the Netherlands. *Journal of Antimicrobial Therapy, 46*, 223-228.

Goldstein, F.W. (2000). Antibiotic susceptibility of bacterial strains from patients with community-acquired urinary tract infections in France. *European Journal of Clinical Microbiology & Infectious Diseases, 19*, 112-117.

Geerlings, S.E., Stolk, R.P., Camps, M.J., Netten, P.M., Hoekstra, J.B., Bouter, K.P. et al. (2000). Asymptomatic bacteriuria may be considered a complication in women with diabetes. *Diabetes Care, 23*, 744-749.

Gray, M. L. (1992). *Genitourinary disorders* (pp. 52-63). St. Louis: Mosby.

Gray, M. L. (1997). Genitourinary system. In S. M. Thompson, G. K. MacFarland, J. E. Hirsh, & S. Tucker (Eds.), *Clinical Nursing* (pp. 1007-1014). St. Louis: Mosby.

Hassay, K. A. (1995). Effective management or urinary discomfort. *Nurse Practitioner, 20*(36), 39-40, 41-44.

Leiner, S. (1995). Recurrent urinary tract infection in otherwise healthy adult women. Rational strategies for work-up and management. *Nurse Practitioner, 20*, 48, 51-52, 54-56.

Loening-Bacucke, V. (1997). Urinary incontinence and urinary tract infection and their resolution with treatment of chronic constipation of childhood. *Pediatrics, 100*, 228-232.

Mikhail, M. S., & Anyaegbunam, A. (1995). Lower urinary tract dysfunction in pregnancy: A review. *Obstetrical and Gynecological Survey, 50*, 675-683.

Millar, L. K., & Cox, S. M. (1997). Urinary tract infections complicating pregnancy. *Infectious Disease Clinics of North America, 11*, 13-26.

Molander, U., Arvidsson, L., Milsom, I., & Sandberg, T. (2000). A longitudinal study of elderly women with urinary tract infection. *Maturatis, 34*, 127-131.

Mouton, C. P., Bazaldua, O. V., Pierce, B., & Espino, D. V. (2001). Common infections in older adults. *American Family Physician, 63*, 257-268.

Nicolle, L. E. (1997). A practical guide to the management of complicated urinary tract infection. *Drugs, 53*, 583-592.

Raz, R., Gennesin, Y., Wasser, J., Stolzer, Z., Rosenfeld, S., Rottensterich, E., & Stamm, W. E. (2000). Recurrent urinary tract infections in postmenopausal women. *Clinical Infectious Diseases, 30*, 152-156.

Sale, P. G. (1995). Genitourinary infection in older women. *Journal of Obstetric, Gynecologic, and Neonatal Nursing, 24*, 769-775.

Schaeffer, A. J. (1996). Urinary tract infections. In J. Y. Gillenwater, J. T. Grayuhack, S. S. Howards, & J. D. Duckett (Eds.), *Adult and pediatric urology* (pp. 219-288). St. Louis: Mosby.

Schaeffer, A. J. (1998). Infections of the urinary tract. In P. C. Walsh, A. B. Retik, E. D. Vaughan, & A. J. Wein (Eds.), *Campbell's urology* (pp. 533-613). Philadeliphia: Saunders.

Schonwald, S., Begovac, J., & Skerek, V. (1999). Urinary tract infections in HIV disease. *International Journal of Antimicrobial Agents, 11*, 309-311.

Stamm, W. E., & Raz, R. (1999). Factors contributing to susceptibility of postmenopausal women to recurrent urinary tract infections. *Clinical Infectious Diseases, 28*, 723-725.

Stapleton, A. (1999). Host factors in susceptibility to urinary tract infections. *Advances in Experimental Medicine and Biology, 462*, 351-358.

Webb, J. A. (1997). The role of imaging in adult acute urinary tract infection. *European Radiology, 7*, 837-843.

Case Study*

Urinary Tract Infection

INITIAL HISTORY

- 27-year-old woman.
- Symptoms of urgency to urinate, frequent urination, and urethral burning during urination has persisted for 48 hours.
- She awoke from sleep with urgency and suprapubic discomfort 2 nights ago.
- Urine now has strong odor and cloudy appearance.

Question 1   What is your differential diagnosis based on the information you have now?

Question 2   What other questions would you like to ask now?

ADDITIONAL HISTORY

- Recurring urinary tract infections since she married at age 22 years.
- Prior UTI associated with similar symptoms.
- Denies history of febrile or hemorrhagic UTI.
- Three previous episodes over past 2 years.
- May be associated with strenuous physical exertion and sexual intercourse.
- No other medical history.
- She reports an allergy to penicillin that causes a "rash" and "trouble breathing."

_____

***Mikel Gray contributed this case study.**

Question 3 Now what do you think of her history?

PHYSICAL EXAMINATION
- Well-nourished female experiencing mild discomfort.
- Tenderness on palpation of abdominal pelvic area; physical examination otherwise unremarkable.
- T = 98.6 orally; BP = 114/64; P = 68; RR = 12 BPM.

Question 4 What laboratory studies are indicated in this patient?

LABORATORY RESULTS
- Dipstick urinalysis
  - Color: dark yellow
  - Specific gravity = 1.030
  - pH = 6.5
  - Protein: negative
  - Glucose: negative
  - Ketones: negative
  - Bilirubin: negative
  - Trace occult blood
  - Leukocytes: large amount
  - Nitrates: positive
  - Urobilinogen: negative

- Microscopic examination
  - WBC: too numerous to count (TNTC)/HPF (high power field)
  - Bacteria: TNTC
  - RBC: 3 to 4/HPF
  - Casts: negative
- Urine culture
  - *Escherichia coli*: >104 cfu/ml
  - Microorganism sensitive to ampicillin, nitrofurantoin, TMX-SMZ, ciprofloxacin, cephalexin

Question 5   What additional studies are indicated in this patient?

Question 6   Based on these findings, what therapy would you initiate?

Question 7   What measures would you recommend to reduce the risk of a recurrence?

15

Peptic Ulcer Disease

DEFINITION

- Peptic ulcer disease (PUD) is defined as defects in the gastrointestinal (GI) mucosa extending through the muscularis mucosae occurring in the esophagus, stomach, or duodenum.
- Peptic ulcers are associated with a number of conditions, however, there are two common forms:
    - Those associated with *Helicobacter pylori* (*H. pylori*) infection.
    - Those associated with nonsteroidal antiinflammatory drug (NSAID) intake.
- NSAIDS and alcohol may exacerbate ulcers of *H. pylori* origin.
- Other less common forms occur with acid hypersecretory syndromes (gastrinoma, mastocytosis), herpes simplex virus (HSV) type I, cytomegalovirus (CMV), duodenal obstruction, vascular insufficiency, and radiation and chemotherapy-associated ulcers.

EPIDEMIOLOGY

- Lifetime prevalence of PUD is 5% to 10%; there is increasing risk with age.
- Duodenal ulcer (DU) is more common than gastric ulcer (GU) and occurs in younger patients; it affects males more often than females.
- Gastric ulcers have a peak incidence at age 55 to 65 and are rare before age 40; they occur in men at the same rate as women.
- Hospitalization rates for PUD are declining but complication rates (perforation, hemorrhage, and death) are relatively stable.
- Genetics appear to play a role with clear familial aggregation but definite specific genetic markers have yet to be identified.
- *H. pylori* can be identified in 95% of DU and 80% to 85% of GU.
    - In developed countries, seroprevalence is directly correlated with increasing age (85% by age 60) and is inversely correlated with socioeconomic status (lowest income class = 100% prevalence; highest = <1%).
    - In the U.S., the prevalence of *H. pylori* is higher in African Americans and Hispanics.
    - The spread of infection through unsanitary conditions is recognized but the specific mode of transmission is unknown.
    - In addition to increasing the risk of PUD, *H. pylori* infection confers up to a 9-fold increase in risk for gastric adenocarcinoma.
- In the U.S., NSAID use is estimated to cause 100,000 hospitalizations and 10,000 to 20,000 deaths per year due to NSAID-related gastrointestinal (GI) complications.
- The risk of gastric and duodenal ulceration ranges from 11% to 30% for patients on daily NSAIDS; it is much higher if patients are also on corticosteroids; also increases risk for upper gastrointestinal bleeding 4-fold, particularly in the elderly.

- Psychological stress has been associated with increased gastric acid secretion, acute gastric erosions, and PUD.

- Cigarette smoking is a risk factor for PUD and has been shown to decrease gastric mucus production.

- Other risk factors include type O blood group, alcohol, chronic pulmonary disease, reflux esophagitis, cirrhosis, and renal failure and transplantation.

PATHOPHYSIOLOGY

- Ulcers form when there is a breakdown in the mucosal defense and repair mechanisms that normally protect the stomach and duodenum from the acid and peptic environment of the upper GI tract.

- Defense mechanisms:

  - A layer of mucus and bicarbonate over the surface of the mucosa provides a buffer and prevents pepsin diffusion into the mucosal layer.

  - A mucosal barrier of tight cellular junctions, growth factors, and membrane transport systems removes excess ions, preventing back-diffusion of hydrogen ions into the mucosa.

  - A vigorous supply of blood to the mucosa removes excess hydrogen ion and maintains nutrient flow for normal cellular function and repair.

- *H. pylori* and NSAIDs cause tissue injury resulting in defects in one or more of these defense mechanisms with subsequent exposure of the mucosa to acid and pepsin.

- *H. pylori* causes tissue injury through:

  - Production of lipopolysaccharide (LPS, endotoxin), other toxic proteins (VacA).

  - Stimulation of the release of inflammatory mediators (IL-1, IL-8, TNF).

  - Induction of chronic active gastritis and atrophic gastritis.

  - Increasing gastrin, pepsin, and acid secretion.

- NSAIDs cause cyclooxygenase-1 (COX-1) inhibition resulting in decreased synthesis of the prostaglandins responsible for GI mucosal protection (the selective cyclooxygenase-2 [COX-2] inhibitors cause less GI toxicity). Risk for PUD is increased because NSAIDS:

  - Inhibit bicarbonate secretion from the gastric and duodenal mucosa.

  - Decreased mucus cell secretion.

  - Inhibit mucosal proliferation and healing.

  - Cause microvascular ischemia.

  - Inhibit physiologic regulation of acid secretion.

  - Stimulate neutrophil adhesion to the splanchnic endothelium.

- NSAIDs and their metabolites also cause local mucosal injury by trapping hydrogen ions in cells and by promoting gastric and pepsin penetration through the gastric mucus lining.

- Gastric ulcers can occur in the absence of hyperacidity, whereas duodenal ulcers occur only in association with hyperacidity and are associated with both increased basal and postprandial acid secretion.

- Gastric hypermotility and duodenal hypomotility have been implicated in DU, whereas gastric hypomotility and pyloric reflux have been associated with GU.

- PUD can be complicated by bleeding, perforation and peritonitis, penetration into surrounding tissues such as pancreas and colon, and pyloric obstruction.

PATIENT PRESENTATION

History

Family history of PUD; smoking; alcohol; stress; older age; low socioeconomic status; NSAID use; chronic pulmonary hepatic, or renal disease.

Uncomplicated symptoms

Epigastric burning or "hunger" sensation occurring 2 to 3 hours after meals and at night temporarily relieved with antacids, food, and milk; occasionally the epigastric discomfort is exacerbated rather than relieved by eating; "irritable stomach" to certain foods; belching; bloating; nausea; vomiting; regurgitation; fatty food intolerance; early satiety; weight loss or weight gain; MOST patients with NSAID-associated ulcers have no dyspepsia prior to the development of serious GI complications.

Complicated symptoms

Severe unremitting pain; pain radiating to the back; projectile vomiting; hematemesis; melena; fever; hypotension.

Examination

Exam often nonspecific and unrevealing in uncomplicated PUD with only epigastric tenderness; guarding, decreased bowel sounds, fever, heme + stools indicate complications.

DIFFERENTIAL DIAGNOSIS

- Gastroesophageal reflux disease (GERD)
- Cholelithiasis/cholecystitis
- Pancreatitis
- Diverticulitis
- Appendicitis
- Gastric carcinoma
- Drug-induced dyspepsia
- Intestinal ischemia
- Infectious gastritis (HSV, CMV, tuberculous, strongyloidiasis, giardiasis)

KEYS TO ASSESSMENT

- Complete blood cell (CBC) count, liver function tests (LFTs), amylase, bilirubin, and chemistries including calcium stool guaiac.
- Assessment should follow two basic pathways:
  - Patients younger than 50 years old with dyspepsia and no history of NSAID use should undergo noninvasive *H. pylori* testing (blood or fecal serology or urea breath test) and therapy if indicated.
  - Patients over the age of 50 or any patient with "alarm" markers (anemia, gastrointestinal bleeding, anorexia, early satiety, weight loss) should undergo upper gastrointestinal endoscopy with biopsy and rapid urease test.
- Upper gastrointestinal endoscopy allows for diagnosis of PUD and differentiation of benign from malignant gastric ulceration; radiography is less sensitive and specific than endoscopy.

KEYS TO MANAGEMENT

- Prevention

    - Smoking cessation; decrease alcohol consumption.

    - Avoid milk and foods that give dyspeptic symptoms (does not induce or prevent ulcers but decreases symptoms and is recommended by virtually every reference as part of a nonpharmacologic ulcer prevention regimen).

    - Avoid nonselective NSAIDs if possible; if not add a proton pump inhibitor (PPI) (ex. omeprazole) which has been shown to be more effective than misoprostol in reducing NSAID-induced ulcers.

    - Selective cyocloxygenase-2 inhibitors (celecoxib, rofecoxib) have been shown to be significantly safer than older NSAIDs and should be considered as an alternative, although their cost is high.

    - New drugs in clinical trials include NSAIDs that contain nitric oxide inducers which may oppose the negative effects of COX-2 inhibition.

- Pharmacologic management of PUD

    - *H. pylori* negative ulcers

        1) Proton pump inhibitors (PPI) (omeprazole, lansoprazole, pantoprazole rabeprazole) provide better 24-hour acid inhibition, and have the highest rate of ulcer healing at 2 to 4 weeks. Recent studies indicate that they are safe even for long-term (months to years) use.

        2) Histamine-2 (H2) receptor blockers (cimetidine, ranitidine, famotidine, nizatidine) reduce gastric pH and are effective for healing acute ulcers but may result in tolerance and rebound hyperacidity in some patients.

        3) Liquid and tablet antacids are effective in ulcer healing, but have much lower rates of patient adherence and have more side effects than either H2 blockers or PPIs.

        4) Sucralfate has similar healing rates to cimetidine and is well tolerated, but it requires qid dosing.

        5) Recurrences are common and full-dose therapy should be continued for 4 to 6 weeks followed by a maintenance regimen of half-therapeutic doses at bedtime for up to 5 years.

    - *H. pylori* positive ulcers

        1) Currently, triple-drug therapy is recommended for documented *H. pylori* infections and can result in eradication of the microorganism in 80% to 95% of patients.

        2) The most effective therapies include a combination of PPI plus two antibiotics (ex. clarithromycin, tetracycline, or metronidazole).

        3) Unfortunately, patient symptoms after therapy do not always correlate with eradication success, and follow-up should include repeat serologic testing or urease breath testing.

        4) If triple therapy fails to eradicate the microorganism, quadruple therapy adding bismuth citrate is indicated.

        5) Ulcer recurrence rates in cases where *H. pylori* has been eradicated are as low as 4% to 6%, compared to 59% to 67% of patients who remain positive for the microorganisms.

- Treatment of ulcer complications

    - Acute upper gastrointestinal bleeding from PUD requires rapid patient stabilization and possible transfusion while preparing for emergent endoscopy and medical or surgical intervention.

    - PUD perforation or penetration is a surgical emergency. Surgery for complicated or refractory ulcers includes vagotomy (truncal or selective) and a variety of gastric and duodenal resection procedures; complications include gastric hypomotility, reflux esophagitis, dumping syndrome, and diarrhea.

Pathophysiology → Clinical Link

What is going on in the disease process that influences how the patient presents and how he or she should be managed?

What should you do now that you understand the underlying pathophysiology?

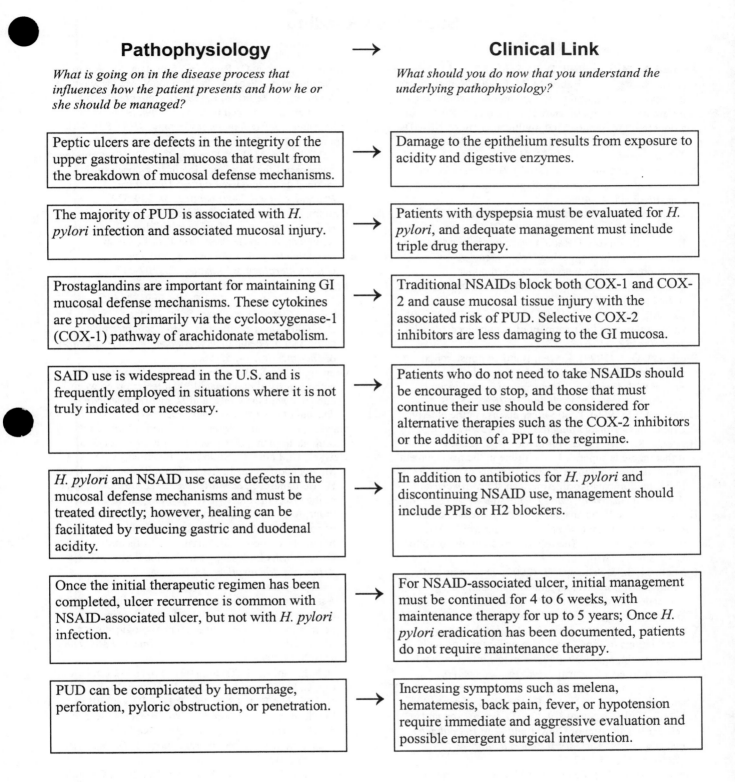

Pathophysiology	Clinical Link
Peptic ulcers are defects in the integrity of the upper gastrointestinal mucosa that result from the breakdown of mucosal defense mechanisms.	Damage to the epithelium results from exposure to acidity and digestive enzymes.
The majority of PUD is associated with *H. pylori* infection and associated mucosal injury.	Patients with dyspepsia must be evaluated for *H. pylori*, and adequate management must include triple drug therapy.
Prostaglandins are important for maintaining GI mucosal defense mechanisms. These cytokines are produced primarily via the cyclooxygenase-1 (COX-1) pathway of arachidonate metabolism.	Traditional NSAIDs block both COX-1 and COX-2 and cause mucosal tissue injury with the associated risk of PUD. Selective COX-2 inhibitors are less damaging to the GI mucosa.
SAID use is widespread in the U.S. and is frequently employed in situations where it is not truly indicated or necessary.	Patients who do not need to take NSAIDs should be encouraged to stop, and those that must continue their use should be considered for alternative therapies such as the COX-2 inhibitors or the addition of a PPI to the regimine.
H. pylori and NSAID use cause defects in the mucosal defense mechanisms and must be treated directly; however, healing can be facilitated by reducing gastric and duodenal acidity.	In addition to antibiotics for *H. pylori* and discontinuing NSAID use, management should include PPIs or H2 blockers.
Once the initial therapeutic regimen has been completed, ulcer recurrence is common with NSAID-associated ulcer, but not with *H. pylori* infection.	For NSAID-associated ulcer, initial management must be continued for 4 to 6 weeks, with maintenance therapy for up to 5 years; Once *H. pylori* eradication has been documented, patients do not require maintenance therapy.
PUD can be complicated by hemorrhage, perforation, pyloric obstruction, or penetration.	Increasing symptoms such as melena, hematemesis, back pain, fever, or hypotension require immediate and aggressive evaluation and possible emergent surgical intervention.

Suggested Reading

Agrawal, N. M., Campbell, D. R., Safdi, M. A., Lukasik, N. L., Huang, B., & Haber, M. M. (2000). Superiority of lansoprazole vs ranitidine in healing nonsteroidal anti-inflammatory drug-associated gastric ulcers: Results of a double-blind, randomized, multicenter study. NSAID-Associated Gastric Ulcer Study Group. *Archives of Internal Medicine, 160,* 1455-1461.

Anderson, J., & Gonzalez, J. (2000). *H pylori* infection. Review of the guideline for diagnosis and treatment. *Geriatrics, 55,* 44-49.

Archimandritis, A., Tzivras, M., Sougioultzis, S., Papaparaskevas, I., Apostolopoulos, P., Avlami, A., & Davaris, P. S. (2000). Rapid urease test is less sensitive than histology in diagnosing *Helicobacter pylori* infection in patients with non-variceal upper gastrointestinal bleeding. *Journal of Gastroenterology & Hepatology, 15,* 369-373.

Asaka, M., Sugiyama, T., Kato, M., & Takeda, H. (2000). Current topics in the treatment of peptic ulcer. *Internal Medicine, 39,* 339-342.

Bjorkman, D. J. (1999). Current status of nonsteroidal anti-inflammatory drug (NSAID) use in the United States: Risk factors and frequency of complications. *American Journal of Medicine, 107*(6A), 3S-8S.

Borum, M. L. (1999). Peptic-ulcer disease in the elderly. *Clinics in Geriatric Medicine, 15*(3), 457-471.

Breiter, J. R., Riff, D., & Humphries, T. J. (2000). Rabeprazole is superior to ranitidine in the management of active duodenal ulcer disease: Results of a double-blind, randomized North American study. *American Journal of Gastroenterology, 95,* 936-942.

Brown, G. J., & Yeomans, N. D. (1999). Prevention of the gastrointestinal adverse effects of nonsteroidal anti-inflammatory drugs: The role of proton pump inhibitors. *Drug Safety, 21*(6), 503-512.

Cappell, M. S., & Schein, J. R. (2000). Diagnosis and treatment of nonsteroidal anti-inflammatory drug-associated upper gastrointestinal toxicity. *Gastroenterology Clinics of North America, 29,* 97-124.

Carmel, R., Aurangzeb, I., & Qian, D. (2001). Associations of food-cobalamin malabsorption with ethnic origin, age, *Helicobacter pylori* infection, and serum markers of gastritis. *American Journal of Gastroenterology, 96,* 63-70.

Chan, F. K., To, K. F., Ng, Y. P., Lee, T. L., Cheng, A. S., Leung, W. K., & Sung, J. J. (2001). Expression and cellular localization of COX-1 and -2 in *Helicobacter pylori* gastritis. *Alimentary Pharmacology & Therapeutics, 15,* 187-193.

Chung, S. C. (2001). Peptic ulcer bleeding. *American Journal of Gastroenterology, 96,* 1-3.

Day, A. S., Jones, N. L., Lynett, J. T., Jennings, H. A., Fallone, C. A., Beech, R., & Sherman, P. M. (2000). cagE is a virulence factor associated with *Helicobacter pylori*-induced duodenal ulceration. *Journal of Infectious Diseases, 181,* 1370-1375.

Di Leo, A., Messa, C., Russo, F., Linsalata, M., Amati, L., Caradonna, L., Pece, S., Pellegrino, N. M., Caccavo, D., Antonaci, S., & Jirillo, E. (1999). *Helicobacter pylori* infection and host cell responses. *Immuno-pharmacology & Immunotoxicology, 21*(4), 803-846.

Donnelly, M. T., Goddard, A. F., Filipowicz, B., Morant, S. V., Shield, M. J., & Hawkey, C. J. (2000). Low-dose misoprostol for the prevention of low-dose aspirin-induced gastroduodenal injury. *Alimentary Pharmacology & Therapeutics, 14,* 529-534.

Drumm, B., Koletzko, S., & Oderda, G. (2000). *Helicobacter pylori* infection in children: A consensus statement. European Paediatric Task Force on *Helicobacter pylori*. *Journal of Pediatric Gastroenterology & Nutrition, 30,* 207-213.

Felig, D. M., & Carafa, C. J. (2000). Stress ulcers of the stomach. *Gastrointestinal Endoscopy, 51,* 596.

Ge, Z. Z., Zhang, D. Z., Xiao, S. D., Chen, Y., & Hu, Y. B. (2000). Does eradication of *Helicobacter pylori* alone heal duodenal ulcers? *Alimentary Pharmacology & Therapeutics, 14,* 53-58.

Graham, D. Y., & Osato, M. S. (2000). *H. pylori* in the pathogenesis of duodenal ulcer: Interaction between duodenal acid load, bile, and *H. pylori*. *American Journal of Gastroenterology, 95,* 87-91.

Hawkey, C. J. (2000). Nonsteroidal anti-inflammatory drug gastropathy. *Gastroenterology, 119,* 521-535.

Hawkey, C., Laine, L., Simon, T., Beaulieu, A., Maldonado-Cocco, J., Acevedo, E., Shahane, A., Quan, H., Bolognese, J., & Mortensen, E. (2000). Comparison of the effect of rofecoxib (a cyclooxygenase 2 inhibitor), ibuprofen, and placebo on the gastroduodenal mucosa of patients with osteoarthritis: A randomized, double-blind, placebo-controlled trial. The Rofecoxib Osteoarthritis Endoscopy Multinational Study Group. *Arthritis & Rheumatism, 43,* 370-377.

Hernandez-Diaz, S., & Rodriguez, L. A. (2000). Association between nonsteroidal anti-inflammatory drugs and upper gastrointestinal tract bleeding/perforation: An overview of epidemiologic studies published in the 1990s. *Archives of Internal Medicine, 160,* 2093-2099.

Hsu, P. I., Lai, K. H., Tseng, H. H., Lo, G. H., Lo, C. C., Lin, C. K., Cheng, J. S., Chan, H. H., Ku, M. K., Peng, N. J., Chien, E. J., Chen, W., & Hsu, P. N. (2001). Eradication of *Helicobacter pylori* prevents ulcer development in patients with ulcer-like functional dyspepsia. *Alimentary Pharmacology & Therapeutics, 15,* 195-201.

Houben, M. H., Van Der, B. D., Hensen, E. F., Craen, A. J., Rauws, E. A., & Tytgat, G. N. (1999). A systematic review of *Helicobacter pylori* eradication therapy—The impact of antimicrobial resistance on eradication rates. *Alimentary Pharmacology & Therapeutics, 13*(8), 1047-1055.

Katelaris, P. H., Adamthwaite, D., Midolo, P., Yeomans, N. D., Davidson, G., & Lambert, J. (2000). Randomized trial of omeprazole and metronidazole with amoxycillin or clarithromycin for *Helicobacter pylori* eradication, in a region of high primary metronidazole resistance. *Alimentary Pharmacology & Therapeutics, 14,* 751-758.

Konturek, P. C., Bielanski, W., Konturek, S. J., & Hahn, E. G. (1999). *Helicobacter pylori* associated gastric pathology. *Journal of Physiology & Pharmacology, 50*(5), 695-710.

Laine, L., Ahnen, D., McClain, C., Solcia, E., & Walsh, J. H. (2000). Review article: Potential gastrointestinal effects of long-term acid suppression with proton pump inhibitors. *Alimentary Pharmacology & Therapeutics, 14,* 651-668.

Manes, G., Balzano, A., Iaquinto, G., Ricci, C., Piccirillo, M. M., Giardullo, N., Todisco, A., Lioniello, M., & Vaira, D. (2001). Accuracy of the stool antigen test in the diagnosis of *Helicobacter pylori* infection before treatment and in patients on omeprazole therapy. *Alimentary Pharmacology & Therapeutics, 15,* 73-79.

McCarthy, D. M. (1999). Comparative toxicity of nonsteroidal anti-inflammatory drugs. *American Journal of Medicine, 107*(6A), 37S-46S.

Michopoulos, S., Tsibouris, P., Bouzakis, H., Balta, A., Vougadiotis, J., Broutet, N., & Kralios, N. (2000). Randomized study comparing omeprazole with ranitidine as anti-secretory agents combined in quadruple second-line *Helicobacter pylori* eradication regimens. *Alimentary Pharmacology & Therapeutics, 14,* 737-744.

Mitchell, H. M. (1999). The epidemiology of *Helicobacter pylori*. *Current Topics in Microbiology & Immunology, 241,* 11-30.

Oderda, G., Rapa, A., Marinello, D., Ronchi, B., & Zavallone, A. (2001). Usefulness of *Helicobacter pylori* stool antigen test to monitor response to eradication treatment in children. *Alimentary Pharmacology & Therapeutics, 15,* 203-206.

Overmier, J. B., & Murison, R. (2000). Anxiety and helplessness in the face of stress predisposes, precipitates, and sustains gastric ulceration. *Behavioural Brain Research, 110,* 161-174.

Perri, F., Festa, V., Clemente, R., Villani, M. R., Quitadamo, M., Caruso, N., Bergoli, M. L., & Andriulli, A. (2001). Randomized study of two "rescue" therapies for *Helicobacter pylori*-infected patients after failure of standard triple therapies. *American Journal of Gastroenterology, 96,* 58-62.

Phull, P. S., & Jacyna, M. R. (1999). The management of young dyspeptic patients in the era of *Helicobacter pylori*. *International Journal of Clinical Practice, 53*(5), 373-375.

Raskin, J. B. (1999). Gastrointestinal effects of nonsteroidal anti-inflammatory therapy. *American Journal of Medicine, 106*(5B), 3S-12S.

Savarino, V., Vigneri, S., & Celle, G. (1999). The 13C urea breath test in the diagnosis of *Helicobacter pylori* infection. *Gut, 45*(Suppl 1), I18-I22.

Scheiman, J. M., Bandekar, R. R., Chernew, M. E., & Fendrick, A. M. (2001). *Helicobacter pylori* screening for individuals requiring chronic NSAID therapy: A decision analysis. *Alimentary Pharmacology & Therapeutics, 15,* 63-71.

Spinzi, G. C., Boni, F., Bortoli, A., Colombo, E., Ballardini, G., Venturelli, R., & Minoli, G. (2000). Seven-day triple therapy with ranitidine bismuth citrate or omeprazole and two antibiotics for eradication of *H. pylori* in duodenal ulcer: A multicentre, randomized, single-blind study. *Alimentary Pharmacology & Therapeutics, 14,* 325-330.

Stanghellini, V., Tosetti, C., De Giorgio, R., Barbara, G., Salvioli, B., & Corinaldesi, R. (1999). How should *Helicobacter pylori* negative patients be managed? *Gut, 45*(Suppl 1), I32-I35

Talley, N. J. (1999). How should *Helicobacter pylori* positive dyspeptic patients be managed? *Gut, 45*(Suppl 1), I28-I31.

To, K. F., Chan, F. K., Cheng, A. S., Lee, T. L., Ng, Y. P., & Sung, J. J. (2001). Up-regulation of cyclooxygenase-1 and -2 in human gastric ulcer. *Alimentary Pharmacology & Therapeutics, 15,* 25-34.

Unge, P. (1999). Antibiotic treatment of *Helicobacter pylori* infection. *Current Topics in Microbiology & Immunology, 241,* 261-300.

Veldhuyzen van zanten, S. J., & Lee, A. (1999). The role of *Helicobacter pylori* infection in duodenal and gastric ulcer. *Current Topics in Microbiology & Immunology, 241,* 47-56.

Westblom, T. U., & Bhatt, B. D. (1999). Diagnosis of *Helicobacter pylori* infection. *Current Topics in Microbiology & Immunology, 241,* 215-235.

Williams, M. P., & Pounder, R. E. (1999*). Helicobacter pylori*: From the benign to the malignant. *American Journal of Gastroenterology, 94*(11 Suppl), S11-S16.

Wolfe, M. M., & Sachs, G. (2000). Acid suppression: Optimizing therapy for gastroduodenal ulcer healing, gastroesophageal reflux disease, and stress-related erosive syndrome. *Gastroenterology, 118,* S9-31.

Wolfe, M. M., Lichtenstein, D. R., & Singh, G. (1999). Gastrointestinal toxicity of nonsteroidal antiinflammatory drugs. *New England Journal of Medicine, 340*(24), 1888-1899.

Xia, H. H., & Talley, N. J. (1999). *Helicobacter pylori* eradication in patients with non-ulcer dyspepsia. *Drugs, 58*(5), 785-792.

Xia, H. H., & Talley, N. J. (2001). Apoptosis in gastric epithelium induced by *Helicobacter pylori* infection: Implications in gastric carcinogenesis. *American Journal of Gastroenterology, 96,* 16-26.

Zullo, A., Rinaldi, V., Winn, S., Meddi, P., Lionetti, R., Hassan, C., Ripani, C., Tomaselli, G., & Attili, A. F. (2000). A new highly effective short-term therapy schedule for *Helicobacter pylori* eradication. *Alimentary Pharmacology & Therapeutics, 14,* 715-718.

Case Study

Peptic Ulcer Disease

INITIAL HISTORY

- 58-year-old male complaining of 3-week history of increasing epigastric pain.
- Has had dyspepsia in the past for which he took "Tums" but this is much worse and only partially relieved with chewable antacids.

Question 1 What is your differential diagnosis based on this limited history?

Question 2 What questions would you like to ask this patient about his symptoms?

ADDITIONAL HISTORY

- Pain has a burning quality.
- Relieved with eating, especially drinking milk, but recurs about 2 hours later.
- Denies radiation to his back, melena, hematemesis, or fever.
- Denies early satiety, anorexia, or weight loss.
- Denies fatty food intolerance or change in stools.
- Denies jaundice, increasing abdominal girth, or easy bruising.
- Denies shortness of breath or pain with exercise.

Question 3   What questions would you like to ask about his recent and past medical history?

MORE HISTORY
- Has been taking ibuprofen for the past 2 months for a sore knee.
- Drinks approximately 3 mixed drinks each day.
- Smokes 2 pack of cigarettes a day.
- Has had recent job change with a great deal of stress.
- Has been feeling a little tired lately but no recent illnesses or hospitalization.
- Has a history of mild hypertension treated with diet.
- No medications or allergies.

PHYSICAL EXAMINATION
- Thin white male in no acute distress.
- T = 37 orally; P = 90 and regular; RR = 16 and unlabored; BP = 148/96 sitting right arm.

HEENT, Neck
- PERRLA, fundi without vascular changes.
- Pharynx clear.
- No thyromegaly.
- No bruits.
- No adenopathy.

Lungs, Cardiac
- Lungs clear to auscultation and percussion.
- Cardiac with RRR without murmurs or gallops.

Abdomen
- Abdomen not distended.
- Bowel sounds present.
- Liver percusses to 8 cm at the midclavicular line, one fingerbreadth below the right costal margin.
- Epigastric tenderness without rebound or guarding.
- Spleen not palpable.

Rectal
- No hemorrhoids seen or felt.
- Prostate not enlarged and soft.
- Stool grossly normal but weakly heme+.

Extremities, Neurological
- No edema.
- Pulses full, no bruits.
- Oriented x4.
- Normal strength, sensation, and DTR.

Question 4   What are the pertinent positives and negatives on the physical exam?

Question 5   What initial diagnostic tests would you obtain now?

LABORATORY RESULTS
- Chemistries including calcium and BUN/Cr normal.
- WBC = 9000 with normal differential.
- HCT = 45%.
- Liver function test including bilirubin normal.
- Serum and urine amylase and lipase normal.
- ECG = normal sinus rhythm without evidence of ischemic changes.

Question 6   What test should be chosen to best evaluate for peptic ulcer disease in this patient?

ENDOSCOPY RESULTS

- Normal esophageal mucosa.
- Gastric mucosa with superficial gastritis without ulceration.
- 0.5 cm duodenal ulcer with evidence of recent bleeding, but no acute hemorrhage and no visible vessels in the ulcer crater.
- *H. pylori* testing negative.

Question 7   What management would you recommend?

16

Hepatitis B and C

DEFINITION

- Inflammation of the liver due to viral infection with the hepatitis B or hepatitis C virus.
- Epidemiology, pathophysiology, and clinical manifestations are dependent on the causative virus and the host inflammatory and immunologic response to infection.

EPIDEMIOLOGY

- Hepatitis B (HBV)
    - 2 billion people in the world are infected with HBV.
    - Over 1 million people in the United States have chronic HBV infection; overall prevalence of HBV infection is .5% to 1% but prevalence is significantly greater in Alaskan native population and in African-Americans.
    - Other high prevalence groups include intravenous (IV) drug users, first generation immigrants from endemic areas such as Southeast Asia, men having sex with men, household contacts and sexual partners of HBV carriers, heterosexuals with multiple partners, people requiring hemodialysis, patients in custodial institutions, and health care workers.
    - Incidence has decreased by almost 50% over the past 10 years (in the U.S., vaccination for Hepatitis B is recommended for all infants).
    - Risk of developing chronic HBV infection varies inversely with age at infection (90% of infants infected by birth become carriers; approximately 5% if older than 5 years). Males are affected more than females; peak age is 10 to 29.
    - Alcohol is a cofactor for the development of chronic disease.
    - There are no known risk factors in 30% to 40% of cases.
    - It is spread by parenteral transmission of virus via blood or blood products, sexual contact, or prenatal exposure.
- Hepatitis C (HCV)
    - 3.9 million Americans are infected with HCV; prevalence is much higher in Asia and the Middle East.
    - HCV is the most common blood-born infection in the U.S., and has surpassed alcoholic cirrhosis as the predominant chronic liver disease in this country.
    - It is associated with IV drug use, multiple transfusions, individuals with needle-stick injury, persons with hemophilia, people requiring hemodialysis, health care workers, HIV infected persons, liver and renal transplant patients, and household and sexual contacts of chronically infected persons.

- Alcohol is a cofactor for the development and progression of chronic disease.

- There are no known risk factors in 40% of cases.

- It is spread by direct parenteral inoculation, sexual contact, transplantation of an infected organ, or perinatal exposure.

PATHOPHYSIOLOGY

- Hepatitis B

  - The HBV is a DNA virus that replicates via an RNA intermediate in the nucleus and cytoplasm of the hepatocyte.

  - Hepatocyte injury is mediated by the immune response, rather than direct cytopathic effects by the virus.

  - Hepatocyte injury is mediated by CD8 lymphocyte (T cytotoxic cell) killing of infected cells and by release of inflammatory cytokines.

  - A vigorous immune response will increase symptoms and cause more hepatocellular necrosis, but is crucial to clearing the virus. Patients with less effective immune responses are less symptomatic with the acute infection, but are more likely to develop chronic hepatitis or the carrier state.

  - The inflammatory cytokines tumor necrosis factor alpha (TNF-α) and interferon gamma (INF-γ) are vital to clearance of HBV (prevent HBV reproduction).

  - Circulating antigen-antibody complexes may result in a serum sickness-like syndrome with angioneurotic edema, polyarteritis nodosa, systemic vasculitis with bowel ischemia, renal disease, neuropathy, and arthritis.

  - Although most acute infections resolve without sequelae, approximately 5% to 10% of patients will develop chronic infection with varying degrees of ongoing hepatocyte injury; the risk of complications can approach 90% in infants.

    1) Chronic active hepatitis with active viral replication, widespread inflammation, and sustained increases in aspartate aminotransferase (AST); 15% to 20% of these will develop cirrhosis within 5 years.

    2) Chronic persistent hepatitis in which the inflammation is limited to portal areas and long-term prognosis is very good.

    3) True carrier state is characterized by normal liver enzymes and normal liver histology; only about 2% of these patients will develop progressive disease.

  - The mechanism of long-term asymptomatic carrier state is believed to be immunologic tolerance to the virus—the virus is not cleared but hepatocyte injury is minimal and the carrier state is life-long; this is especially common in infants in whom the immune system is immature and unable to eradicate the virus.

  - Chronic HBV infection is associated with a 10- to 100-fold risk of hepatocellular carcinoma.

- Hepatitis C

  - HCV is a small envelope virus containing RNA and has multiple genotypes with varying phenotypic disease expressions.

  - Direct viral cytopathicity is the primary mode of hepatocyte injury, and the viral load positively correlates with the amount of inflammation seen on liver biopsy.

  - CD8 lymphocyte-mediated cellular destruction of infected cells is the primary means of effective immune response to HCV. The virus can evade humoral immunity by its rapid mutation rate, thus it quickly develops resistant strains to antibodies.

- Autoimmune hepatitis is also commonly associated with HCV infection. Many patients develop anti-liver-kidney microsomal antibodies that can destroy uninfected hepatocytes. This autoimmune component of HCV results in multiple extrahepatic manifestations of the disease including membranous glomerulonephritis, cryoglobulinemia, vasculitis, dermatitis, pulmonary fibrosis, and rheumatoid arthritis.

- Recent studies suggest that only 15% of infected patients are able to completely eradicate the virus. Approximately 70% will develop chronic hepatitis; disease progression is usually clinically silent and characterized by ongoing inflammation.

- Cirrhosis occurs in 20% of chronic HCV infections and may be evident as early as 15 months after the acute infection, although the average time to cirrhosis is 20 years. Cofactors in the development of cirrhosis include increasing age, alcoholism, co-infection with HIV and co-infection with HBV.

- Hepatocellular carcinoma (HCC) occurs in 1% to 5% of patients with chronic HCV infection. The pathogenesis of HCC related to the high level of hepatocellular regeneration seen with chronic HCV hepatitis (mitogenesis), as well as possible mutagenic effects of the virus.

PATIENT PRESENTATION

History

Needle-stick injury; hemodialysis; blood transfusion; organ transplant; homosexual contact with an infected individual; alcohol abuse.

Symptoms

Acute infection is often asymptomatic with both HBV and HCV (50% to 80%); incubation periods from time of exposure to development of symptoms can be 5 to 8 weeks or as long as 6 months; if acute symptoms occur, they include fatigue, fever, myalgias and arthralgias, jaundice, anorexia, abdominal discomfort, and nausea; some cases of acute HBV, infection will present with fulminant hepatic failure, including encephalitis, coagulopathy, and ascites; symptoms of chronic infection are most common in HCV and include fatigue, nausea, anorexia, coagulopathy, ascites, encephalopathy, and gastrointestinal bleeding; extra hepatic manifestations of both HBV and HCV may occur including rashes, severe abdominal pain, renal dysfunction, dyspnea , joint pain, and Raynaud phenomenon.

Examination

The examination is often normal in the absence of significant hepatic failure; when liver dysfunction is severe, exam findings may include asterixis, decreased mental status, jaundice, ecchymoses, ascites, edema, pectoral alopecia, palmer erythema, spider angiomata, gynecomastia, and heme+ stools; evidence of extraarticular disease may be seen in HCV including skin lesions, arthritic changes, pulmonary crackles, and corneal ulcers.

DIFFERENTIAL DIAGNOSIS

- Hepatitis A, D, E, or G
- Hepatitis due to other viruses (Epstein-Barr [EBV], cytomegalovirus [CMV], herpes, coxsackievirus)
- Alcoholic hepatitis or cirrhosis
- Autoimmune hepatitis
- α_1-antitrypsin deficiency
- Biliary cirrhosis
- Toxins or drugs (isoniazid, rifampin, acetaminophen)

- Hemochromatosis
- Sclerosing cholangitis

KEYS TO ASSESSMENT

- History of exposures is important, but the incubation period is long and the acute infection is usually asymptomatic, so that even a careful history may not pinpoint the time or source of initial infection.
- The examination will be relatively unrevealing until late in the course of the disease; diagnosis prior to hepatic failure is dependent on serologic testing.
- Serologic testing:
  - HBV
    1) Three viral antigens and three antibodies can be detected: HBsAg, HBcAg, and HBeAg; and anti-HBs, anti-HBc (IgM or IgG), and anti-Hbe.
    2) In acute infection, HBsAg is positive but could represent a previous carrier state; the diagnosis of acute HBV infection is confirmed with a positive HBeAg and IgM anti-HBc antibody.
    3) Chronic infection is diagnosed by the presence of HBsAg in serum for 6 months or longer after initial detection; IgG anti-HBc are usually present and anti-HBs and anti-HBe are present in most, but not all, cases and may take months to become detectable.
    4) HBV deoxyribonucleic acid (DNA) by polymerase chain reaction (PCR) testing is now available and can detect active viral replication in both acute and chronic infection; it is used primarily to follow response to treatment for research protocols.
  - HCV
    1) HCV screening is indicated for:
       a) Persons who received blood products prior to 1991
       b) Persons with hemophilia
       c) Dialysis patients
       d) Children born to HCV+ mothers
       e) IVDA
       f) Donors for transplants
    2) PCR testing for viral RNA detects presence of the virus (acute or chronic).
    3) Anti-HCV testing has evolved rapidly and the "second and third generation" testing techniques have fewer problems with specificity and sensitivity than did the older assays; antibody titers become detectable weeks to months after the original infection.
- Serum alanine aminotransferase (ALT) and aspartate aminotransferase (AST) levels usually rise 2 to 3 months after the initial infection.
- Diagnosis of liver failure is evidenced by increased bilirubin, prolonged coagulation times, decreased albumin, and evidence of ascites and portal hypertension with the possibility of finding esophageal varices on endoscopy.

KEYS TO MANAGEMENT

- Prevention
    - HBV
        1) Behavior changes in sexual practices, universal precautions in health care, and discontinuation of IV drug use.
        2) Passive immunoprophylaxis is recommended for:
            a) Perinatal exposure to an infected mother.
            b) Prolonged contact of a less than 12-month-old infant with an infected primary care deliverer.
            c) Needle-stick from an infected patient.
            d) Sexual exposure to an infected individual.
            e) Organ transplant if infected prior to transplantation.
        3) Hepatitis B immunoglobulin (HBIG) is given within 12 hours of delivery or 14 days of other exposures followed by the three-dose vaccination series.
        4) Active immunoprophylaxis is recommended for all children and for other high risk groups such as health care workers and IV drug users; a three-dose regimen at 0, 1, and 6 months results in 95% of patients developing antibody with a subsequent rate of HBV infection of 3.2% compared to 26% in controls.
    - HCV
        1) Changes in sexual behavior as with HBV.
        2) Trials of passive immunoprophylaxis have not been effective thus far.
        3) Vaccine development is difficult due to the high mutation rate of the virus.
- Pharmacologic treatment
    - HBV
        1) Interferon-alpha (INF-α) with our without lamivudine.
        2) Combined regimen has higher response rates than either drug alone.
        3) Side effects are frequent and include an influenza-like illness with fever, chills, myalgias, and headache 4 to 8 hours after injection; fatigue; myalgias; anorexia; weight loss; bone marrow suppression; psychological side effects such anxiety, depression, and irritability; and autoimmune phenomena such as autoimmune thyroiditis, hemolytic anemia, and collagen vascular disease.
        4) Patients with HBV may experience a "flare" of their disease with interferon treatment characterized by a dramatic rise in ALT. This is a good prognostic sign indicating an increased likelihood of response; this is not seen with HCV.
    - HCV
        1) Interferon alpha (INF-α) plus ribavirin.
        2) Combined regimen has higher response rates than either drug alone (response rates 30% to 40%).
        3) Side effects similar to HBV regimen.
        4) Indicated for patients with acute or chronic HCV infection, including those with cirrhosis.
        5) Contraindicated in patients with severe depression, active alcoholism or substance abuse, severe autoimmune disease, or severe pancytopenia; controversial use in HIV+ patients or those with normal serum ALT.

6) New therapies include pegylated INF-α, protease inhibitors, RNA polymerase inhibitors, and DNA vaccines.

- Liver transplant

  - Survival rates are now 70% to 85% at 5 years.

  - Indications include severe symptoms, decreased quality of life, and sustained jaundice and coagulopathy.

  - HBV is associated with a high risk of recurrence after transplantation (close to 100% in some studies) unless the patient is also treated with HBIG; postoperative treatment with lamivudine further improves outcomes with overall results now equivalent to all other indications for liver transplant.

  - HCV accounts for about one-third of all liver transplants performed in the United States; recurrence after transplant is 100%, but it is usually associated with only mild increases in ALT. Postoperative survival is excellent.

Pathophysiology → # Clinical Link

What is going on in the disease process that influences how the patient presents and how he or she should be managed?

What should you do now that you understand the underlying pathophysiology?

Pathophysiology	Clinical Link
HBV causes liver injury primarily through immune-dependent mechanisms rather than through direct viral cytopathicity.	Patients with an effective immune response are less likely to become carriers but will present with a more fulminant clinical presentation and a high ALT.
Some patients are immunologically tolerant to HBV and will have persistent viral replication and chronic hepatitis.	HBV carrier state occurs in approximately 5% of patients and is associated with persistent infectivity, chronic liver damage, and a risk of hepatocellular carcinoma.
Treatment of HBV with INF-α and lamivudine may result in a transient flare in immunologic activity that indicates effective HBV killing.	Patients may experience an increase in ALT and experience a flu-like illness after therapy.
Both active and passive immunoprophylaxis for HBV are effective in preventing infection.	Postexposure HBIG and vaccination with the three-dose regimen are effective in preventing active infection.
HCV mutates rapidly and can avoid the immune system and can develop resistance to vaccines.	Chronic HCV infection is common, and both passive and active immunoprophylaxis have been ineffective so far.
HCV has direct cytopathicity on the hepatocytes with significant hepatocellular injury and necrosis.	HCV is associated with a significant risk of cirrhosis and hepatocellular carcinoma.
HCV is associated with autoantibodies that can attack the kidney, the skin, joints, and the thyroid.	HCV infection may be associated with membranous glomerulonephritis, rashes, collagen vascular disease, and an autoimmune thyroiditis.

Suggested Reading

Aach, R. D., Yomtovian, R. A., & Hack, M. (2000). Neonatal and pediatric posttransfusion hepatitis C: A look back and a look forward. *Pediatrics, 105,* 836-842.

Anonymous. (1999). EASL International Consensus Conference on hepatitis C. Paris, 26-27 February 1999. Consensus statement. *Journal of Hepatology, 31*(Suppl 1), 3-8.

Ansaldi, F., Torre, F., Bruzzone, B. M., Picciotto, A., Crovari, P., & Icardi, G. (2001). Evaluation of a new hepatitis C virus sequencing assay as a routine method for genotyping. *Journal of Medical Virology, 63,* 17-21.

Baffis, V., Shrier, I., Sherker, A. H., & Szilagyi, A. (1999). Use of interferon for prevention of hepatocellular carcinoma in cirrhotic patients with hepatitis B or hepatitis C virus infection. *Annals of Internal Medicine, 131*(9), 696-701.

Baid, S., Cosimi, A. B., Tolkoff-Rubin, N., Colvin, R. B., Williams, W. W., & Pascual, M. (2000). Renal disease associated with hepatitis C infection after kidney and liver transplantation. *Transplantation, 70,* 255-261.

Boyer, N., & Marcellin, P. (2000). Pathogenesis, diagnosis and management of hepatitis C. *Journal of Hepatology, 32,* 98-112.

Buffington, J., Rowel, R., Hinman, J. M., Sharp, K., & Choi, S. (2001). Lack of awareness of hepatitis C risk among persons who received blood transfusions before 1990. *American Journal of Public Health, 91,* 47-48.

Chisari, F. V. (2000). Rous-Whipple Award Lecture. Viruses, immunity, and cancer: Lessons from hepatitis B. *American Journal of Pathology, 156,* 1117-1132.

Degos, F. (1999). Hepatitis C and alcohol. *Journal of Hepatology, 31*(Suppl 1), 113-118.

Dervite, I., Hober, D., & Morel, P. (2001). Acute hepatitis B in a patient with antibodies to hepatitis B surface antigen who was receiving rituximab. *New England Journal of Medicine, 344,* 68-69.

Diaz, T., Des, J., Vlahov, D., Perlis, T. E., Edwards, V., Friedman, S. R., Rockwell, R., Hoover, D., Williams, I. T., & Monterroso, E. R. (2001). Factors associated with prevalent hepatitis C: Differences among young adult injection drug users in lower and upper Manhattan, New York City. *American Journal of Public Health, 91,* 23-30.

Di Bisceglie, A. M. (2000). Natural history of hepatitis C: Its impact on clinical management. *Hepatology, 31,* 1014-1018.

Eckels, D. D., Wang, H., Bian, T. H., Tabatabai, N., & Gill, J. C. (2000). Immunobiology of hepatitis C virus (HCV) infection: The role of CD4 T cells in HCV infection. *Immunological Reviews, 174,* 90-97.

Eng, M. A., Kallemuchikkal, U., & Gorevic, P. D. (2000). Hepatitis C virus, autoimmunity and lymphoproliferation. *Mount Sinai Journal of Medicine, 67,* 120-132.

European Consensus Group. (2000) Are booster immunisations needed for lifelong hepatitis B immunity? European Consensus Group on Hepatitis B Immunity. *Lancet, 355,* 561-565.

Fabrizi, F., & Martin, P. (2000). Hepatitis B virus infection in dialysis patients. *American Journal of Nephrology, 20,* 1-11.

Fanning, L. J., Levis, J., Kenny-Walsh, E., Whelton, M., O'Sullivan, K., & Shanahan, F. (2001). HLA class II genes determine the natural variance of hepatitis C viral load. *Hepatology, 33,* 224-230.

Feitelson, M. A. (1999). Hepatitis B virus in hepatocarcinogenesis. *Journal of Cellular Physiology, 181*(2), 188-202.

Feng, X. (1999). Hepatitis C infection: A review. *Lippincott's primary care practice, 3*(3), 345-353.

Ferrari, C., Urbani, S., Penna, A., Cavalli, A., Valli, A., Lamonaca, V., Bertoni, R., Boni, C., Barbieri, K., Uggeri, J., & Fiaccadori, F. (1999). Immunopathogenesis of hepatitis C virus. *Journal of Hepatology, 31*(Suppl 1), 31-38.

Flint, M., & McKeating, J. A. (2000). The role of the hepatitis C virus glycoproteins in infection. *Reviews in Medical Virology, 10,* 101-117.

Glacken, M., Kernohan, G., & Coates, V. (2001). Diagnosed with hepatitis C: A descriptive exploratory study. *International Journal of Nursing Studies, 38,* 107-116.

Houghton, M. (2000). Strategies and prospects for vaccination against the hepatitis C viruses. *Current Topics in Microbiology & Immunology, 242,* 327-329.

Hunt, C. M., McGill, J. M., Allen, M. I., & Condreay, L. D. (2000). Clinical relevance of hepatitis B viral mutations. *Hepatology, 31,* 1037-1044.

Jefferson, T., Demicheli, V., Deeks, J., MacMillan, A., Sassi, F., & Pratt, M. (2000). Vaccines for preventing hepatitis B in health-care workers. *Cochrane Database of Systematic Reviews [computer file]* CD000100.

Jirillo, E., Pellegrino, N. M., Piazzolla, G., Caccavo, D., & Antonaci, S. (2000). Hepatitis C virus infection: Immune responsiveness and interferon-alpha treatment. *Current Pharmaceutical Design, 6,* 169-180.

Kim, W. R., Gross, J. B., Poterucha, J. J., Locke, G. R., & Dickson, E. R. (2001). Outcome of hospital care of liver disease associated with hepatitis C in the United States. *Hepatology, 33,* 201-206.

Koziel, M. J. (1999). Cytokines in viral hepatitis. *Seminars in Liver Disease, 19*(2), 157-169.

Lai, M. M., & Ware, C. F. (2000). Hepatitis C virus core protein: Possible roles in viral pathogenesis. *Current Topics in Microbiology & Immunology, 242,* 117-134.

Lawrence, S. P. (2000). Advances in the treatment of hepatitis C. *Advances in Internal Medicine, 45,* 65-105.

Liang, T. J., Rehermann, B., Seeff, L. B., & Hoofnagle, J. H. (2000). Pathogenesis, natural history, treatment, and prevention of hepatitis C. *Annals of Internal Medicine, 132,* 296-305.

Loayza, T. (1999). Hepatitis C. *Journal of the American Academy of Nurse Practitioners, 11*(9), 407-412.

Lok, A. S. (2000). Hepatitis B infection: Pathogenesis and management. *Journal of Hepatology, 32,* 89-97.

Lorvick, J., Kral, A. H., Seal, K., Gee, L., & Edlin, B. R. (2001). Prevalence and duration of hepatitis C among injection drug users in San Francisco, California. *American Journal of Public Health, 91,* 46-47.

Malay, S., Tizer, K., & Lutwick, L. I. (2000). Current update of pediatric hepatitis vaccine use. *Pediatric Clinics of North America, 47,* 395-406.

Manns, M. P., & Rambusch, E. G. (1999). Autoimmunity and extrahepatic manifestations in hepatitis C virus infection. *Journal of Hepatology, 31*(Suppl 1), 39-42.

McKiernan, S., & Kelleher, D. (2000). Immunogenetics of hepatitis C. *Journal of Viral Hepatitis, 7*(Suppl 1), 13-14.

Mondelli, M. U., & Silini, E. (1999). Clinical significance of hepatitis C virus genotypes. *Journal of Hepatology, 31*(Suppl 1), 65-70.

Muir, A. J. (2000). The natural history of hepatitis C viral infection. *Seminars in Gastrointestinal Disease, 11,* 54-61.

Pawlotsky, J. M. (1999). Diagnostic tests for hepatitis C. *Journal of Hepatology, 31*(Suppl 1), 71-79.

Pessoa, M. G., & Wright, T. L. (1999). Overview of HBV therapy. *Advances in Experimental Medicine & Biology, 458,* 1-10.

Pol, S., Samuel, D., Cadranel, J., Legendre, C., Bismuth, H., Brechot, C., & Kreis, H. (2000). Hepatitis and solid organ transplantation. *Transplantation Proceedings, 32,* 454-457.

Rehermann, B., & Chisari, F. V. (2000). Cell mediated immune response to the hepatitis C virus. *Current Topics in Microbiology & Immunology, 242,* 299-325.

Rosenberg, W. (1999). Mechanisms of immune escape in viral hepatitis. *Gut, 44*(5), 759-764.

Rosenberg, S. D., Goodman, L. A., Osher, F. C., Swartz, M. S., Essock, S. M., Butterfield, M. I., Constantine, N. T., Wolford, G. L., & Salyers, M. P. (2001). Prevalence of HIV, hepatitis B, and hepatitis C in people with severe mental illness. *American Journal of Public Health, 91,* 31-37.

Sarbah, S. A., & Younossi, Z. M. (2000). Hepatitis C: An update on the silent epidemic. *Journal of Clinical Gastroenterology, 30,* 125-143.

Schiff, E. R. (2000). Lamivudine for hepatitis B in clinical practice. *Journal of Medical Virology, 61,* 386-391.

Seeger, C., & Mason, W. S. (2000). Hepatitis B virus biology. *Microbiology & Molecular Biology Review (Washington, DC), 64,* 51-68.

Soriano, V., Garcia-Samaniego, J., Rodriguez-Rosado, R., Gonzalez, J., & Pedreira, J. (1999). Hepatitis C and HIV infection: Biological, clinical, and therapeutic implications. *Journal of Hepatology, 31*(Suppl 1), 119-123.

Sulkowski, M. S., Mast, E. E., Seeff, L. B., & Thomas, D. L. (2000). Hepatitis C virus infection as an opportunistic disease in persons infected with human immunodeficiency virus. *Clinical Infectious Diseases, 30*(Suppl 1), S77-S84.

Sullivan, J. S. (2001). Links between the HLA system and hepatitis C infections. *Transfusion Medicine Reviews, 15,* 77-81.

Theodore, D., & Fried, M. W. (2000). Natural history and disease manifestations of hepatitis C infection. *Current Topics in Microbiology & Immunology, 242,* 43-54.

Thio, C. L., Thomas, D. L., & Carrington, M. (2000). Chronic viral hepatitis and the human genome *Hepatology, 31,* 819-827.

Thomas, D. L. (2000). Hepatitis C epidemiology. *Current Topics in Microbiology & Immunology, 242,* 25-41.

Torresi, J., & Locarnini, S. (2000). Antiviral chemotherapy for the treatment of hepatitis B virus infections. *Gastroenterology, 118,* S83-103.

Valiante, N. M., D'Andrea, A., Crotta, S., Lechner, F., Klenerman, P., Nuti, S., Wack, A., & Abrignani, S. (2000). Life, activation and death of intrahepatic lymphocytes in chronic hepatitis C. *Immunological Reviews, 174,* 77-89.

van der Poel, C. L. (1999). Hepatitis C virus and blood transfusion: Past and present risks. *Journal of Hepatology, 31*(Suppl 1), 101-106.

Wejstal, R. (1999). Sexual transmission of hepatitis C virus. *Journal of Hepatology, 31*(Suppl 1), 92-95.

Zanetti, A. R., Tanzi, E., & Newell, M. L. (1999). Mother-to-infant transmission of hepatitis C virus. *Journal of Hepatology, 31*(Suppl 1), 96-100.

Zarski, J. P., & Leroy, V. (1999). Counselling patients with hepatitis C. *Journal of Hepatology, 31*(Suppl 1), 136-140.

Zdilar, D., Franco-Bronson, K., Buchler, N., Locala, J. A., & Younossi, Z. M. (2000). Hepatitis C, interferon alfa, and depression. *Hepatology, 31,* 1207-1211.

Zein, N. N. (2000). Clinical significance of hepatitis C virus genotypes. *Clinical Microbiology Reviews, 13,* 223-235.

Zuckerman, A. J. (2000). Effect of hepatitis B virus mutants on efficacy of vaccination. *Lancet, 355,* 1382-1384.

Case Study

Hepatitis B and C

INITIAL HISTORY
- 37-year-old IV drug abuser.
- Several days of increasing fatigue and anorexia.
- Now with fever, abdominal discomfort, and myalgias.

Question 1   What questions would you like to ask this patient about his symptoms?

ADDITIONAL HISTORY
- Discomfort is dull and located over the right upper quadrant.
- Patient denies jaundice, easy bruising, increasing abdominal birth, edema, or confusion.
- Stools are normal; no bloody or dark stools.
- No rashes; no hot, swollen joints.
- No dyspnea; no decrease in urination.

Question 2   What questions would you like to ask this patient about his lifestyle or past medical history?

MORE HISTORY

- Patient lived in Philadelphia and has used IV drugs for years; he was in a needle exchange program.
- Moved to this area 6 months ago; no needle exchange program is available here.
- Lives alone, has not had a sexual encounter since moving here.
- Doesn't know of anyone who has had hepatitis.
- No dyspnea; no decrease in urination.
- Denies history of significant illnesses or any hospitalizations except for drug rehabilitation.
- Drinks alcohol "occasionally."
- On no medications; no allergies.

PHYSICAL EXAMINATION

- Ill appearing alert male in mild distress.
- T = 38 orally; P = 90 and regular; RR = 18 and unlabored; BP = 128/82 right arm sitting.

HEENT, Neck, Skin

- PERRLA, fundi without lesions.
- Nares clear.
- No mouth lesions.
- Pharynx clear without erythema or exudate.
- No thyromegaly.
- No adenopathy.
- Nonicteric.
- No rashes; no petechia or ecchymoses.

Lungs, Cardiac

- Lungs clear to auscultation and percussion.
- Cardiac exam with regular rate and rhythm without murmurs or gallops.

Abdomen

- Nondistended.
- Bowel sounds present.
- Liver percusses to 12 cm at the midclavicular line.
- Tenderness over the right upper quadrant without guarding or rebound.
- Spleen not palpable.

Rectal

- No hemorrhoids felt.
- Prostate not enlarged or tender.
- Stool heme negative.

Extremities

- No edema.
- No joint swelling or erythema.

Neurological

- Alert and oriented.
- No sensory or motor deficits.
- DTR 2+ and symmetrical.

Question 3 What are the pertinent positives and negatives on examination?

Question 4 What is the differential diagnosis based on the history and physical examination?

Question 5 What laboratory assessment would you do now?

LABORATORY RESULTS

- WBC = 15,000 with a mild increase in lymphocytes.
- Chemistries normal including albumin.
- PT/PTT normal.
- ALT >700 and AST >300 IU/L.
- Total bilirubin upper limit of normal, alkaline phosphatase mildly elevated.
- Serum ferritin normal.
- HBsAg positive, IgM anti-HBc positive, HBeAg positive.
- IgM anti-HAV negative, HCV RNA negative by polymerase chain reaction (PCR) testing.
- HIV RNA by PCR negative, anti-HIV ELSIA negative.

Question 6 What do these laboratory results mean?

Question 7   What should you do for the patient now?

RETURN VISIT 8 MONTHS LATER

- Patient states he recovered slowly without therapy; finally feeling back to "normal" 3 months after his initial visit.
- Did not see why he needed to return for follow-up (as instructed) until now.
- Heard he might still be infectious and wants to be checked.
- Has no complaints at this time; has been sexually active for the past 2 months.

Question 8   What tests would you do now?

LABORATORY RESULTS

- AST and ALT upper limit of normal.
- Total bilirubin normal.
- HIV ELISA negative.
- HBsAg still positive.
- HBV DNA (PCR) low level.

Question 9   What does this mean and what should you tell the patient?

17

Alcoholic Hepatic Cirrhosis and Portal Hypertension

DEFINITION

- Alcoholic cirrhosis
  - A chronic disease of the liver caused by alcohol intake characterized by steatosis (fatty infiltration), inflammation, and fibrosis.
  - Destroys normal hepatic architecture and results in fibrous bands of connecting tissue separating lobules with nodules of regenerating liver cells unrelated to the normal vasculature.
- Portal hypertension
  - Increased pressure in the portal system due to increased portal blood flow and increased resistance to hepatic perfusion.
  - Results in dilation of collateral veins and is associated with liver dysfunction, splenomegaly, and fluid and electrolyte imbalances.

EPIDEMIOLOGY

- There are an estimated 15.3 million alcoholics in the United States.
- In the U.S., alcoholic cirrhosis has been surpassed recently by chronic hepatitis C infection as the most common cause of chronic liver disease.
- Cirrhosis requires a cumulative intake of approximately 600 kg of ethanol for men and 150 to 300 kg for women; however, of those who consume this much alcohol, only 40% develop cirrhosis.
- Additional cofactors for alcoholic cirrhosis include genetic polymorphisms of the enzymes responsible for ethanol metabolism, female gender (although males tend to have a more rapid progression of their cirrhosis once it is established), poor nutrition, body mass index, and viral hepatitis (hepatitis B or C).
- In the United States, portal hypertension is most commonly the result of alcoholic cirrhosis, followed by chronic viral hepatitis (especially hepatitis C).
- Patients with alcoholic cirrhosis and portal hypertension, 30% will bleed from esophageal varices with a mortality of nearly 50%; if the patient survives the first episode, there is a 60% chance of recurrence.

PATHOPHYSIOLOGY

- Alcoholic cirrhosis
  - Ethanol is metabolized by several enzymes. When alcohol intake is excessive, these enzymatic reactions result in the release of toxic oxygen radicals; in addition, alcohol intake reduces the activity of endogenous antioxidants (vitamins E and A, glutathione). Oxygen radicals cause hepatocyte lipid peroxidation and deoxyribonucleic acid (DNA) damage.

- Ethanol increases intestinal permeability leading to alcohol-associated endotoxemia and further inflammation of the liver with recruitment of polymorphonucleocytes (PMN). Hepatocyte apoptosis and degeneration with PMN infiltration is common.

- Ethanol and hepatic injury stimulates production of inflammatory cytokines including IL-1, IL-6, IL-8, and tumor necrosing factor (TNF) released primarily from the hepatic macrophages (Kupffer cells); these result in further hepatocyte injury.

- One of the major metabolites of ethanol is acetaldehyde, which affects protein synthesis and can stimulate hepatic fibrosis.

- Ethanol also directly affects mitochondria with intrahepatocyte accumulation of microvesicular fat described as alcoholic foamy steatosis. This process is reversible with discontinuation of alcohol intake and does not necessarily lead to cirrhosis.

- Fibrosis results from activation of the hepatic stellate cells, which proliferate and produce large amounts of collagen.

- The pathologic characteristics of established alcoholic cirrhosis include steatosis, ballooning degeneration of hepatocytes, Mallory bodies (crescent shaped bunches of intracellular filaments), neutrophilic inflammation, and pericellular fibrosis.

- Hepatocyte injury results in loss of the normal hepatic functions resulting in the risk for many complications including encephalopathy, jaundice, ascites, coagulopathy, pancytopenia, hypoalbuminemia (with resultant edema), and hyperestrinism (decreased estrogen metabolism leads to increased circulating estrogen levels).

- Portal Hypertension
  - Increased portal pressure results from resistance to portal flow into the liver, and from increased portal blood flow.
  - Increased resistance:
    1) Alcoholic cirrhosis with inflammation causes hepatocyte swelling and collagen deposition with obstruction of the hepatic sinusoids.
    2) Myofibroblasts (found in cirrhotic livers) have some contractile function; their constriction further obstructs portal inflow to the sinusoids (and provides some response to vasodilator therapy).
    3) Intrahepatic vasoactive mediators, such as endothelin and nitric oxide, cause further changes in hepatic resistance to portal blood flow.
  - Increased portal blood flow:
    1) A complex interaction of neurohumoral factors (sympathetic nervous system, glucagon, serotonin, adenosine, angiotensin, atrial natriuretic factor, adenosine, and nitric oxide).
    2) Results in splanchnic vasodilation, increased cardiac output, decreased systemic peripheral resistance, and sodium retention.
  - The result of all of these interactions is increased pressure in the portal system, with a systemic hyperdynamic state (increased cardiac output and tachycardia but decreased systemic arterial pressure).
  - Once portal pressure exceeds a level of 10 mmHg to 12 mmHg above the pressure in the hepatic vein, portal collaterals begin shunting portal blood.
    1) Portal hypertension persists due to further increases in portal flow and increases in collateral resistance modulated by serotonin and nitric oxide.
    2) The major portal collaterals include those around the esophagus, stomach, rectum, and umbilicus; patients that have undergone previous abdominal surgery may also have collaterals around the small and large bowel.

3) Dilation of these collaterals (esophageal and gastric varices, caput medusa, and hemorrhoids) results in considerable risk for serious hemorrhage.

– Increased portal pressure, plus the likely associated increases in aldosterone and decreases in serum albumin, result in ascites and edema.

– Ascites and relative immune compromise (decreased T cell activity) from cirrhosis and portal hypertension creates a risk for spontaneous bacterial peritonitis.

PATIENT PRESENTATION

History

Alcohol abuse (40 to 80 g of ethanol a day, or about 2 to 4 drinks); female gender; poor diet; history of hepatitis.

Symptoms

Confusion; jaundice; easy bruising; increasing abdominal girth; decreased exercise tolerance; hematemesis; hematochezia; melena; anorexia; weight loss; edema.

Examination

Hepatomegaly; hard nodular surface to the liver; splenomegaly; jaundice; ascites; encephalopathy; asterixis; fever; edema; ecchymoses; gynecomastia; palmar erythema; testicular atrophy; spider nevi; caput medusae; hemorrhoids; heme-positive stools.

DIFFERENTIAL DIAGNOSIS

- Viral or toxic hepatitis
- Nonalcoholic steatohepatitis (NASH)
    - Parenteral nutrition
    - Obesity
    - Diabetes
    - Diethylstilbestrol
    - Glucocorticoids
    - Amiodarone
- Hemochromatosis
- Primary biliary fibrosis
- Hepatic carcinoma
- Portal vein thrombosis
- Polycystic liver

KEYS TO ASSESSMENT

- Laboratory findings include macrocytic anemia, leukocytosis, modest elevations in aspartate aminotransferase (AST) and alanine aminotransferase (ALT) with an AST/ALT ratio >2, increased bilirubin, elevated prothrombin time (PT) and partial thromboplastin time (PTT), and decreased albumin.

- Other markers of alcoholic cirrhosis include laminin, hyaluronan, type III procollagen, type IV collagen, tissue inhibitor of metalloproteinase, and prolyl hydroxylase (these are not used clinically at this time).

- Patients at high risk for early mortality: 4.6X[PT(seconds) - control] + bilirubin (mg/dL) >32 indicates a 1-month mortality of 50%.

- Liver biopsy is indicated for clinical evidence of cirrhosis with a minimal alcohol intake.

- Abdominal computed tomography (CT) should be considered for evaluation of possible hepatic carcinoma.

- Ultrasound and pulsed doppler are used to evaluate biliary tree and portal vein blood flow if suspected portal hypertension.

- If portal hypertension is present, endoscopy is indicated to evaluate for varices.

- Magnetic resonance angiography can be used to further evaluate the portal vein if surgery is contemplated.

- Direct portal vein pressure measurements of the portal circulation are rarely needed, but can be done in selected cases prior to surgical intervention.

KEYS TO MANAGEMENT

Management of cirrhosis

- Abstinence is the most important intervention and can improve survival in most patients; it does not guarantee improvement, but must be present for improvement to occur.

- Malnutrition is correlated with poor prognosis in alcoholic cirrhosis, and although nutritional supplementation has not been clearly shown to improve outcomes, it is reasonable to provide some nutritional support to malnourished and anorexic patients. Protein supplements are important to raise albumin levels, but must be given with caution in patients with a history of encephalopathy.

- Bedrest with *careful* administration of diuretics can improve edema and ascites; however, high doses of diuretics can result in intravascular hypovolemia, hypotension, and renal toxicity.

- Pharmacologic intervention includes propylthiouracil, corticosteroids, colchicine, and antioxidants, which reduce hepatic inflammation and fibrosis. All of these have shown some benefit in alcoholic cirrhosis, but results are not dramatic and side effects are common.

- Liver transplant for alcoholic cirrhosis requires evaluation for strict preoperative criteria including 6 months confirmed abstinence; survival rates after transplant are equivalent for nonalcoholic liver disease and recidivism is less than 10%.

- Hepatorenal syndrome develops in a significant number of patients with cirrhosis and has a poor prognosis. Although liver transplantation is the only proven therapy, avoidance of nephrotoxic drugs and hypovolemia is indicated.

- Hepatic encephalopathy ranges from mild confusion to deep coma and is often precipitated by associated insults such as gastrointestinal bleeding or surgery. Treatment includes lactulose and neomycin; ornithine aspartate and zinc are promising in early trials.

Management of portal hypertension and its complications

- Propranolol has been used in portal hypertension with improvement in portal pressures and decreased risk of variceal bleeding; nitrates can be tried in patients that are intolerant of beta blockade.

- Endoscopic prophylactic ligation of esophageal varices has been recently shown to be superior to propanolol in preventing variceal bleeding in selected patients.

- Management of acute variceal hemorrhage requires emergent endoscopy and sclerotherapy and/or administration of octreotide or vasopressin plus nitroglycerin.

- Balloon tamponade can be used to control bleeding until the patient can undergo one of several surgical interventions, including esophageal devascularization or shunt operations such as a splenorenal shunt.

- A transjugular intrahepatic portosystemic shunt (TIPS) can be placed percutaneously, but this procedure is associated with significant risk of encephalopathy, accelerated liver failure, and restenosis and it has a 15% mortality at 1 month; it should be used only to manage acute and recurrent hemorrhage, not as a prophylactic procedure.

- Ascites can be managed with bedrest (decreases activity of the renin-angiotensin-aldosterone system) with salt and fluid restriction. Spironolactone can be administered carefully to further induce diuresis (furosemide can also be added in patients who have low urinary sodium concentrations). Therapeutic paracentesis is reserved for patients with tense ascites.

- Spontaneous bacterial peritonitis occurs in 10-30% of hospitalized patients with cirrhosis and ascites. Rapid paracentesis for diagnosis and prompt administration of empiric antibiotics is crucial.

- Gastric ulceration is common in portal hypertension, reducing portal pressures with propanolol in addition to usual ulcer therapy is most effective.

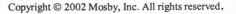

Pathophysiology → Clinical Link

What is going on in the disease process that influences how the patient presents and how he or she should be managed?

What should you do now that you understand the underlying pathophysiology?

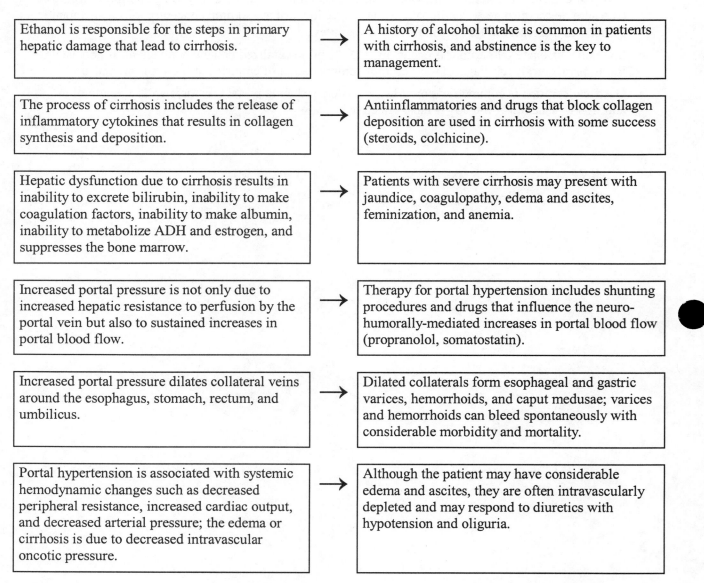

Pathophysiology	Clinical Link
Ethanol is responsible for the steps in primary hepatic damage that lead to cirrhosis.	A history of alcohol intake is common in patients with cirrhosis, and abstinence is the key to management.
The process of cirrhosis includes the release of inflammatory cytokines that results in collagen synthesis and deposition.	Antiinflammatories and drugs that block collagen deposition are used in cirrhosis with some success (steroids, colchicine).
Hepatic dysfunction due to cirrhosis results in inability to excrete bilirubin, inability to make coagulation factors, inability to make albumin, inability to metabolize ADH and estrogen, and suppresses the bone marrow.	Patients with severe cirrhosis may present with jaundice, coagulopathy, edema and ascites, feminization, and anemia.
Increased portal pressure is not only due to increased hepatic resistance to perfusion by the portal vein but also to sustained increases in portal blood flow.	Therapy for portal hypertension includes shunting procedures and drugs that influence the neuro-humorally-mediated increases in portal blood flow (propranolol, somatostatin).
Increased portal pressure dilates collateral veins around the esophagus, stomach, rectum, and umbilicus.	Dilated collaterals form esophageal and gastric varices, hemorrhoids, and caput medusae; varices and hemorrhoids can bleed spontaneously with considerable morbidity and mortality.
Portal hypertension is associated with systemic hemodynamic changes such as decreased peripheral resistance, increased cardiac output, and decreased arterial pressure; the edema or cirrhosis is due to decreased intravascular oncotic pressure.	Although the patient may have considerable edema and ascites, they are often intravascularly depleted and may respond to diuretics with hypotension and oliguria.

Suggested Reading

Binmoeller, K. F., & Borsatto, R. (2000). Variceal bleeding and portal hypertension. *Endoscopy, 32,* 189-199.

Bolondi, L., Sofia, S., Siringo, S., Gaiani, S., Casali, A., Zironi, G., Piscaglia, F., Gramantieri, L., Zanetti, M., & Sherman, M. (2001). Surveillance programme of cirrhotic patients for early diagnosis and treatment of hepatocellular carcinoma: A cost effectiveness analysis. *Gut, 48,* 251-259.

Bonis, P. A., Friedman, S. L., & Kaplan, M. M. (2001). Is liver fibrosis reversible? *New England Journal of Medicine, 344,* 452-454.

Bosch, J., & Garcia-Pagan, J. C. (2000). Complications of cirrhosis. I. Portal hypertension. *Journal of Hepatology, 32,* 141-156.

Chalasani, N., Clark, W. S., Martin, L. G., Kamean, J., Khan, M. A., Patel, N. H., & Boyer, T. D. (2000). Determinants of mortality in patients with advanced cirrhosis after transjugular intrahepatic portosystemic shunting. *Gastroenterology, 118,* 138-144.

Deschenes, M., & Barkun, A. N. (2000). Comparison of endoscopic ligation and propranolol for the primary prevention of variceal bleeding. *Gastrointestinal Endoscopy, 51,* 630-633.

Escorsell, A., Bordas, J. M., Castaneda, B., Llach, J., Garcia-Pagan, J. C., Rodes, J., & Bosch, J. (2000). Predictive value of the variceal pressure response to continued pharmacological therapy in patients with cirrhosis and portal hypertension. *Hepatology, 31,* 1061-1067.

Flisiak, R., Pytel-Krolczuk, B., & Prokopowicz, D. (2000). Circulating transforming growth factor beta(1) as an indicator of hepatic function impairment in liver cirrhosis. *Cytokine, 12,* 677-681.

Fujimoto, M., Uemura, M., Nakatani, Y., Tsujita, S., Hoppo, K., Tamagawa, T., Kitano, H., Kikukawa, M., Ann, T., Ishii, Y., Kojima, H., Sakurai, S., Tanaka, R., Namisaki, T., Noguchi, R., Higashino, T., Kikuchi, E., Nishimura, K., Takaya, A., & Fukui, H. (2000). Plasma endotoxin and serum cytokine levels in patients with alcoholic hepatitis: Relation to severity of liver disturbance. *Alcoholism: Clinical & Experimental Research, 24,* 48S-54S.

Ganne-Carrie, N., Christidis, C., Chastang, C., Ziol, M., Chapel, F., Imbert-Bismut, F., Trinchet, J. C., Guettier, C., & Beaugrand, M. (2000). Liver iron is predictive of death in alcoholic cirrhosis: A multivariate study of 229 consecutive patients with alcoholic and/or hepatitis C virus cirrhosis: A prospective follow up study. *Gut, 46,* 277-282.

Gotzsche, P. C. (2000). Somatostatin or octreotide for acute bleeding oesophageal varices. *Cochrane Database of Systematic Reviews [computer file],* CD000193.

Gough, S. C. (2000). Think cytokines before you drink. *Gut, 46,* 448-449.

Gournay, J., Masliah, C., Martin, T., Perrin, D., & Galmiche, J. P. (2000). Isosorbide mononitrate and propranolol compared with propranolol alone for the prevention of variceal rebleeding. *Hepatology, 31,* 1239-1245.

Green, J. A., Amaro, R., & Barkin, J. S. (2000). Therapeutic face-off: Band ligation versus beta blockage for variceal bleeding. *American Journal of Gastroenterology, 95,* 1358-1359.

Grove, J., Daly, A. K., Bassendine, M. F., Gilvarry, E., & Day, C. P. (2000). Interleukin 10 promoter region polymorphisms and susceptibility to advanced alcoholic liver disease. *Gut, 46,* 540-545.

Hanazaki, K., Kajikawa, S., Shimozawa, N., Shimada, K., Hiraguri, M., Koide, N., Adachi, W., & Amano, J. (2001). Hepatic resection for hepatocellular carcinoma in the elderly. *Journal of the American College of Surgeons, 192,* 38-46.

Hanck, C., Glatzel, M., Singer, M. V., & Rossol, S. (2000). Gene expression of TNF-receptors in peripheral blood mononuclear cells of patients with alcoholic cirrhosis. *Journal of Hepatology, 32,* 51-57.

Helton, W. S., Maves, R., Wicks, K., & Johansen, K. (2001). Transjugular intrahepatic portasystemic shunt vs surgical shunt in good-risk cirrhotic patients: A case-control comparison. *Archives of Surgery, 136,* 17-20.

Hou, M. C., Lin, H. C., Lee, F. Y., Chang, F. Y., & Lee, S. D. (2000). Recurrence of esophageal varices following endoscopic treatment and its impact on rebleeding: Comparison of sclerotherapy and ligation. *Journal of Hepatology, 32,* 202-208.

Jalan, R., Lui, H. F., Redhead, D. N., & Hayes, P. C. (2000). TIPSS 10 years on. *Gut, 46,* 578-581.

Junquera, F., Lopez-Talavera, J. C., Mearin, F., Saperas, E., Videla, S., Armengol, J. R., Esteban, R., & Malagelada, J. R. (2000). Somatostatin plus isosorbide 5-mononitrate versus somatostatin in the control of acute gastro-oesophageal variceal bleeding: A double blind, randomised, placebo controlled clinical trial. *Gut, 46,* 127-132.

Kerr, W. C., Fillmore, K. M., & Marvy, P. (2000). Beverage-specific alcohol consumption and cirrhosis mortality in a group of English-speaking beer-drinking countries [see comments]. *Addiction, 95,* 339-346.

Khaitiyar, J. S., Luthra, S. K., Prasad, N., Ratnakar, N., & Daruwala, D. K. (2000). Transjugular intrahepatic portosystemic shunt versus distal splenorenal shunt. *Hepato-Gastroenterology, 47,* 492-497.

Kitano, S., & Dolgor, B. (2000). Does portal hypertension contribute to the pathogenesis of gastric ulcer associated with liver cirrhosis? *Journal of Gastroenterology, 35*(2), 79-86.

Kramer, L., Tribl, B., Gendo, A., Zauner, C., Schneider, B., Ferenci, P., & Madl, C. (2000). Partial pressure of ammonia versus ammonia in hepatic encephalopathy. *Hepatology, 31,* 30-34.

Kravetz, D., Bildozola, M., Argonz, J., Romero, G., Korula, J., Munoz, A., Suarez, A., & Terg, R. (2000). Patients with ascites have higher variceal pressure and wall tension than patients without ascites. *American Journal of Gastroenterology, 95,* 1770-1775.

Kuschner, W. G. (2000). Massive esophageal variceal hemorrhage triggered by complicated endotracheal intubation. *Journal of Emergency Medicine, 18,* 317-322.

Lieber, C. S. (2000). Alcohol and the liver: Metabolism of alcohol and its role in hepatic and extrahepatic diseases. *Mount Sinai Journal of Medicine, 67,* 84-94.

Ludwig, D., Schadel, S., Bruning, A., Schiefer, B., & Stange, E. F. (2000). 48-hour hemodynamic effects of octreotide on postprandial splanchnic hyperemia in patients with liver cirrhosis and portal hypertension: Double-blind, placebo-controlled study. *Digestive Diseases & Sciences, 45,* 1019-1027.

Makino, N., Suematsu, M., Sugiura, Y., Morikawa, H., Shiomi, S., Goda, N., Sano, T., Nimura, Y., Sugimachi, K., & Ishimura, Y. (2001). Altered expression of heme oxygenase-1 in the livers of patients with portal hypertensive diseases. *Hepatology, 33,* 32-42.

Martin, P. Y., Gines, P., & Schrier, R. W. (1998). Nitric oxide as a mediator of hemodynamic abnormalities and sodium and water retention in cirrhosis. *New England Journal of Medicine, 339*(8), 533-541.

McCullough, A. J., & Bugianesi, E. (1997). Protein-calorie malnutrition and the etiology of cirrhosis. *American Journal of Gastroenterology, 92*(5), 734-738.

Menon, K. V., & Kamath, P. S. (2000). Managing the complications of cirrhosis. *Mayo Clinic Proceedings, 75,* 501-509.

Merkel, C., Marin, R., Sacerdoti, D., Donada, C., Cavallarin, G., Torboli, P., Amodio, P., Sebastianelli, G., Bolognesi, M., Felder, M., Mazzaro, C., & Gatta, A. (2000). Long-term results of a clinical trial of nadolol with or without isosorbide mononitrate for primary prophylaxis of variceal bleeding in cirrhosis. *Hepatology, 31,* 324-329.

Moloney, M., & Wilkinson, M. (2000). Early administration of somatostatin and efficacy of sclerotherapy in acute oesophageal variceal bleeds: The European Acute Bleeding Oesophageal Variceal Episodes (ABOVE) randomised trial. *Gastrointestinal Endoscopy, 51,* 372-374.

Nikolic, J. A., Todorovic, V., Bozic, M., Tosic, L., Bulajic, M., Alempijevic, T., Nedic, O., & Masnikosa, R. (2000). Serum insulin-like growth factor (IGF)-II is more closely associated with liver dysfunction than is IGF-I in patients with cirrhosis. *Clinica Chimica Acta, 294,* 169-177.

Okazaki, I., Watanabe, T., Hozawa, S., Arai, M., & Maruyama, K. (2000). Molecular mechanism of the reversibility of hepatic fibrosis: With special reference to the role of matrix metalloproteinases. *Journal of Gastroenterology & Hepatology, 15*(Suppl), D26-D32.

Ong, J. P., Sands, M., & Younossi, Z. M. (2000). Transjugular intrahepatic portosystemic shunts (TIPS): A decade later. *Journal of Clinical Gastroenterology, 30*(1), 14-28.

Rockey, D. (1997). The cellular pathogenesis of portal hypertension: Stellate cell contractility, endothelin, and nitric oxide [review, 43 refs]. *Hepatology, 25*(1), 2-5.

Rockey, D. C. (2000). Vasoactive agents in intrahepatic portal hypertension and fibrogenesis: Implications for therapy. *Gastroenterology, 118*(6), 1261-1265.

Romero, G., Kravetz, D., Argonz, J., Bildozola, M., Suarez, A., & Terg, R. (2000). Terlipressin is more effective in decreasing variceal pressure than portal pressure in cirrhotic patients. *Journal of Hepatology, 32,* 419-425.

Rosa, H., Silverio, A. O., Perini, R. F., & Arruda, C. B. (2000). Bacterial infection in cirrhotic patients and its relationship with alcohol. *American Journal of Gastroenterology, 95,* 1290-1293.

Santolaria, F., Perez-Manzano, J. L., Milena, A., Gonzalez-Reimers, E., Gomez-Rodriguez, M. A., Martinez-Riera, A., Aleman-Valls, M. R., & Vega-Prieto, M. J. (2000). Nutritional assessment in alcoholic patients. Its relationship with alcoholic intake, feeding habits, organic complications and social problems. *Drug & Alcohol Dependence, 59,* 295-304.

Sarin, S. K., Lamba, G. S., Kumar, M., Misra, A., & Murthy, N. S. (1999). Comparison of endoscopic ligation and propranolol for the primary prevention of variceal bleeding. *New England Journal of Medicine, 340*(13), 988-993.

Savolainen, V. T., Pajarinen, J., Perola, M., Penttila, A., & Karhunen, P. J. (1997). Polymorphism in the cytochrome P450 2E1 gene and the risk of alcoholic liver disease. *Journal of Hepatology, 26*(1), 55-61.

Schirren, C. A., Jung, M. C., Zachoval, R., Diepolder, H., Hoffmann, R., Riethmuller, G., & Pape, G. R. (1997). Analysis of T cell activation pathways in patients with liver cirrhosis, impaired delayed hypersensitivity and other T cell-dependent functions. *Clinical and Experimental Immunology, 108*(1), 144-150.

Sekiyama, T., Komeichi, H., Nagano, T., Ohsuga, M., Terada, H., Katsuta, Y., Satomura, K., & Aramaki, T. (1997). Effects of the alpha-/beta-blocking agent carvedilol on hepatic and systemic hemodynamics in patients with cirrhosis and portal hypertension. *Arzneimittel-Forschung, 47*(4), 353-355.

Spahr, L., Villeneuve, J. P., Tran, H. K., & Pomier-Layrargues, G. (2001). Furosemide-induced natriuresis as a test to identify cirrhotic patients with refractory ascites. *Hepatology, 33,* 28-31.

Takahashi, T., So-Wan, T., Kamimura, T., & Asakura, H. (2000). Infiltrating polymorphonuclear leukocytes and apoptotic bodies derived from hepatocytes but not from ballooning hepatocytes containing Mallory bodies show nuclear DNA fragmentation in alcoholic hepatitis. *Alcoholism: Clinical & Experimental Research, 24,* 68S-73S.

Uemura, M., Lehmann, W. D., Schneider, W., Seitz, H. K., Benner, A., Keppler-Hafkemeyer, A., Hafkemeyer, P., Kojima, H., Fujimoto, M., Tsujii, T., Fukui, H., & Keppler, D. (2000). Enhanced urinary excretion of cysteinyl leukotrienes in patients with acute alcohol intoxication. *Gastroenterology, 118,* 1140-1148.

Ueno, T., Hashimoto, O., Kimura, R., Torimura, T., waguchi, T., Nakamura, T., Sakata, R., Koga, H., & Sata, M. (2001). Relation of type II transforming growth factor-beta receptor to hepatic fibrosis and hepatocellular carcinoma. *International Journal of Oncology, 18,* 49-55.

Vlachogiannakos, J., Goulis, J., Patch, D., & Burroughs, A. K. (2000). Review article: Primary prophylaxis for portal hypertensive bleeding in cirrhosis. *Alimentary Pharmacology & Therapeutics, 14*(7), 851-860.

Zeigler, F. (2000). Managing patients with alcoholic cirrhosis. *Dimensions of Critical Care Nursing, 19,* 23-30.

Zoli, M., Merkel, C., Magalotti, D., Gueli, C., Grimaldi, M., Gatta, A., & Bernardi, M. (2000). Natural history of cirrhotic patients with small esophageal varices: A prospective study. *American Journal of Gastroenterology, 95,* 503-508.

Zuberi, B. F., & Baloch, Q. (2000). Comparison of endoscopic variceal sclerotherapy alone and in combination with octreotide in controlling acute variceal hemorrhage and early rebleeding in patients with low-risk cirrhosis. *American Journal of Gastroenterology, 95,* 768-771.

Case Study*

Alcoholic Cirrhosis and Portal Hypertension

INITIAL HISTORY

- 59-year-old male.
- Brought into the emergency department by wife who noticed increased confusion over last 3 days.
- Dark stools all week.
- Increased abdominal girth and tenderness.

Question 1   What is your differential diagnosis based on initial information?

Question 2   What additional history would you obtain?

ADDITIONAL HISTORY (from wife)

- No recent infections, fever, illnesses, falls.
- Drinks 8 to 12 beers/day and more on weekends (±25 years); had last beer 2 days ago.
- Smoking: 20 pack/year history.
- Has had a "beer belly" for about 10 years, getting bigger over the last month (tender for 3 to 4 days).
- Confusion over the last 3 to 4 days.
- Occasional use of Advil or Tylenol for headache; no known use of prescription or illicit drugs.
- No history to suggest prior cardiac or gallbladder disease; no previous history of hepatitis.

_____

*Suzanne M. Burns contributed this case study.

Question 3 Now what do you think?

PHYSICAL EXAMINATION

- Confused; knows his name and his wife's name; restless in bed, lying on side.
- T = 36.7 orally; P = 120 beats/minute and regular; RR = 24 breaths/minute, slightly labored; BP = 138/80 lying, 120/75 sitting.

HEENT, Skin, Neck

- Slight scleral icterus.
- No bruises, masses, deformities on head.
- Nystagmus with lateral gaze.
- Pupils 3 mm, reactive to light.
- Funduscopy without lesions.
- Ears: cerumen in left ear canal.
- Spider angiomas over upper chest and abdomen.
- Palmar erythema.
- Slightly diaphoretic.
- Mild jaundice.
- Several bruises on lower extremities.
- Supple.
- No adenopathy, thyromegaly, bruits.

Lungs, Chest

- Clear to auscultation.
- Poor diaphragmatic excursions (rapid, shallow breathing pattern).
- Gynecomastia.

Cardiac

- Tachycardia
- Grade II systolic ejection murmur.
- No gallops, rubs, or clicks.

Abdomen

- Large, distended.
- Hyperactive bowel sounds (has just passed large, dark maroon stool, and vomited about 100 cc blood).
- Diffusely tender to palpation.
- No aortic, iliac, renal bruits.
- Positive fluid wave, shifting dullness, difficult to ascertain liver border.
- Splenomegaly.

Extremities
- Good capillary refill.
- Trace to +1 edema of feet.

Neurological
- Oriented to person only; confused, muttering.
- Cranial nerves: II-XII grossly intact (exception noted cranial nerve VI).
- Sensory: extremities grossly intact to pinprick and light touch.
- Reflexes: hyperreflexic.
- Asterixis.

Rectal
- Hemorrhoids (no visible bleeding).
- Passing dark maroon stool.

Question 4 What are the pertinent positives and significant negatives on the exam and what do they suggest?

Question 5 What diagnostic studies and/or therapeutic interventions do you think are indicated now?

LABORATORY
- SaO_2 = 89%; ABGs: pH = 7.43, $PaCO_2$ = 33 mmHg, PaO_2 = 58 mmHg on room air.
- CBC: HGB/HCT = 9/27, WBC = 12,000, PLTs = 75,000.
- Electrolytes = Na, K, MG, and phosphate decreased.
- Bilirubin (direct) slightly increased.
- AST and ALT both elevated (ratio > 2/1); alkaline phosphatase = normal.
- PT = 20, PTT = 32 (both elevated).
- Serum ammonia = elevated.
- Albumin = low; cholesterol = low.
- Chest x-ray = normal.
- ECG = sinus tachycardia.

Question 6   Which labs are most important for you to act on now and what will you do?

Question 7   Do other labs suggest the etiology of Mr. Z's internal bleeding?

STATUS UPON ICU TRANSFER

- Mr. Z is transferred to ICU.
- Continues to pass maroon colored stools.
- Started on octreotide.
- Mr. Z is still confused and is intubated prior to sclerotherapy for airway protection.
- GI consult service performs endoscopy, which demonstrates both esophageal and gastric varices; esophageal varices (which appear to be the site of active bleeding) are sclerosed.

Question 8   Why is octreotide used?

Question 9   Following sclerotherapy, Mr. Z is more stable (appears to have stopped bleeding). Despite being confused, he is able to protect his airway and is extubated. What other management do you want to consider now?

HOSPITAL COURSE

- Mr. Z does well and is transferred from the ICU to a medical floor within 48 hours of admission.
- PT is corrected; bleeding has stopped.
- Mental status has improved.
- Has not experienced delirium tremens.
- Spontaneous bacterial peritonitis is ruled out.

Question 10 Now what should the plan be?

DAY 4 ON MEDICAL FLOOR/HOSPITALIZATION DAY 6

- Mr. Z is ready to be discharged in the care of his wife.
- Tired but alert and oriented.
- No further bleeding.

Question 11 What instructions and medications should go home with Mr. Z and his wife?

18

Headache

DEFINITION

- Primary headaches refer to those that fit the diagnostic criteria for one of three major categories of headache: migraine, tension-type, or cluster headache.
- Each of these major categories has subtypes as described by the 1988 International Headache Society classification system. Some of the major subtypes of headache are:
  - Migraine
    1) Migraine without aura.
    2) Migraine with aura.
    3) Ophthalmoplegic migraine.
    4) Retinal migraine.
    5) Childhood periodic syndromes that may be precursors to or associated with migraine.
    6) Complications of migraine.
    7) Migrainous disorder not fulfilling above criteria.
  - Tension-type headache
    1) Episodic tension-type headache associated with disorder of pericranial muscles.
    2) Episodic tension-type headache unassociated with disorder of pericranial muscles.
    3) Chronic tension-type headache associated with disorder of pericranial muscles.
    4) Chronic tension-type headache unassociated with disorder of pericranial muscles.
    5) Headache of the tension-type not fulfilling above criteria.
  - Cluster headache
    1) Episodic cluster headache.
    2) Chronic cluster headache.
    3) Chronic paroxysmal hemicrania.
    4) Cluster headache-like disorder not fulfilling the above criteria.
- Secondary headaches refer to those that are associated with an identified underlying cause such as drug-induced, cerebrovascular disease, sinusitis, ophthalmologic or otic disease, trauma and postconcussion syndrome, trigeminal neuralgia and many others.

EPIDEMIOLOGY

- 90% to 95% of the people in the United States have unprovoked headaches annually.
- It is the number one reason for seeking health care in this country.
- 35% to 40% of patients seeking treatment have chronic daily headache (CDH), meaning headache for at least 4 hours per day for at least 25 days per month.

- Many patients with CDH have both migrainous and tension-type headaches.
- Migraine:
  - Prevalence is 18% for females, and 6% for males; prevalence is increasing.
  - Onset is often in the teens; peak prevalence is in ages 35 to 45.
  - Over 70% of migraine patients have a positive family history, with a possible association with mitochondrial deoxyribonucleic acid (DNA) and chromosome 19.
- Tension-type:
  - It is the most common type of primary headache; overall prevalence of episodic headache is 38.3%, including 47% of women aged 30 to 39; incidence increases with educational level.
  - Overall prevalence of CHD is 2.2%; most CDH patients have a preceding history of episodic tension-type headaches.
- Cluster:
  - It is much less common than migraine or tension-type; incidence is <1%.
  - The male to female ratio is 5:1.
  - The incidence is highest in the late 20s or early 30s.

PATHOPHYSIOLOGY

- Migraine (there are many theories of pathogenesis; a few consistent features are being identified)
  - Triggers include fasting, alcohol intake, oral contraceptives, menstruation, hormone replacement, stress, caffeine withdrawal, sleep disturbance, bright lights, scents, smoke, certain foods (chocolate, aged cheese, nitrites, aspartame, citrus), and trauma.
  - Many patients experience symptoms of mood change, hunger, or drowsiness during the 24 hours prior to headache, and the onset of headache is often associated with circadian rhythms, thus suggesting a central site for initiation of migraine near the hypothalamus.
  - Preceding the headache, there is a reduction in blood flow (oligemia) and resultant cortical depression that spreads across the hemicortex at a rate of 2 mm to 3 mm per minute. This may or may not be associated with the symptoms of an aura including scintillating scotoma, paraesthesias, blurred vision, or other focal neurologic signs.
  - As the headache progresses, trigeminal ganglion stimulation appears to be an important step in migraine pathogenesis causing intracerebral and extracerebral vasodilation, thus resulting in what has been called trigeminovascular pain.
  - Neurons that arise in the trigeminal ganglion produce a variety of neurohumoral cytokines (e.g., substance P and calcitonin gene-related peptide [CGRP]) that cause perivascular neurogenic inflammation, mast cell degranulation, and changes in serotonin that further promote migraine progression.
  - Decreased serotonin appears to be important in migraine pathogenesis. Serotonin agonists cause vasoconstriction, reduce neurogenic inflammation, and reduce pain transmission through the trigeminal system.
  - Other proposed mechanisms include dopamine receptor hypersensitivity and parasympathetic hypofunction.
  - In premenopausal women, cyclic estrogen withdrawal contributes to changes in serotonin and other neurotransmitters and causes a rise in serum prostaglandins that promote migraine pathogenesis (menstrual migraine).

- Tension-type
  - There has been a long-standing appreciation for the presence of pericranial muscle spasm and headache in many patients, but it is clear that there are many patients who fit the criteria for tension-type headache that do not have these muscle spasms.
  - In those patients with pericranial muscle spasms, there is increased electromyographic activity in pericranial muscles, decreased blood flow and muscle ischemia especially of the temporalis muscle, and tenderness upon palpation of the head and neck muscles.
  - It has been postulated that there are several possible central mechanisms for tension-type headaches that are not associated with pericranial muscle spasms, but these are poorly understood. Recent evidence shows that serotonin levels are reduced in patients with chronic tension-type headache. Increased CNS nitric oxide has also been implicated.
- Cluster
  - In susceptible individuals, alterations in seasonal photoperiod may contribute to "cluster periods" lasting 2 to 4 months and affecting hypothalamic function.
  - Hypothalamic dysfunction leads to changes in chemoreceptor responses to hypoxemia, impaired autoregulation, and neuroendocrine dysfunction.
  - With "triggering" (hypoxemia, alcohol, histamine, vasodilators), unilateral extra and intracranial vasodilation occurs with increased intracerebral blood flow resulting in compression of the sympathetic plexus and release of serotonin and histamine.
  - Patients may exhibit nasal stuffiness, lacrimation, rhinorrhea, miosis, ptosis, sweating, and eyelid edema.

PATIENT PRESENTATION

- Criteria for diagnosis of each type of primary headache are listed in Box 18-1.

Box 18-1 Criteria for Diagnosis of Each Type of Primary Headache

DIAGNOSTIC CRITERIA FOR MIGRAINE WITHOUT AND WITH AURA

Migraine without Aura
A. At least five attacks fulfilling B-D
B. Headache attacks lasting 4 to 72 hours (untreated or unsuccessfully treated)
C. Headache has at least two of the following characteristics
   1. Unilateral location
   2. Pulsating quality
   3. Moderate or severe intensity (inhibits or prohibits daily activities)
   4. Aggravation by walking stairs or similar routine physical activity
D. During headache, at least one of the following are present
   1. Nausea and/or vomiting
   2. Photophobia and phonophobia.
E. At least one of the following are present
   1. History and physical and neurologic examinations do not suggest headaches secondary to organic or systemic metabolic disease
   2. History and/or physical and/or neurologic examinations do suggest such disorder, but it is ruled out by appropriate investigations
   3. Such disorder is present, but migraine attacks do not occur for the first time in close temporal relation to the disorder

Migraine with Aura
A. At least two attacks fulfilling B
B. At least three of the following four characteristics are present
   1. One or more fully reversible aura symptoms indicating focal cerebral cortical and/or brain stem dysfunction
   2. At least one aura symptom develops gradually over more than 4 minutes or two or more symptoms occur in succession

Continued.

Box 18-1 continued

    3. No aura symptom lasts more than 60 minutes; if more than one aura symptom is present, accepted duration is proportionally increased

    4. Headache follows aura with a free interval of less than 60 minutes (it may also begin before or simultaneously with the aura)

  C. At least one of the following are present

    1. History and/or physical and/or neurologic examinations do not suggest headaches secondary to organic or systemic metabolic disease

    2. History and physical and/or neurologic examinations do suggest such disorder but it is ruled out by appropriate investigations

CRITERIA FOR VARIOUS FORMS OF TENSION-TYPE HEADACHE

Tension-type Headache

  A. At least two of the following pain characteristics are present

    1. Pressing/tightening (nonpulsing quality)

    2. Mild or moderate intensity (may inhibit but does not prohibit activities)

    3. Bilateral location

    4. No aggravation by walking stairs or similar routine physical activity

  B. Both of the following occur

    1. No nausea or vomiting (anorexia may occur); and

    2. Photophobia and phonophobia are absent; or one but not the other is present

  C. At least one of the following occur

    1. History and physical and neurological examinations do not suggest headaches secondary to organic or systemic metabolic disease.

    2. History and/or physical and/or neurological examinations do suggest such disorders, but it is ruled out by appropriate investigations

    3. Such disorder is present, but tension-type headache does not occur for the first time in close temporal relation to the disorder

Episodic Tension-type Headache

  A. Diagnostic criteria includes

    1. At least 10 previous headache episodes; number of days with such headache is 180 per year ($<$15 per month)

    2. Headache lasting from 30 minutes to 7 days

Chronic tension-type Headache

  A. Diagnostic criteria includes

    1. Average headache frequency $\geq$15 days per month ($\geq$180 days per year) for $\geq$6 months

Tension-type Headache Associated with Disorder of Pericranial Muscles

  A. At least one of the following is present

    1. Increased tenderness of pericranial muscles demonstrated by manual palpation or pressure algometer

    2. Increased electromyographic activity of pericranial muscles at rest or during physiologic tests

Tension-type Headache Unassociated with Disorder of Pericranial Muscles

  A. There is no increased tenderness of pericranial muscles; if studied, electromyography of pericranial muscles shows normal levels of activity

DIAGNOSTIC CRITERIA FOR CLUSTER HEADACHE

  A. At least five attacks fulfilling B-D

  B. Severe unilateral orbital, supraorbital, and/or temporal pain lasting 15 to 180 minutes untreated

  C. Headache is associated with at least one of the following signs, which have to be present on the pain side

    1. Conjuncival injection

    2. Lacrimation

    3. Nasal congestion

    4. Rhinorrhea

    5. Forehead and facial swelling

    6. Meiosis

    7. Ptosis

    8. Eyelid edema

  D. Frequency of attacks: from 1 every other day to 8 per day

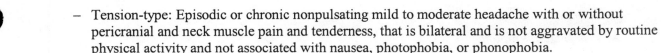

Box 18-1 continued

E. At least one of the following occurs
  1. History and physical and neurologic examinations do not suggest headaches secondary to organic or systemic metabolic disease
  2. History and/or physical neurologic examinations do not suggest such disorder, but it is ruled out by appropriate investigations
  3. Such disorder is present but migraine attacks do not occur for the first time in close temporal relation to the disorder
F. Cluster headache; periodicity undetermined
G. Episodic cluster headache attacks occur in periods lasting 7 days to 1 year separated by pain-free periods lasting ≥14 days
H. Chronic cluster headache: attacks occur for more than 1 year without remission or with remissions lasting ≥14 days

Adapted from the 1988 International Headache Society Classification System. In Solomon, S. (1997). Diagnosis of primary headache disorders. Validity of the International Headache Society criteria in clinical practice [review]. *Neurologic Clinics, 15*(1), 15-26.

- Each type of primary headache is characterized by several classic features:
  - Migraine: Unilateral (can be bilateral in up to 40%), pulsating headache of severe intensity associated with nausea, photophobia, phonophobia, and aggravated by physical activity lasting 4 to 72 hours; some will be preceded (less than 1 hour prior to onset of headache) by one or more fully reversible aura symptoms indicating focal cerebral cortical or brainstem dysfunction (e.g., visual blurring or scotoma, paresthesias, focal weakness or numbness); common in women in their 30s and 40s (e.g., often in association with menses); often a positive family history of migraine can be elicited.

  - Tension-type: Episodic or chronic nonpulsating mild to moderate headache with or without pericranial and neck muscle pain and tenderness, that is bilateral and is not aggravated by routine physical activity and not associated with nausea, photophobia, or phonophobia.

  - Cluster: Episodic clustered attacks of excruciating unilateral periorbital headache with associated conjunctival injection, lacrimation, nasal congestion and rhinorrhea, facial sweating, miosis, and ptosis, occurring up to 8 times a day lasting 15 to 180 minutes, and often awakening the patient from sleep; more common in men and may be triggered by alcohol, histamine, or vasodilators.

DIFFERENTIAL DIAGNOSIS

- Cerebrovascular accident
- Tumor
- Temporal arteritis
- Sinusitis
- Meningitis
- Subarachnoid hemorrhage
- Posttraumatic headache
- Hypertensive headache
- Medication-induced headache
- Benign exertional or cough headache
- High altitude headache
- Idiopathic stabbing headache
- Cold stimulus headache (ice cream headache); nitrate/nitrite-induced headache (hot dog headache); monosodium glutamate (MSG) headache

- Temporomandibular joint disease
- Cervical arthritis
- Cranial neuralgias
- Ophthalmologic pain (eyestrain, ophthalmoplegia with diplopia, spasm of the near reflex, corneal or conjunctival disease, glaucoma, uveitis)
- Otalgia (otitis media, mastoiditis, neoplasms)
- Oral or pharyngeal pain (toothache, aphthous ulcers, carcinomas)

KEYS TO ASSESSMENT

History

- History should identify the pattern of symptoms that may help identify the cause:
    - Onset
    - Frequency
    - Duration
    - Intensity
    - Location
    - Quality
    - Precipitators and exacerbators
    - Ameliorators
    - Associated symptoms
    - Neurologic accompaniments
- Past medical history about childhood and adult illnesses, injuries, immunizations, medications, and allergies:
    - Family history
    - Lifestyle and social history
    - Systems review

Examination

- General appearance and activity (e.g., migraine patients usually lie still, cluster patients are often restless).
- Look for fever and hypertension.
- Do a careful physical examination for signs of infection, neoplasm, or vascular disease.
- Perform a head exam for scalp or facial tenderness and vascular bruits.
- Check the eyes, ears and temporomandibular joints.
- Check the neck for mobility and tenderness.
- Perform a careful neurologic exam for focal neurologic findings.

Diagnostics

- Further studies would be indicated based on any specific findings on the physical exam.
- If the patient has a normal examination, no more studies may be indicated.

- Magnetic resonance imaging (MRI) or computed tomography (CT) are indicated for focal neurologic signs, altered consciousness, nuchal rigidity, severe headache or first headache in a person over age 50, worsening headache while under observation, or inconsistent pattern.

- If meningitis or subarachnoid hemorrhage are suspected, lumbar puncture is indicated.

- Other suspected causes of secondary headache should be evaluated as appropriate.

KEYS TO MANAGEMENT

- Migraine

  - Avoid precipitating factors.

  - Modify diet (e.g., decrease caffeine, highly seasoned foods, and chocolate).

  - Maintain a regular sleeping schedule.

  - Avoid alcohol.

  - Maximize stress coping mechanisms.

  - Avoid oral contraceptives.

- Acute migraine

  - **"Triptans"** (sumatriptan, zolmitriptan, naratriptan, rizatriptan): serotonin agonists with effective and rapid relief (>80% respond) and well tolerated. Contraindications include coronary artery disease, Prinzmetal's angina, uncontrolled hypertension, liver disease, or neurologic deficits with the headache.

  - **Dihydroergotamine** (DHE): intravenous (IV) or intramuscular (IM) injection gives rapid and effective relief (up to 90% respond); may require repeated injections; useful if patient does not respond to sumatriptan; may cause coronary spasm but less so than ergotamine.

  - **Ergotamine** (usually in combination with caffeine): <50% respond; also has a significant risk for coronary spasm.

  - **Nonsteroidal anti inflammatories** (ibuprofen, Ketoralac, etc.): for mild to moderate HA.

  - **Steroids**: Dexamethasone sometimes given for very severe headache.

  - **Others**: Intranasal lidocaine; intravenous chlorpromazine or prochlorperazine; narcotics.

  - **Future**: Substance P antagonists, nitric oxide synthetase inhibitors, CGRP inhibitors.

- Migraine prophylaxis is indicated when attack frequency is between 2 and 8 per month and are severe enough to impair normal life, or when patient is intolerant to abortive therapies due to side effects.

  - β-blockers (propranolol, metoprolol, atenolol, nadolol, and timolol only) are the first choice with 10% to 15% of patients having side effects.

  - **Amitriptyline or nortriptyline** are useful in patients with both migraine and tension-type headaches, but also has significant side effects.

  - **Calcium antagonists** (flunarizine) have frequent side effects that limit use.

  - **Valproate or divalproex sodium** are effective, but have frequent side effects.

  - **Nonsteroidal antiinflammatory drugs (NSAIDS)** are useful in some patients who do not tolerate β-blockers.

  - **Methysergide** should be used only for severe refractory cases due to high risk of serious side effects such as abdominal pain, nausea, and retroperitoneal fibrosis.

- Tension-type
  - Episodic headaches can usually be managed with over-the-counter (OTC) drugs, such as aspirin, acetaminophen, or nonsteroidal antiinflammatory agents, in combination with caffeine.
  - CDH should be treated with antidepressants: tricyclic antidepressants have the longest track record. Selective serotonin reuptake inhibitors (SSRIs) are being used effectively in many patients. Rebound headache from an overuse of OTCs can be a serious problem.
  - Physical therapy including proper attention to posture (especially at work) and daily exercises to loosen up the neck and shoulder muscles can be very helpful.
  - Stress management and relaxation therapy can also be effective, sometimes in combination with biofeedback or percutaneous electrical nerve stimulation (PENS).
  - Obtain a referral for a psychological evaluation if indicated.
- Cluster
  - Avoidance of triggers.
    1) Avoid alcohol, histamine, and vasodilators.
    2) Avoid prolonged contact with solvents, gasoline and oil-based paints.
    3) Prophylaxis prior to airplane or high altitude travel.
  - Acute cluster headache
    1) Oxygen inhalation (aborts 90% of attacks) should be started immediately at 7 L/min.
    2) Sublingual, medihaler, or IM ergotamine or DHE.
    3) Intranasal lidocaine and sumatriptan are also used with some success.
  - Cluster headache prophylaxis
    1) Ergotamine daily during attack periods.
    2) Verapamil daily (70% respond).
    3) Lithium if resistant to ergotamine-verapamil (70% respond).
    4) Methysergide, histamine desensitization, prednisone trigeminal ganglion surgery or ablation of the greater superficial petrosal nerve in highly refractory cases.

Pathophysiology $\rightarrow$ Clinical Link

What is going on in the disease process that influences how the patient presents and how he or she should be managed?

What should you do now that you understand the underlying pathophysiology?

Pathophysiology	Clinical Link
Migraine is possibly associated with changes in mitochondrial DNA.	Migraine is more common in females and has a familial tendency, especially from mothers to daughters.
Migraines are associated with vasoconstriction followed by vasodilation and inflammation with activation of the trigeminal ganglion and disturbances in neurotransmitters, especially serotonin.	Many migraines are preceded by an aura of neurologic symptoms such as scotoma paresthesias, followed by severe pulsating headache; serotonin agonists and vasoconstrictor medications can be used to abort an attack, and anti inflammatories help some patients.
Estrogen withdrawal just prior to menses is associated with changes in neurotransmitters in the central nervous system (CNS), especially serotonin.	Migraines are often associated with the menstrual cycle or the use of exogenous hormones.
Tension-type headaches are often associated with pericranial muscle spasms, but some are not, and there appears to be a central mechanism that may also be related to serotonin.	Many tension-type headaches are associated with poor posture and stress-related muscle tension and will respond to physical therapy and relaxation techniques; other patients have features of both tension-type and migraine and may respond to antidepressants and/or serotonin agonists.
Cluster headaches are associated with hypothalamic dysfunction, cerebral hypoxemia, and neuroendocrine dysfunction with release of histamine; intracranial vasodilation may compress the sympathetic plexus.	Seasonal "clusters" of headaches are related to changes in photoperiod; headaches are associated with nasal stuffiness and lacrimation as well as miosis and ptosis.
There are many structures in the head that can cause cranial pain such as sinuses, eyes, ears, mouth, etc., but most are associated with positive findings on physical exam.	The differential diagnosis of headache is extensive, but a primary headache is common, and patients with a normal exam do not require extensive diagnostic testing.

Suggested Reading

Aguirre, J., Gallardo, R., Pareja, J. A., & Perez-Miranda, M. (2000). Cluster of MMPI personality profiles in chronic tension-type headache and predictable response to Fluoxetine. *Cephalalgia, 20*(1), 51-56.

Ahmed, H. E., White, P. F., Craig, W. F., Hamza, M. A., Ghoname, E. S., & Gajraj, N. M. (2000). Use of percutaneous electrical nerve stimulation (PENS) in the short-term management of headache. *Headache, 40*(4), 311-315.

Ashina, M., Bendtsen, L., Jensen, R., & Olesen, J. (2000). Nitric oxide-induced headache in patients with chronic tension-type headache. *Brain, 123*(Pt 9), 1830-1837.

Ashina, M., Bendtsen, L., Jensen, R., Sakai, F., & Olesen, J. (1999). Muscle hardness in patients with chronic tension-type headache: Relation to actual headache state. *Pain, 79*(2-3), 201-205.

Ashina, M., Lassen, L. H., Bendtsen, L., Jensen, R., & Olesen, J. (1999). Effect of inhibition of nitric oxide synthase on chronic tension-type headache: A randomised crossover trial. *Lancet, 353*(9149), 287-289.

Aube, M. (1999). Migraine in pregnancy. *Neurology, 53*(4 Suppl 1), S26-S28.

Bahra, A., Gawel, M. J., Hardebo, J. E., Millson, D., Breen, S. A., & Goadsby, P. J. (2000). Oral zolmitriptan is effective in the acute treatment of cluster headache. *Neurology, 54*(9), 1832-1839.

Bartleson, J. D. (1999). Treatment of migraine headaches. *Mayo Clinic Proceedings, 74*(7), 702-708.

Berliner, R., Solomon, S., Newman, L. C., & Lipton, R. B. (1999). Migraine: Clinical features and diagnosis. *Comprehensive Therapy, 25*(8-10), 397-402.

Bove, G. M., & Nilsson, N. (1999). Pressure pain threshold and pain tolerance in episodic tension-type headache do not depend on the presence of headache. *Cephalalgia, 19*(3), 174-178.

Boyle, C. A. (1999). Management of menstrual migraine. *Neurology, 53*(4 Suppl 1), S14-S18.

Chase, S. (1999). Treatment of migraine headache. *Lippincott's Primary Care Practice, 3*(3), 259-267.

Chervin, R. D., Zallek, S. N., Lin, X., Hall, J. M., Sharma, N., & Hedger, K. M. (2000). Sleep disordered breathing in patients with cluster headache. *Neurology, 54*(12), 2302-2306.

Dahlof, C. G. (1999). Current concepts of migraine and its treatment. *Neurologia, 14*(2), 67-77.

Dalessio, D. J. (2001). Relief of cluster headache and cranial neuralgias. Promising prophylactic and symptomatic treatments. *Postgraduate Medicine, 109,* 69-72.

de Tommaso, M., Sciruicchio, V., Guido, M., Sasanelli, G., & Puca, F. (1999). Steady-state visual-evoked potentials in headache: Diagnostic value in migraine and tension-type headache patients. *Cephalalgia, 19*(1), 23-26.

Deleu, D., & Hanssens, Y. (2000). Current and emerging second-generation triptans in acute migraine therapy: A comparative review. *Journal of Clinical Pharmacology, 40*(7), 687-700.

DeRaps, P. K. (1999). Migraine management. New approaches focus on serotonin receptors. *Advance for Nurse Practitioners, 7*(5), 51-55.

Diamond, S. (2001). A fresh look at migraine therapy. New treatments promise improved management. *Postgraduate Medicine, 109,* 49-54.

Diamond, S., Balm, T. K., & Freitag, F. G. (2000). Ibuprofen plus caffeine in the treatment of tension-type headache. *Clinical Pharmacology & Therapeutics, 68*(3), 312-319.

Diener, H. C., & Limmroth, V. (1999). Acute management of migraine: Triptans and beyond. *Current Opinion in Neurology, 12*(3), 261-267.

Fettes, I. (1999). Migraine in the menopause. *Neurology, 53*(4 Suppl 1), S29-S33.

Goadsby, P. J. (1999). Cluster headache: New perspectives. *Cephalalgia, 19*(Suppl 25), 39-41.

Goadsby, P. J. (2001). Migraine, aura, and cortical spreading depression: Why are we still talking about it? *Annals of Neurology, 49,* 4-6.

Goadsby, P. J., Bahra, A., & May, A. (1999). Mechanisms of cluster headache. *Cephalalgia, 19*(Suppl 23), 19-21.

Hand, P. J., & Stark, R. J. (2000). Intravenous lignocaine infusions for severe chronic daily headache. *Medical Journal of Australia, 172*(4), 157-159.

Hargreaves, R. J., & Shepheard, S. L. (1999). Pathophysiology of migraine—New insights. *Canadian Journal of Neurological Sciences, 26*(Suppl 3), S12-S19.

Hering-Hanit, R., & Gadoth, N. (2000). Baclofen in cluster headache. *Headache, 40*(1), 48-51.

Holroyd, K. A., Stensland, M., Lipchik, G. L., Hill, K. R., O'Donnell, F. S., & Cordingley, G. (2000). Psychosocial correlates and impact of chronic tension-type headaches. *Headache, 40*(1), 3-16.

Jensen, R. (1999). Pathophysiological mechanisms of tension-type headache: A review of epidemiological and experimental studies. *Cephalalgia, 19*(6), 602-621.

Jensen, R. (1999). The tension-type headache alternative. Peripheral pathophysiological mechanisms. *Cephalalgia, 19*(Suppl 25), 9-10.

Jensen, R., & Olesen, J. (2000). Tension-type headache: An update on mechanisms and treatment. *Current Opinion in Neurology, 13*(3), 285-289.

Jorge, R. E., Leston, J. E., Arndt, S., & Robinson, R. G. (1999). Cluster headaches: Association with anxiety disorders and memory deficits. *Neurology, 53*(3), 543-547.

Kors, E. E., Haan, J., & Ferrari, M. D. (1999). Genetics of primary headaches. *Current Opinion in Neurology, 12*(3), 249-254.

Leone, M., D'Amico, D., Frediani, F., Moschiano, F., Grazzi, L., Attanasio, A., & Bussone, G. (2000). Verapamil in the prophylaxis of episodic cluster headache: A double-blind study versus placebo. *Neurology, 54*(6), 1382-1385.

Lobo, B. L., Cooke, S. C., & Landy, S. H. (1999). Symptomatic pharmacotherapy of migraine. *Clinical Therapeutics, 21*(7), 1118-1130.

Logemann, C. D., & Rankin, L. M. (2000). Newer intranasal migraine medications. *American Family Physician, 61*(1), 180-186.

Montagna, P. (2000). Molecular genetics of migraine headaches: A review. *Cephalalgia, 20*(1), 3-14.

Nahab, F. B., Worrell, G. A., & Weinshenker, B. G. (2001). 25-year-old man with recurring headache and confusion. *Mayo Clinic Proceedings, 76,* 75-78.

Neufeld, J. D., Holroyd, K. A., & Lipchik, G. L. (2000). Dynamic assessment of abnormalities in central pain transmission and modulation in tension-type headache sufferers. *Headache, 40*(2), 142-151.

Nicolodi, M., & Sicuteri, F. (1999). Triptans. A support to the central link between serotonin and acetylcholine in migraine. *Advances in Experimental Medicine & Biology, 467,* 183-189.

Oguzhanoglu, A., Sahiner, T., Kurt, T., & Akalin, O. (1999). Use of amitriptyline and fluoxetine in prophylaxis of migraine and tension headaches. *Cephalalgia, 19*(5), 531-532.

Pauwels, P. J., & John, G. W. (1999). Present and future of 5-HT receptor agonists as antimigraine drugs. *Clinical Neuropharmacology, 22*(3), 123-136.

Rambihar, V. S. (2001). Headache angina. *Lancet, 357,* 72.

Remahl, I. N., Waldenlind, E., Bratt, J., & Ekbom, K. (2000). Cluster headache is not associated with signs of a systemic inflammation. *Headache, 40*(4), 276-282.

Rollnik, J. D., Tanneberger, O., Schubert, M., Schneider, U., & Dengler, R. (2000). Treatment of tension-type headache with botulinum toxin type A: A double-blind, placebo-controlled study. *Headache, 40*(4), 300-305.

Rossi, L. N., Cortinovis, I., Menegazzo, L., Brunelli, G., Bossi, A., & Macchi, M. (2001). Classification criteria and distinction between migraine and tension-type headache in children. *Developmental Medicine & Child Neurology, 43,* 45-51.

Saper, J. R. (2000). Headache disorders. *Medical Clinics of North America, 83*(3), 663-690.

Schwartz, B. S., Stewart, W. F., Simon, D., & Lipton, R. B. (1998) Epidemiology of tension-type headache. *Journal of the American Medical Association, 279(5),* 381-383.

Silberstein, S. D., Niknam, R., Rozen, T. D., & Young, W. B. (2000). Cluster headache with aura. *Neurology, 54*(1), 219-221.

Smetana, G. W. (2000). The diagnostic value of historical features in primary headache syndromes: A review. *Archives of Internal Medicine, 160*(18), 2729-2737.

Spierings, E. L., Ranke, A. H., Schroevers, M., & Honkoop, P. C. (2000). Chronic daily headache: A time perspective. *Headache, 40*(4), 306-310.

Spinhoven, P., & ter Kuile, M. M. (2000). Treatment outcome expectancies and hypnotic susceptibility as moderators of pain reduction in patients with chronic tension-type headache. *International Journal of Clinical & Experimental Hypnosis, 48*(3), 290-305.

Tfelt-Hansen, P., Saxena, P. R., Dahlof, C., Pascual, J., Lainez, M., Henry, P., Diener, H., Schoenen, J., Ferrari, M. D., & Goadsby, P. J. (2000). Ergotamine in the acute treatment of migraine: A review and European consensus. *Brain, 123*(Pt 1), 9-18.

Tietjen, G. E. (2000). The relationship of migraine and stroke. *Neuroepidemiology, 19*(1), 13-19.

Vernon, H., McDermaid, C. S., & Hagino, C. (1999). Systematic review of randomized clinical trials of complementary/alternative therapies in the treatment of tension-type and cervicogenic headache. *Complementary Therapies in Medicine, 7*(3), 142-155.

Weitzel, K. W., Thomas, M. L., Small, R. E., & Goode, J. V. (1999). Migraine: A comprehensive review of new treatment options. *Pharmacotherapy, 19*(8), 957-973.

Case Study*

Headache

INITIAL HISTORY

- 34-year-old female presents with headache.
- 2-day history of dull pain over the top of her head.
- Unrelieved by aspirin or acetaminophen.
- Admits to previous headaches of a similar nature.
- Notes that they are becoming increasingly frequent.

Question 1   What is the differential diagnosis based on this history alone?

Question 2   What further questions would you like to ask her to complete her review of symptoms?

ADDITIONAL HISTORY

- Headache is generalized around the entire head.
- The pain sometimes wakes her from sleep but does not interfere with her daily activities.
- She denies nausea, vomiting, fever, chills, numbness or tingling, or visual changes.
- She had some neck and shoulder pain, but no neck stiffness.
- She denies photosensitivity or decreased level of consciousness.
- She has no nasal or postnasal drainage.

_____

*Leslie Buchanan contributed this case study.

Question 3 What other questions would you like to ask about her past medical, family, and social history?

MORE HISTORY

- Patient denies any head injury.
- She admits to experiencing a great deal of stress recently.
- She drinks 3 to 4 beers each evening.
- Her mother had similar headaches occasionally, but nothing serious.
- Her last menstrual period was 3 weeks ago.
- She does not take oral contraceptives (OCPs) or estrogens.

PHYSICAL EXAMINATION

- Alert, well-developed, well nourished female in no acute distress.
- BP = 140/90; P = 80 and regular; RR = 16 and unlabored; T = 37.2 orally.
- Skin is warm and dry; no rashes.

HEENT

- No scalp tenderness.
- Face nontender; no pain with percussion of the sinus cavities.
- Tympanic membranes noninjected; no bulging or retraction.
- Extraocular movements full; visual acuity sharp (20/20 OU with corrective lenses).
- PERRL; no photosensitivity; conjunctiva clear; funduscopic demonstrates sharp disks and no hemorrhages.
- Nasal mucosa pink; no drainage.
- Throat noninjected without postnasal drainage.

Neck

- Supple with full range of motion.
- No palpable lymphadenopathy in the anterior or posterior chains.
- No bruits heard.

Lungs, Cardiovascular

- Lungs clear to auscultation and percussion.
- Cardiac with RRR without murmurs or gallops.

Abdomen, Extremities

- Abdomen without tenderness or masses.
- Extremities with good pulses, no edema.

Neurological
- Oriented x3, memory recent and remote clear.
- No focal motor or sensory deficits.
- Cranial nerves in tact.
- Deep tendon reflexes +2 in all groups.
- Negative Kernig and Brudzinski sign.
- Negative Romberg.

Question 4　What are the pertinent positive and negative findings on examination?

Question 5　What laboratory studies are indicated at this time?

Question 6　What is your diagnosis?

Question 7 What should your treatment plan encompass?

MANAGEMENT

- Patient was given appropriate pharmacologic suggestions (for OTC medication).
- Patient was referred for physical therapy.
- Patient was referred for stress management therapy.

Question 8 What further care would you recommend?

19

Stroke

DEFINITION

- A stroke (cerebrovascular accident [CVA]) is defined as a focal neurological disorder developing suddenly because of a pathophysiological process in blood vessels.
    - Acute brain infarction (ABI)
    - Intracerebral hemorrhage (ICH)
    - Subarachnoid hemorrhage (SAH)

EPIDEMIOLOGY

- Third leading cause of death in the United States; 10.6% of all deaths, 600,000 strokes/year.
- **ABI**
    - 75% of all strokes; risk increases with age.
    - Strong association with coronary artery disease; both share many risk factors.
        1) Hypertension (especially systolic) is the most important modifiable risk factor.
        2) Smoking increases risk by 2- to 3-fold.
        3) Other factors include age >67, diabetes, hyperlipidemia, hyperhomocystinemia male sex or a female after menopause, family history, African-American race, and recent myocardial infarction.
    - Atrial fibrillation carries a 5% to 6 % per year risk of embolic stroke.
    - Arteriolar obstruction and hypercoagulability: polycythemia, sickle cell disease, oral contraceptives, inherited thrombotic disorders, migraine.
- **ICH**
    - 15% of all strokes: mortality is high (35% to 50% at one month), especially if there is severe coma upon presentation.
    - Risk factors include hypertension, alcohol abuse, coagulopathies, cocaine or amphetamine abuse, blood dyscrasia, and iatrogenic anticoagulation.
- **SAH**
    - 10% of all strokes (25% of all stroke deaths): incidence is higher in young adults and in women.
    - Risk factors include congenital saccular aneurysms, migraine, hypertension, smoking, polycystic kidney, Marfan's syndrome, fibromuscular dysplasia, and sickle cell disease.

PATHOPHYSIOLOGY

- **Cerebral circulation:**
    - In the normal brain, cerebral blood flow (CBF) is maintained despite changes in mean arterial pressure (MAP) or intracranial pressure (ICP) due to regulation of cerebrovascular resistance (CVR) called **autoregulation** (CBF= MAP-ICP/CVR). In the injured brain, autoregulation is lost such that small changes in MAP or ICP will affect cerebral blood flow.

- There are many collaterals for cerebral perfusion (Circle of Willis) so that the obstruction of a vessel may not lead to infarction of distal tissue and deficits can be unpredictable.

- **Transient ischemic attack (TIA)** describes a sudden loss of neurologic function usually due to atheroemboli from extracranial arteries or due to cardioemboli (see below) that resolves within 24 hours. Most resolve within 5 minutes. Over 40% of patients with TIA will have an ABI within 5 years.

- **ABI**

  - There are four main classifications:

    1) Atherothrombotic occlusion of extracranial (especially at the carotid bifurcation) or intracranial arteries.

    2) Cardioembolic due to atrial fibrillation, recent myocardial infarction with ventricular aneurysm, congestive heart failure, or valvular disease.

    3) Lacunar due to deep cerebral infarcts of the lenticulostriate arteries.

    4) Hemodynamic due to decreased global cerebral perfusion.

  - The neural cellular response to ischemia includes inflammation, release of excitotoxins, cell membrane injury, and both acute and delayed cell death (Fig. 19-1).

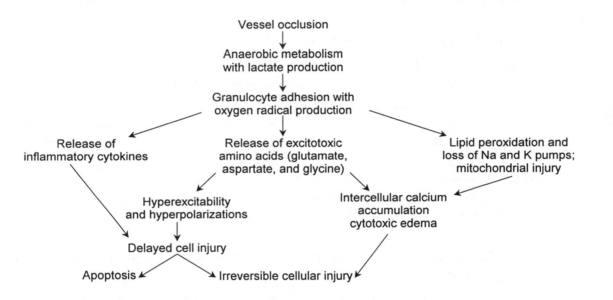

Fig. 19-1 Neural Response to Ischemia

  - Patterns of ischemic neuronal injury, sparing, and healing:

    1) An area of dense infarction and necrosis forms at the center of ischemic brain tissue.

    2) Spontaneous or therapeutic reperfusion results in the limitation of infarct size but also contributes to oxygen radical production (reperfusion injury).

    3) Selective neuronal necrosis: some neurons and glial cells survive, especially if reperfused with 12 hours; sparing may be maximized by rapid perfusion and neuroprotective therapy.

  - Penumbra: tissue at the periphery of the ischemic zone:

    1) Cerebral blood flow (CBF) approximately 20 ml/100 gm/min: neurons are viable but there is no synaptic function; they may be salvageable if perfusion is restored 90 minutes to several hours after initial event.

2) Ischemic tissue contains high extracellular potassium causing multiple repetitive depolarizations leading to ATP depletion and delayed cell death; new therapies are aimed at blocking peri infarct depolarizations.

– Delayed neuronal death:

1) Inflammation, granulocyte adhesion, oxygen radical production, and cytokine release cause not only acute neuronal damage but also delayed effects with T lymphocytes and macrophages infiltrating up to 2 weeks after the initial insult.

2) Cytokines (TNFα, TGFβ) also induce the activation of cellular endonucleases that cleave neuronal deoxyribonucleic acid (DNA) (apoptosis); this may continue for 2 weeks after infarct.

– Healing and functional recovery:

1) The brain surrounding the infarct is hypermetabolic; it underscores the need for maximal oxygen and nutrient delivery during the peri infarction time period.

2) Polypeptide growth factors (neurotrophins, fibroblast growth factors) result in dendritic sprouting and new axonal growth, and they are protective against delayed neuronal injury. Trials with basic fibroblast growth factor (bFGF) are encouraging.

– Systemic responses to cerebral ischemia:

1) Arrhythmias (tachy or brady, arrhythmias, ST-T wave changes, increased creatinine phosphokinase MB [CPK-MB], and wall motion abnormalities) are believed to be due to a burst of catecholamines.

2) Neurogenic pulmonary edema (acute respiratory distress syndrome [ARDS]).

3) Peptic ulcer disease (Cushing ulcer).

4) Endocrine abnormalities (syndrome of inappropriate antidiuretic hormone [SIADH]).

- **ICH**

– Rupture of artery or arteriole with hematoma formation under arterial pressure.

– Once thought to be caused by microaneurysms (Charcot-Bouchard) but recent studies discount this; some are caused by congenital saccular aneurysms in the fissures (see SAH).

– Cerebral amyloid angiopathy is a common cause in patients over age 65 and is associated with pathologic brain changes and dementia similar to Alzheimer disease. Vascular malformations and angiomas cause hemorrhage in children and young adults.

– Mechanisms of brain injury in ICH:

1) Direct trauma to neurons by ejection of blood into brain tissue.

2) Mass effect with mechanical compression of surrounding tissues.

a) Hematoma is surrounded by an ischemic penumbra; ischemic changes of intracellular calcium accumulation, excitotoxic amino acid release, and hyperpolarization will lead to acute and delayed cell death.

b) Extravasation of blood causes vasospasm and worsening ischemia.

c) Mass effect increases ICP, which decreases CBF, and may result in shift of the brain and herniation across the midline or through the foramenae.

d) Evacuation of the hematoma within 2 to 4 hours may reduce brain injury; expansion of the hematoma occurs in 14%, usually within 6 hours, with a poor prognosis.

- **SAH**

– Rupture of congenital saccular (berry) aneurysms: most common at the junction of the anterior cerebral and anterior communicating arteries; 12% to 31% have multiple aneurysms. Acute presentation may be preceded by one or more promontory bleeds.

 – Mechanism of brain injury in SAH:

   1) Extravasation of blood (oxyhemoglobin) over the brain surface and ventricles.

   2) Results in inflammation, release of excitotoxic amino acids, and toxic oxygen radicals.

   3) Causes cerebrospinal fluid outflow obstruction and hydrocephalus; increases ICP.

   4) Delayed vasospasm:

      a) Occurs in 70% of cases; symptomatic in 36%.

      b) Occurs 3 to 21 days after the initial bleed (peak = days 4 to 12).

      c) Increases overall mortality by 3-fold and can result in significant ischemic neuronal damage.

   5) Rebleeding is common (4% per day acutely, 1% to 2% within the first month).

 – Hyponatremia:

   1) Common (10% to 34%); linked to a higher rate of secondary cerebral infarctions.

   2) May be due to the syndrome of inappropriate antidiuretic hormone (SIADH) or cerebral salt wasting syndrome that is mediated by atrial natriuretic factor (ANF).

PATIENT PRESENTATION

Patient presentation varies widely. Generally, ABI tends to be painless with less change in level of consciousness than ICH or SAH. Only 20% to 50% of patients with SAH have the classic "thunderclap headache," and only a little more than half have any prodromal headaches at all.

History

Risk factors; history of drug abuse; recent cardiac event; palpitations; recent change in medications; previous transient painless loss of focal neurologic function (TIA); previous syncope or seizures; recurrent headaches.

Symptoms

Abrupt painless loss of neurologic function (ABI) or severe headache (ICH and SAH); decreased level of consciousness; focal weakness or numbness; difficulty speaking; visual changes; difficulty controlling gait; intention tremor; seizures, nausea and vomiting.

Examination

Decreased level of consciousness; fever; pupillary asymmetry and decreased reactiveness; papilledema; meningismus; aphasia or dysarthria; focal motor or sensory deficit; flaccid or spastic muscle tone; asymmetrical deep tendon reflexes; Babinski reflex; ataxia; other specialized neurologic test abnormalities; ventilatory abnormalities (e.g., Cheyne-Stokes respirations); tachycardia; premature beats or arrhythmias; carotid bruits; decreased peripheral pulses or peripheral bruits; evidence of hematologic disease or coagulopathy (petechiae, ecchymoses).

DIFFERENTIAL DIAGNOSIS

- Primary cardiac event with acute hypotension
- Primary seizure disorder
- Brain tumor
- Metabolic or toxic insult (hypoglycemia, drugs)
- Meningitis
- Trauma

KEYS TO ASSESSMENT

- Monitor vital signs and obtain arterial blood gases.
- Neurological examination (NIH stroke scale).
- Electrocardiogram (ECG) and cardiovascular assessment; continuous blood pressure monitoring.
- Repetitive exams: monitor for stroke in evolution with worsening deficits.
- Serum laboratory studies: arterial blood gases, glucose, electrolytes, coagulation studies, complete blood count (CBC), toxicology screen.
- Computed tomography (CT) scan/magnetic resonance imagery (MRI): most still consider CT scan best but many suggest that high speed diffusion-weighted MRI is better for differentiation of cerebral hemorrhage from infarction acutely.
- Consider lumbar puncture for suspected SAH.
- Vascular studies:
  - Angiography may be indicated urgently in SAH.
  - Noninvasive vascular studies to evaluate cerebral and carotid circulations include:
    1) Carotid duplex ultrasonography
    2) Quantitative oculopneumoplethysmography
    3) Transcranial doppler sonography
    4) MRI or spiral CT angiography
  - Echocardiography: standard or transesophageal to evaluate for cardiac source of emboli.

KEYS TO MANAGEMENT

- **Acute**
  - Oxygen: intubation and mechanical ventilation if hypoxic and/or hypercapnic.
  - Control blood pressure:
    1) Fluid resuscitation increases blood flow and vascular volume in hypotension patient.
    2) Hypertension should be treated carefully, no more than a decrease of 20% in MAP over 1 hour; IV nitroprusside or labetalol.
  - Monitor and control ICP:
    1) Consider ICP bolt placement.
    2) Consider osmotherapy (mannitol).
    3) Consider hyperventilation; watch out for decreased CBF.
  - Monitor and manage electrolyte disturbances.
  - Rapid seizure intervention.
  - Attention to nutrition should be begun early (malnutrition results in poorer outcomes).
  - Curling ulcer prophylaxis (sucralfate vs H2 blockers).
  - **ABI**
    1) Reperfusion:
       a) Recombinant tissue plasminogen activator (rt-Pa) has its greatest efficacy with lowest risk of hemorrhagic conversion if given <3 hours after stroke onset. Patient outcomes significantly improved at 3 months.

b) Intra-arterial prourokinase can be given within 6 hours of onset of symptoms in patients with middle cerebral artery occlusion with improved outcomes at 3 months; not as effective as rt-Pa in the first 3 hours after symptom onset.

c) Intravenous ancrod (defibrinogenic agent from pit viper venom) has also improved stroke outcomes if given within 3 hours of stroke onset; also confers a risk of intracranial hemorrhage similar to that of rt-Pa.

d) Heparin and low-molecular-weight heparin are still used in conjunction with thrombolytic therapy, however their use as single agents in treating ABI has declined significantly. They do decrease the risk of deep venous thrombosis.

2) Neuroprotection: despite numerous positive studies in animals and small trials in patients, none of these modalities conclusively improve stroke outcomes; studies are ongoing.

a) N-methyl-D-aspartate (NMDA) receptor/channel antagonists: blocks release of glutamate and aspartate, thus decreasing intracellular calcium influx; examples include dextrorphan, cerestat, dizocilpine, selfotel, and remacemide. Preliminary studies are encouraging and may be used as adjuncts to thrombolysis.

b) Lubeluzole (inhibits presynaptic release of glutamate).

c) Alpha-amino-3-hydroxy-5-methyl-4-isoxazole (AMPA) channel antagonists.

d) Calcium channel blockers: studies are mixed; nimodipine is promising.

e) Gamma: aminobutyric agonists (piracetam may decrease early mortality).

f) Toxic oxygen radical scavengers (tirilazad, ebselen).

g) Monoclonal antibodies against leukocyte adhesion molecules (decrease inflammatory response).

h) Cytokine inhibitors.

i) Nitric oxide donors (L-arginine) and prostacyclin analogues.

j) Methylxanthines (pentoxifylline).

k) Insulin: hyperglycemia worsens stroke injury; it is used to control glucose in neuro ICU, but benefits not proven.

l) Physical cooling.

- **ICH**

1) Bedrest, sedate; consider intubation to control airway, administer oxygen, and ventilate if necessary.

2) Control blood pressure: use labetalol rather than nitrates because it does not cause cerebral vasodilation; balance with fluid administration.

3) Pressure bolt for ICP monitoring: hyperventilate + osmolar therapy if indicated.

4) Surgical decompression in selected patients; <4 hours after event for maximal effect; needle aspiration of hematomas can be successful in selected patients.

5) Seizure and ulcer prophylaxis for most patients.

- **SAH**

1) Monitor for arrhythmias and myocardial ischemia.

2) Darkened room; bedrest with head at 30 degrees.

3) Meperidine or codeine for pain; reassess mental status.

4) Ulcer prophylaxis; stool softeners; seizure prophylaxis controversial.

5) Monitor for adequate cerebral perfusion using transcranial doppler (TCD).

6) Monitor for increased ICP - hyperventilate + osmolar therapy.

7) Prevent rebleeding:

a) Antifibrinolytic drugs: aminocaproic acid or tranexamic given at admission.

b) Perform surgery if in good condition: operate in 1 to 2 days to clip aneurysm (up to 90% successful); if in poor condition delay 7 to 14 days and reconsider (<50% improvement).

c) Intraarterial balloons or platinum coils used to block aneurysm in the necks of selected patients; the results are very encouraging so far.

8) Prevent vasospasm:

a) Monitor for headache, mental status changes, and new deficits.

b) Triple H (hypervolemic/hypertensive/hemodilution) can be used in the absence of increased ICP; improves perfusion pressure and reduces viscosity.

c) Calcium channel blockers: nimodipine, nicardipine, nilvadipine; given IV; they clearly reduce severe neurologic deficits and work more by reducing ischemic intracellular calcium influx than by cerebral vasodilation.

d) Percutaneous transluminal carotid angioplasty (PTCA): helpful in some patients with refractory vasospasm.

e) Monitor with daily transcranial doppler ultrasound.

- **Chronic**

  – Neurologic rehabilitation techniques are varied and of mixed clear therapeutic benefit but all are superior to neglect. Improvements can be seen many months after the acute event.

  – Nutrition is vitally important.

  – Monitor for depression, recurrent cerebrovascular disease, and cardiac disease, especially coronary artery disease. Pneumonia is also a significant cause of post-stroke mortality.

- **Prevention**

  – Hypertension is the single most important modifiable risk factor; over half of strokes could be prevented with hypertension control.

  – Stopping smoking and decreasing alcohol intake can reduce risk.

  – Cholesterol management reduces risk, especially using reductase inhibitors (e.g., pravastatin).

  – Use warfarin therapy for nonvalvular atrial fibrillation.

  – Aspirin (50 mg/day to 325 mg/day) for primary prevention; aspirin plus dipyridamole is the most effective antithrombotic regimen for secondary prevention of stroke; others include clopidogrel and ticlopidine.

  – Management of transient ischemic attacks (TIA).

    1) Medical therapy with antiplatelet drugs is first choice for "noncritical" stenosis.

    2) Use warfarin for a known cardiac source and in atrial fibrillation.

    3) Surgical intervention (carotid endarterectomy) or PTCA with possible stenting is the best choice for critical stenoses. It is indicated for asymptomatic critical carotid obstruction as well as in TIA.

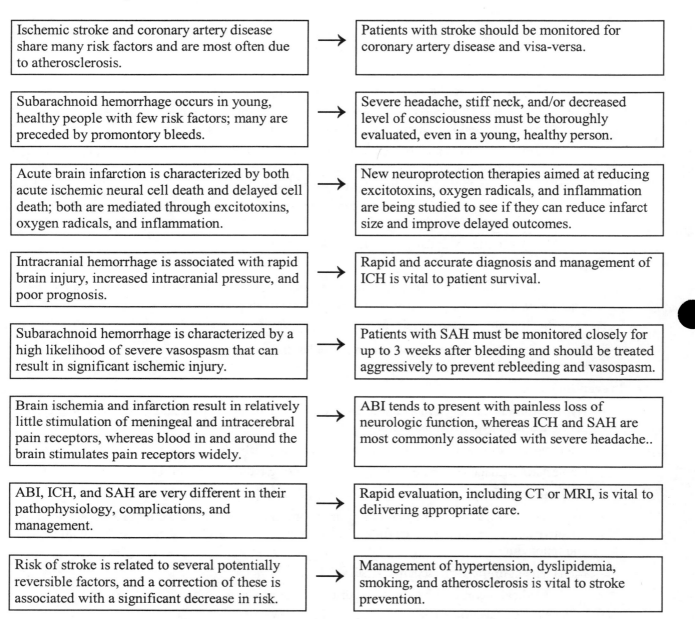

Pathophysiology → Clinical Link

What is going on in the disease process that influences how the patient presents and how he or she should be managed?

What should you do now that you understand the underlying pathophysiology?

Pathophysiology	Clinical Link
Ischemic stroke and coronary artery disease share many risk factors and are most often due to atherosclerosis.	Patients with stroke should be monitored for coronary artery disease and visa-versa.
Subarachnoid hemorrhage occurs in young, healthy people with few risk factors; many are preceded by promontory bleeds.	Severe headache, stiff neck, and/or decreased level of consciousness must be thoroughly evaluated, even in a young, healthy person.
Acute brain infarction is characterized by both acute ischemic neural cell death and delayed cell death; both are mediated through excitotoxins, oxygen radicals, and inflammation.	New neuroprotection therapies aimed at reducing excitotoxins, oxygen radicals, and inflammation are being studied to see if they can reduce infarct size and improve delayed outcomes.
Intracranial hemorrhage is associated with rapid brain injury, increased intracranial pressure, and poor prognosis.	Rapid and accurate diagnosis and management of ICH is vital to patient survival.
Subarachnoid hemorrhage is characterized by a high likelihood of severe vasospasm that can result in significant ischemic injury.	Patients with SAH must be monitored closely for up to 3 weeks after bleeding and should be treated aggressively to prevent rebleeding and vasospasm.
Brain ischemia and infarction result in relatively little stimulation of meningeal and intracerebral pain receptors, whereas blood in and around the brain stimulates pain receptors widely.	ABI tends to present with painless loss of neurologic function, whereas ICH and SAH are most commonly associated with severe headache..
ABI, ICH, and SAH are very different in their pathophysiology, complications, and management.	Rapid evaluation, including CT or MRI, is vital to delivering appropriate care.
Risk of stroke is related to several potentially reversible factors, and a correction of these is associated with a significant decrease in risk.	Management of hypertension, dyslipidemia, smoking, and atherosclerosis is vital to stroke prevention.

Suggested Reading

Abou-Chebl, A., & Furlan, A. J. (2000). Intra-arterial thrombolysis in acute stroke. *Current Opinion in Neurology, 13,* 51-55.

Albers, G. W., Bates, V. E., Clark, W. M., Bell, R., Verro, P., & Hamilton, S. A. (2000). Intravenous tissue-type plasminogen activator for treatment of acute stroke: The standard treatment with alteplase to reverse stroke (STARS) study. *Journal of the American Medical Association, 283*(9), 1145-1150.

Anonymous. (2000). Abciximab in acute ischemic stroke: A randomized, double-blind, placebo-controlled, dose-escalation study. *Stroke, 31*(3), 601-609.

A'Rogvi-Hansen, B., & Boysen, G. (2000). Glycerol for acute ischaemic stroke. *Cochrane Database of Systematic Reviews [computer file],* CD000096.

Asplund, K., Israelsson, K., & Schampi, I. (2000). Haemodilution for acute ischaemic stroke. *Cochrane Database of Systematic Reviews [computer file],* CD000103.

Barnett, H. J., Gunton, R. W., Eliasziw, M., Fleming, L., Sharpe, B., Gates, P., & Meldrum, H. (2000). Causes and severity of ischemic stroke in patients with internal carotid artery stenosis. *Journal of the American Medical Association, 283*(11), 1429-1436.

Baron, J. C. (2001). Mapping the ischaemic penumbra with PET: A new approach. *Brain, 124,* 2-4.

Bath, P. M., & Bath, F. J. (2000). Prostacyclin and analogues for acute ischaemic stroke. *Cochrane Database of Systematic Reviews [computer file],* CD000177.

Bath, P. M., Bath, F. J., & Asplund, K. (2000). Pentoxifylline, propentofylline and pentifylline for acute ischaemic stroke. *Cochrane Database of Systematic Reviews [computer file],* CD000162.

Bath, F. J., Butterworth, R. J., & Bath, P. M. (2000). Nitric oxide donors (nitrates), L-arginine, or nitric oxide synthase inhibitors for acute ischaemic stroke. *Cochrane Database of Systematic Reviews [computer file],* CD000398.

Bath, P. M., Iddenden, R., & Bath, F. J. (2000). Low-molecular-weight heparins and heparinoids in acute ischemic stroke: A meta-analysis of randomized controlled trials. *Stroke, 31*(7), 1770-1778.

Bath, P. M., & Lees, K. R. (2000). ABC of arterial and venous disease. Acute stroke. *British Medical Journal, 320*(7239), 920-923.

Becker, K. (2000). Intensive care unit management of the stroke patient. *Neurologic Clinics, 18,* 439-454.

Benavente, O., Hart, R., Koudstaal, P., Laupacis, A., & McBride, R. (2000). Antiplatelet therapy for preventing stroke in patients with non-valvular atrial fibrillation and no previous history of stroke or transient ischemic attacks. *Cochrane Database of Systematic Reviews [computer file],* CD001925.

Benavente, O., Hart, R., Koudstaal, P., Laupacis, A., & McBride, R. (2000). Oral anticoagulants for preventing stroke in patients with non-valvular atrial fibrillation and no previous history of stroke or transient ischemic attacks. *Cochrane Database of Systematic Reviews [computer file],* CD001927.

Bereczki, D., & Fekete, I. (2000). Vinpocetine for acute ischaemic stroke. *Cochrane Database of Systematic Reviews [computer file],* CD000480.

Berge, E., Abdelnoor, M., Nakstad, P. H., & Sandset, P. M. (2000). Low molecular-weight heparin versus aspirin in patients with acute ischaemic stroke and atrial fibrillation: A double-blind randomised study. HAEST study group: Heparin in acute embolic stroke trial. *Lancet, 355*(9211), 1205-1210.

Berrouschot, J., Barthel, H., Hesse, S., Knapp, W. H., Schneider, D., & von Kummer, R. (2000). Reperfusion and metabolic recovery of brain tissue and clinical outcome after ischemic stroke and thrombolytic therapy. *Stroke, 31*(7), 1545-1551.

Bertram, M., Bonsanto, M., Hacke, W., & Schwab, S. (2000). Managing the therapeutic dilemma: Patients with spontaneous intracerebral hemorrhage and urgent need for anticoagulation. *Journal of Neurology, 247,* 209-214.

Bjorklund, A., & Lindvall, O. (2000). Cell replacement therapies for central nervous system disorders. *Nature Neuroscience, 3,* 537-544.

Brott, T., & Bogousslavsky, J. (2000). Treatment of acute ischemic stroke. *New England Journal of Medicine. 343*(10), 710-722.

Caimi, G., Ferrara, F., Montana, M., Meli, F., Canino, B., Carollo, C., & Presti, R. L. (2000). Acute ischemic stroke: Polymorphonuclear leukocyte membrane fluidity and cytosolic Ca(2+) concentration at baseline and after chemotactic activation. *Stroke, 31*(7), 1578-1582.

Candelise, L., & Ciccone, A. (2000). Gangliosides for acute ischaemic stroke. *Cochrane Database of Systematic Reviews [computer file],* CD000094.

Castillo, J., Rama, R., & Davalos, A. (2000). Nitric oxide-related brain damage in acute ischemic stroke. *Stroke, 31*(4), 852-857.

Chemerinski, E., Robinson, R. G., & Kosier, J. T. (2001). Improved recovery in activities of daily living associated with remission of poststroke depression. *Stroke, 32,* 113-117.

Correia, M., Silva, M., & Veloso, M. (2000). Cooling therapy for acute stroke. *Cochrane Database of Systematic Reviews [computer file],* CD001247.

Counsell, C., & Sandercock, P. (2000). Low-molecular-weight heparins or heparinoids versus standard unfractionated heparin for acute ischaemic stroke. *Cochrane Database of Systematic Reviews [computer file],* CD000119.

del Zoppo, G. J., Ginis, I., Hallenbeck, J. M., Iadecola, C., Wang, X., & Feuerstein, G. Z. (2000). Inflammation and stroke: Putative role for cytokines, adhesion molecules and iNOS in brain response to ischemia. *Brain Pathology, 10,* 95-112.

del Zoppo, G. J., & Hallenbeck, J. M. (2000). Advances in the vascular pathophysiology of ischemic stroke. *Thrombosis Research, 98,* 73-81.

Demchuk, A. M., & Buchan, A. M. (2000). Predictors of stroke outcome. *Neurologic Clinics, 18,* 455-473.

Demchuk, A. M., Burgin, W. S., Christou, I., Felberg, R. A., Barber, P. A., Hill, M. D., & Alexandrov, A. V. (2001). Thrombolysis in brain ischemia (TIBI) transcranial Doppler flow grades predict clinical severity, early recovery, and mortality in patients treated with intravenous tissue plasminogen activator. *Stroke, 32,* 89-93.

Diener, H. C. (2000). Stroke prevention: Anti-platelet and anti-thrombolytic therapy. *Neurologic Clinics, 18,* 343-355.

Diener, H. C., Ringelstein, E. B., von Kummer, R., Langohr, H. D., Bewermeyer, H., Landgraf, H., Hennerici, M., Welzel, D., ve, M., Brom, J., & Weidinger, G. (2001). Treatment of acute ischemic stroke with the low-molecular-weight heparin certoparin: Results of the TOPAS trial. *Stroke, 32,* 22-29.

Dietrich, H. H., & Dacey, R. G., Jr. (2000). Molecular keys to the problems of cerebral vasospasm. *Neurosurgery, 46,* 517-530.

Di Napoli, M., Papa, F., & Bocola, V. (2001). Prognostic influence of increased C-reactive protein and fibrinogen levels in ischemic stroke. *Stroke, 32,* 133-138.

Duncan, P. W., Jorgensen, H. S., & Wade, D. T. (2000). Outcome measures in acute stroke trials: A systematic review and some recommendations to improve practice. *Stroke, 31,* 1429-1438.

Edlow, J. A., & Caplan, L. R. (2000). Avoiding pitfalls in the diagnosis of subarachnoid hemorrhage. *New England Journal of Medicine, 342,* 29-36.

Feigin, V. L., Rinkel, G. J., Algra, A., & van Gijn, J. (2000). Circulatory volume expansion for aneurysmal subarachnoid hemorrhage. *Cochrane Database of Systematic Reviews [computer file],* CD000483.

Feigin, V. L., Rinkel, G. J., Algra, A., Vermeulen, M., & van Gijn, J. (2000). Calcium antagonists for aneurysmal subarachnoid haemorrhage. *Cochrane Database of Systematic Reviews [computer file],* CD000277.

Gebel, J. M., & Broderick, J. P. (2000). Intracerebral hemorrhage. *Neurologic Clinics, 18,* 419-438.

Gillum, L. A., Mamidipudi, S. K., & Johnston, S. C. (2000). Ischemic stroke risk with oral contraceptives: A meta-analysis. *Journal of the American Medical Association, 284*(1), 72-78.

Go, A. S., Hylek, E. M., Phillips, K. A., Borowsky, L. H., Henault, L. E., Chang, Y., Selby, J. V., & Singer, D. E. (2000). Implications of stroke risk criteria on the anticoagulation decision in nonvalvular atrial fibrillation: The Anticoagulation and Risk Factors in Atrial Fibrillation (ATRIA) study. *Circulation, 102*(1), 11-13.

Goldstein, L. B., Adams, R., Becker, K., Furberg, C. D., Gorelick, P. B., Hademenos, G., Hill, M., Howard, G., Howard, V. J., Jacobs, B., Levine, S. R., Mosca, L., Sacco, R. L., Sherman, D. G., Wolf, P. A., & del Zoppo, G. J. (2001). Primary prevention of ischemic stroke: A statement for healthcare professionals from the Stroke Council of the American Heart Association. *Stroke, 32,* 280-299.

Gregson, B. A., Mendelow, A. D., Fernandes, H., Pearson, A. J., & Siddique, M. S. (2000). Surgery for intracerebral hemorrhage. *Stroke, 31,* 791-792.

Gubitz, G., Counsell, C., Sandercock, P., & Signorini, D. (2000). Anticoagulants for acute ischaemic stroke. *Cochrane Database of Systematic Reviews [computer file],* CD000024.

Gubitz, G., & Sandercock, P. (2000). Acute ischaemic stroke. *British Medical Journal, 320*(7236), 692-696.

Gunsilius, E., Petzer, A. L., Stockhammer, G., Kahler, C. M., & Gastl, G. (2001). Serial measurement of vascular endothelial growth factor and transforming growth factor-beta1 in serum of patients with acute ischemic stroke. *Stroke, 32,* 275-278.

Hankey, G. J., Sudlow, C. L., & Dunbabin, D. W. (2000). Thienopyridine derivatives (ticlopidine, clopidogrel) versus aspirin for preventing stroke and other serious vascular events in high vascular risk patients. *Cochrane Database of Systematic Reviews [computer file],* CD001246.

Hankey, G. J., Sudlow, C. L., & Dunbabin, D. W. (2000). Thienopyridines or aspirin to prevent stroke and other serious vascular events in patients at high risk of vascular disease? A systematic review of the evidence from randomized trials. *Stroke, 31*(7), 1779-1784.

Hart, R. G., Halperin, J. L., McBride, R., Benavente, O., Man-Son-Hing, M., & Kronmal, R. A. (2000). Aspirin for the primary prevention of stroke and other major vascular events: Meta-analysis and hypotheses. *Archives of Neurology, 57*(3), 326-332.

Hess, D. C., Demchuk, A. M., Brass, L. M., & Yatsu, F. M. (2000). HMG-CoA reductase inhibitors (statins): A promising approach to stroke prevention. *Neurology, 54,* 790-796.

Hickenbottom, S. L., & Barsan, W. G. (2000). Acute ischemic stroke therapy. *Neurologic Clinics, 18,* 379-397.

Horn, J., & Limburg, M. (2000). Calcium antagonists for acute ischemic stroke. *Cochrane Database of Systematic Reviews [computer file],* CD001928.

Hu, F. B., Stampfer, M. J., Colditz, G. A., Ascherio, A., Rexrode, K. M., Willett, W. C., & Manson, J. E. (2000). Physical activity and risk of stroke in women. *Journal of the American Medical Association, 283*(22), 2961-2967.

Inzitari, D., Eliasziw, M., Gates, P., Sharpe, B. L., Chan, R. K., Meldrum, H. E., & Barnett, H. J. (2000). The causes and risk of stroke in patients with asymptomatic internal-carotid-artery stenosis. North American Symptomatic Carotid Endarterectomy Trial Collaborators. *New England Journal of Medicine. 342*(23), 1693-1700.

Joshi, N., Chaturvedi, S., & Coplin, W. M. (2001). Poor prognosis of acute stroke patients denied thrombolysis due to early CT findings. *Journal of Neuroimaging, 11,* 40-43.

Juurlink, B. H. (2000). Introduction: The role of inflammation in mediating damage following stroke and neurotrauma. *Brain Pathology, 10,* 93-94.

Kario, K., & Pickering, T. G. (2000). Blood pressure levels and risk of stroke in elderly patients. *Journal of the American Medical Association, 284*(8), 959-960.

Keller, E., Wietasch, G., Ringleb, P., Scholz, M., Schwarz, S., Stingele, R., Schwab, S., Hanley, D., & Hacke, W. (2000). Bedside monitoring of cerebral blood flow in patients with acute hemispheric stroke. *Critical Care Medicine, 28*(2), 511-516.

Klungel, O. H., Heckbert, S. R., Longstreth, W. T., Furberg, C. D., Kaplan, R. C., Smith, N. L., Lemaitre, R. N., Leufkens, H. G., de Boer, A., & Psaty, B. M. (2001). Antihypertensive drug therapies and the risk of ischemic stroke. *Archives of Internal Medicine, 161,* 37-43.

Lang, E. W., Diehl, R. R., & Mehdorn, H. M. (2001). Cerebral autoregulation testing after aneurysmal subarachnoid hemorrhage: The phase relationship between arterial blood pressure and cerebral blood flow velocity. *Critical Care Medicine, 29,* 158-163.

Langhorne, P., Stott, D. J., Robertson, L., MacDonald, J., Jones, L., McAlpine, C., Dick, F., Taylor, G. S., & Murray, G. (2000). Medical complications after stroke: A multicenter study. *Stroke, 31*(6), 1223-1229.

Lansberg, M. G., Norbash, A. M., Marks, M. P., Tong, D. C., Moseley, M. E., & Albers, G. W. (2000). Advantages of adding diffusion-weighted magnetic resonance imaging to conventional magnetic resonance imaging for evaluating acute stroke. *Archives of Neurology, 57*(9), 1311-1316.

Lees, K. R., Asplund, K., Carolei, A., Davis, S. M., Diener, H. C., Kaste, M., Orgogozo, J. M., & Whitehead, J. (2000). Glycine antagonist (gavestinel) in neuroprotection (GAIN International) in patients with acute stroke: A randomised controlled trial. GAIN international investigators *Lancet, 355*(9219), 1949-1954.

Lindsberg, P. J., Roine, R. O., Tatlisumak, T., Sairanen, T., & Kaste, M. (2000). The future of stroke treatment. *Neurologic Clinics, 18,* 495-510.

Liu, M., Counsell, C., & Sandercock, P. (2000). Anticoagulants for preventing recurrence following ischaemic stroke or transient ischaemic attack. *Cochrane Database of Systematic Reviews [computer file],* CD000248.

Liu, M., & Wardlaw, J. (2000). Thrombolysis (different doses, routes of administration and agents) for acute ischaemic stroke. *Cochrane Database of Systematic Reviews [computer file],* CD000514.

Lynch, G. F., & Gorelick, P. B. (2000). Stroke in African Americans. *Neurologic Clinics, 18,* 273-290.

Malarcher, A. M., Giles, W. H., Croft, J. B., Wozniak, M. A., Wityk, R. J., Stolley, P. D., Stern, B. J., Sloan, M. A., Sherwin, R., Price, T. R., Macko, R. F., Johnson, C. J., Earley, C. J., Buchholz, D. W., & Kittner, S. J. (2001). Alcohol intake, type of beverage, and the risk of cerebral infarction in young women. *Stroke, 32,* 77-83.

McCarron, M. O., & Nicoll, J. A. (2000). Apolipoprotein E genotype and cerebral amyloid angiopathy-related hemorrhage. *Annals of the New York Academy of Sciences, 903,* 176-179.

Meiklejohn, D. J., Vickers, M. A., Dijkhuisen, R., & Greaves, M. (2001). Plasma homocysteine concentrations in the acute and convalescent periods of atherothrombotic stroke. *Stroke, 32,* 57-62.

Nieuwkamp, D. J., de Gans, K., Rinkel, G. J., & Algra, A. (2000). Treatment and outcome of severe intraventricular extension in patients with subarachnoid or intracerebral hemorrhage: A systematic review of the literature. *Journal of Neurology, 247,* 117-121.

Palmer, B. F. (2000). Hyponatraemia in a neurosurgical patient: Syndrome of inappropriate antidiuretic hormone secretion vs cerebral salt wasting. *Nephrology, Dialysis, Transplantation, 15,* 262-268.

Pereira, A. C., & Warburton, E. (2000). Heparin vs aspirin in acute ischaemic stroke *Lancet, 356*(9223), 73.

Perry, H. M., Jr., Davis, B. R., Price, T. R., Applegate, W. B., Fields, W. S., Guralnik, J. M., Kuller, L., Pressel, S., Stamler, J., & Probstfield, J. L. (2000). Effect of treating isolated systolic hypertension on the risk of developing various types and subtypes of stroke: The systolic hypertension in the elderly program (SHEP). *Journal of the American Medical Association, 284,* 465-471.

Polidori, M. C., Cherubini, A., Senin, U., & Mecocci, P. (2001). Hyperhomocysteinemia and oxidative stress in ischemic stroke. *Stroke, 32,* 275-278.

Ringelstein, E. B., & Nabavi, D. (2000). Long-term prevention of ischaemic stroke and stroke recurrence. *Thrombosis Research, 98,* 83-96.

Rodgers, H. (2000). The scope for rehabilitation in severely disabled stroke patients. *Disability & Rehabilitation, 22,* 199-200.

Roos, Y. B., Rinkel, G. J., Vermeulen, M., Algra, A., & van Gijn, J. (2000). Antifibrinolytic therapy for aneurysmal subarachnoid haemorrhage. *Cochrane Database of Systematic Reviews [computer file],* CD001245.

Rosenson, R. S. (2000). Biological basis for statin therapy in stroke prevention. *Current Opinion in Neurology, 13,* 57-62.

Sacco, R. L., & Elkind, M. S. (2000). Update on antiplatelet therapy for stroke prevention. *Archives of Internal Medicine, 160,* 1579-1582.

Sadamitsu, D., Kuroda, Y., Nagamitsu, T., Tsuruta, R., Inoue, T., Ueda, T., Nakashima, K., Ito, H., & Maekawa, T. (2001). Cerebrospinal fluid and plasma concentrations of nitric oxide metabolites in postoperative patients with subarachnoid hemorrhage. *Critical Care Medicine, 29,* 77-79.

Sarasin, F. P., Gaspoz, J. M., & Bounameaux, H. (2000). Cost-effectiveness of new antiplatelet regimens used as secondary prevention of stroke or transient ischemic attack. *Archives of Internal Medicine. 160*(18), 2773-2778.

Schmulling, S., Grond, M., Rudolf, J., & Heiss, W. D. (2000). One-year follow-up in acute stroke patients treated with rtPA in clinical routine. *Stroke, 31*(7), 1552-1554.

Sherman, D. G., Atkinson, R. P., Chippendale, T., Levin, K. A., Ng, K., Futrell, N., Hsu, C-Y., & Levy, D. E. (2000). Intravenous ancrod for treatment of acute ischemic stroke: The STAT study: A randomized controlled trial. Stroke treatment with ancrod trial. *Journal of the American Medical Association, 283(18),* 2395-2403.

Singer, A. (2000). Treatment and secondary prevention of stroke. *Lancet, 355*(9200), 321.

Stern, S., Altkorn, D., & Levinson, W. (2000). Anticoagulation for chronic atrial fibrillation. *Journal of the American Medical Association, 283*(22), 2901-2903.

Suter, P. M. (2000). Effect of vitamin E, vitamin C, and beta-carotene on stroke risk. *Nutrition Reviews, 58,* 184-187.

Tatu, L., Moulin, T., El Mohamad, R., Vuillier, F., Rumbach, L., & Czorny, A. (2000). Primary intracerebral hemorrhages in the Besancon stroke registry. Initial clinical and CT findings, early course and 30-day outcome in 350 patients. *European Neurology, 43,* 209-214.

Thomson, R., Parkin, D., Eccles, M., Sudlow, M., & Robinson, A. (2000). Decision analysis and guidelines for anticoagulant therapy to prevent stroke in patients with atrial fibrillation. *Lancet, 355*(9208), 956-962.

Wardlaw, J. M., del Zoppo, G., & Yamaguchi, T. (2000). Thrombolysis for acute ischaemic stroke. *Cochrane Database of Systematic Reviews [computer file],* CD000213.

Wardlaw, J. M., Warlow, C. P., Sandercock, P. A., Dennis, M. S., & Lindley, R. I. (2000). Neuroprotection disappointment yet again. *Lancet, 356*(9229), 597.

White, H. D., Simes, R. J., Anderson, N. E., Hankey, G. J., Watson, J. D., Hunt, D., Colquhoun, D. M., Glasziou, P., MacMahon, S., Kirby, A. C., West, M. J., & Tonkin, A. M. (2000). Pravastatin therapy and the risk of stroke. *New England Journal of Medicine, 343,* 317-326.

Williams, L. S., Yilmaz, E. Y., & Lopez-Yunez, A. M. (2000). Retrospective assessment of initial stroke severity with the NIH Stroke Scale. *Stroke, 31*(4), 858-862.

Wityk, R. J., & Beauchamp, N. J., Jr. (2000). Diagnostic evaluation of stroke. *Neurologic Clinics, 18,* 357-378.

Wong, K. S., Mok, V., Lam, W. W., Kay, R., Tang, A., Chan, Y. L., & Woo, J. (2000). Aspirin-associated intracerebral hemorrhage: Clinical and radiologic features. *Neurology, 54,* 2298-2301.

Yoon, B. W., Bae, H. J., Kang, D. W., Lee, S. H., Hong, K. S., Kim, K. B., Park, B. J., & Roh, J. K. (2001). Intracranial cerebral artery disease as a risk factor for central nervous system complications of coronary artery bypass graft surgery. *Stroke, 32,* 94-99.

Case Study*
Stroke

INITIAL HISTORY
- 76-year-old man.
- Describes symptoms starting 30 minutes ago.
- Sudden onset of difficulty getting his mouth to form words; speech is slurred.
- Face and mouth numb; tongue felt "thick."
- Unable to hold his coffee cup in his right hand.
- Right leg weak; needs to hold onto the table to stand.

Question 1   What is your differential diagnosis based on the information you have now?

Question 2   What other questions would you like to ask?

ADDITIONAL HISTORY
- History of essential hypertension.
- Has not been taking his thiazide diuretic because it makes him feel "bad."
- Was told he has high cholesterol but has not returned to see his primary care provider.
- Has experienced several brief spells of right-sided weakness which resolved in a few minutes; thought this was his arm falling asleep.
- No head trauma or recent infections.
- Family history: mother died of stroke, father died of acute myocardial infarction (AMI).
- Smokes 1 pack/day for past 30 years.
- Sedentary lifestyle.

---

*Gail L. Kongable contributed this case study.

Question 3 Now what do you think?

PHYSICAL EXAMINATION

- Alert and anxious white male.
- Slurred speech, uses appropriate words.
- T = 37 C, orally; RR = 16 and regular; HR = 86 and irregular; BP = 190/120 mmHg standing

HEENT

- Conjunctiva is clear without exudate or lesions.
- Fundi is without lesions, nicking, or cotton tufts.
- Nasal mucosa is pink without drainage.
- Oral mucous membranes are moist.
- Pharynx is pink without lesions or exudate.

Skin, Neck

- Pale with senile lentigines, no lesions or bruises.
- No lesions or bruises, no tenting; dry and flaky.
- Supple, no lymphadenopathy or thyromegaly.
- Bruit auscultated over left carotid artery.

Lungs

- Chest expansion is symmetric and full.
- Diaphragmatic excursion is equal at 4 cm.
- Lung sounds are clear to auscultation.

Cardiac

- Heart sounds: irregular; irregular rate and rhythm.
- No murmurs, gallops, or clicks.

Abdomen

- Nondistended; bowel sounds are present and not hyperactive.
- Liver percusses 2 cm below right costal margin but overall 12 cm in size.
- No tenderness or masses.

Extremities

- Cool but good capillary refill at 3 seconds.
- 1+ pitting edema of bilateral ankles.
- Radial artery pulses full and equal; anterior pedal pulses diminished but equal.
- No clubbing.

Neurological
- Alert and oriented.
- Facial droop on right, with loss of nasolabial fold.
- Diminished gag reflex.
- Strength 3/5 in the right upper extremity and 4/5 in the right lower extremity; 5/5 in the left upper and lower extremities.
- Deep tendon reflexes (DTRs) 1+ on right, 2+ on left.
- Sensory intact to touch; no neglect.

Question 4   What studies would you initiate now while preparing your interventions?

Question 5   What therapies would you initiate immediately while awaiting results of the lab studies?

LABORATORY
- ECG; atrial fibrillation.
- Serum glucose 130 mg%.
- PT = 12.5 seconds; PTT = 28 seconds.
- Platelet count 220,000/cubic mm.
- Head CT without contrast was normal.

EMERGENCY ROOM COURSE
- Risks and benefits of thrombolytic therapy are explained to patient and family.
- Patient does not improve neurologically.
- BP responds to labetalol.

PHYSICAL EXAM NOW

- Vital signs
  - BP = 170/86; HR = 100, irregular.
- Neurological exam
  - Alert and oriented.
  - Follows commands.
  - Right hemiparesis worsening; strength is now 2/5 in both the upper and lower extremities on the right, still 5/5 on the left.
  - Moderate dysarthria.
  - Decreased sensation on right.

Question 6   What do you think is happening? Why is the hemiparesis worsening? What does his CT scan mean? Should you continue to treat his hypertension to bring it down to normal?

Question 7   What interventions should be initiated now?

Question 8   Now what should be done and what can the patient expect?

HOSPITAL COURSE

- Patient does well with digoxin 0.125 mg PO daily for atrial fibrillation. He converts to normal sinus rhythm; P = 82, regular.
- Total cholesterol = 270; HDL = 25, ratio 6.6.
- Antihypertensive therapy with an ACE inhibitor is initiated.
- Antiplatelet therapy; aspirin 325 mg PO QID.
- He has not smoked while hospitalized.
- Cardiac echo was normal (no mural thrombus); carotid doppler showed <40% stenosis on right and <50% stenosis on the left with no hemodynamic changes (not a candidate for carotid endarterectomy at this point).

Question 9   What instructions and medication should this patient go home with?

Question 10   What steps can he take to prevent future attacks?

20

Alzheimer Disease

DEFINITION

- Alzheimer disease (AD) is defined as a gradual onset and continuing decline of cognitive function from a previously higher level, resulting in impairment of social and occupational function.
- Impairment of recent memory occurs and at least one of the following:
    - Language disturbances.
    - Word-finding difficulties.
    - Disturbances of praxis.
    - Visual agnosia.
    - Constructional disturbances.
    - Disturbances of executive function, including abstract reasoning and concentration.
- Cognitive deficits are not due to other psychiatric, neurologic, or systemic diseases.
- Cognitive deficits do not exclusively occur in the setting of delirium.

EPIDEMIOLOGY

- Most common dementia of the elderly; 15% lifetime risk in the United States.
- Over the age or 65, 4% to 8% of the population is affected; over the age of 80, 20% of the population is affected.
- Over 4 million people in the United States have AD.
- There are 100,000 deaths per year.
- Risk factors:
    - Increasing age.
    - Female gender.
    - Genetics:
        1) There is an increased risk in siblings; an even greater risk in identical twins.
        2) Most people with trisomy 21 (Down syndrome) will develop AD after age 40.
        3) Several genes have been identified so far:
            a) Abeta-amyloid precursor protein gene (APP) on chromosome 21 (Abeta-amyloid protein fragments found in structural lesions commonly seen in AD brain tissue) (see below).
            b) Presenilin 1 gene (PS1) on chromosome 14; associated with early onset dementia in particular families.
            c) Presenilin 2 gene (PS2) on chromosome 1; associated with early onset dementia in particular families.

   d) Epsilon 4 allele on the apolipoprotein E (ApoE) gene of chromosome 19; heterozygous mutation doubles the risk of AD and occurs in 34% to 65% of people with AD but also occurs in 24% to 31% of people without AD; results in abnormal binding of ApoE protein to tau protein of neurofibrillary tangles and to amyloid-beta proteins of senile plaques (see Fig. 20-1).

   4) There is also evidence for a probable gene locus on chromosome 12 that has yet to be identified.

   5) The primary genetic defect for sporadic AD may be located in the mitochondrial deoxyribonucleic acid (DNA) with defects in intracellular calcium regulation and premature cell death.

 − Head trauma with a loss of consciousness results in a 3-fold increase in risk; the latest studies suggest this is only true if ApoE allele is also present.

 − Estrogen deficiency in postmenopausal women may be a contributing factor to the development of AD. Estrogen replacement improves cognitive function and protects against AD in older women.

 − Other associated risk factors include alcohol abuse, depression, and sleep disturbance.

 − Recent studies have found chlamydia in brain tissue of AD patients at autopsy.

PATHOPHYSIOLOGY

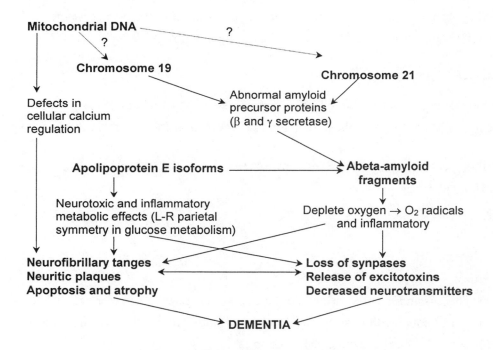

Fig. 20-1 Theories of Alzheimer Pathogenesis

 • There are several structural abnormalities common to AD brain tissue:

 − Neurofibrillary tangles: bundles of filamentous tau proteins in the cytoplasm of neurons.

 − Neuritic plaques: clusters of degenerating nerve-terminals with Abeta-amyloid protein fragments that occur in greatest numbers in the parietal-temporal region and hippocampus (memory).

 − Degeneration of cholinergic neurons.

- Inflammation with the production of toxic oxygen radicals clearly plays a role, and there is some evidence for an autoimmune contribution to the disease process (increased T lymphocytes).

- Excitotoxins (glutamate and aspartate) are found in high levels in the structural lesions of AD, and are known to damage cells.

- Several neurotransmitters are altered; the most important change is a 40% to 90% decrease in choline acetyltransferase with decreased levels of acetylcholine (ACH) occurring even in the first year of dementia symptoms.

- Metabolic changes include decreased parietal glucose metabolism.

- Decreased cerebral perfusion and nitric oxide levels may also play a role.

PATIENT PRESENTATION

History

Often obtained from family; patient may be unaware of changes; family history; history of head trauma; absence of other causes such as heavy alcohol abuse, nutritional deficits, and drug use (illicit or prescribed); seizures; other neurologic complaints (focal weakness or numbness; cerebral or meningeal infections; syphilis; thyroid disease.

Symptoms

Insidious and gradually progressive loss of memory with apraxias, aphasias, and visual and cognitive disturbances; clear consciousness with absence of hallucinations and delusions until late in the disease course; absence of asterixis or tremor.

Examination

Cognitive memory deficits without focal neurologic findings or evidence of delirium or systemic disease as the cause of mental status changes.

DIFFERENTIAL DIAGNOSIS

- Other forms of idiopathic dementia such as Dementia Associated with Lewy Bodies (DLB)
- Depression
- Vascular dementia
- Alcohol and/or drug use
- Pernicious anemia
- Mass lesions
- Thyroid disorders
- Huntington chorea, Creutzfeldt-Jacob disease
- Chronic infection (syphilis, viral [HIV], fungal)
- Toxins (lead)
- Chronic subdural hematoma
- Normal pressure hydrocephalus
- Parkinson disease
- Anoxic brain injury

KEYS TO ASSESSMENT

- Establish dementia using the DSM IV criteria: Use established mental-status tests, such as Information-Orientation-Concentration Test, Mini-Mental State Examination (MMSE), Dementia Rating Scale, Mattis, Blessed Scale, etc.

- Determine "Alzheimer Score" to document severity.

- Rule out treatable causes of dementia:
    - Magnetic resonance imaging (MRI)
    - Electroencephalogram (EEG)
    - B_{12}, thyroid
    - Toxin screens
    - Serology
    - Lumbar puncture (measure CSF Abeta-amyloid and tau proteins, and look for evidence of chronic infection)
    - Review drugs
    - Rule out depression (pseudodementia)

- Differentiate from delirium which has a sudden onset, fluctuating course, reduced consciousness, globally oriented attention, visual hallucinations, fleeting delusions, complete disorientation, reduced or greatly exaggerated activity, incoherent speech, and asterixis or tremor.

- The family is an important source of information about the underlying disease process and for identifying the key issues in patient management.

- Establish the stage of AD progression:
    - Stage I: forget where things are placed, get lost, forget appointments (both recent and remote memory), depression, and anxiety.
    - Stage II: language trouble, spatial disorientation, poor problem solving, confusion, denial.
    - Stage III: aimlessness, hallucinations, agitation, aphasia.

KEYS TO MANAGEMENT

- Prevention and early intervention
    - Although nothing has been proven to prevent Alzheimer's disease, controlling hypertension, preventing and treating cerebrovascular disease, and active participation in cognitive activities, such as reading, have been associated with a decreased risk for dementia.
    - Hormone replacement therapy and the use of nonsteroidal antiinflammatory medications may also decrease risk; studies are ongoing.

- Nonpharmacologic
    - Involve the family early and assess the "caregiver burden" to decide on the need for alternative living options and for monitoring changes in the patient with therapy.
    - Obtain patient participation in drafting advance directives and power of attorney while the patient is still competent.
    - Maintain the socialization of the patient. Walking daily with a care provider has been shown to improve AD patient's cognitive abilities.
    - Prevent injury, especially in later stages when disorientation worsens.

- Maintain good nutrition and exercise.
- Refer families to support organizations.
- Pharmacologic
  - Treating primary cognitive deficits
    1) Tacrine, donepezil, and galanthamine are cholinesterase inhibitors that increase acetylcholine; they provide some improvements in memory, orientation, and ability to care for self, but it is not clear how well these improvements are maintained. The drugs are associated with fatigue, insomnia, and significant gastrointestinal (GI) distress including nausea and diarrhea. Newer cholinergic drugs awaiting approval in the US include rivastigmine, metrifonate, trichlorfon, and physostigmine salicylate.
    2) Nicotine administration has been associated with improved cognition in AD and is being evaluated in studies.
  - Slowing disease progression
    1) N-methyl-D-aspartate (NMDA) antagonists (block the excitotoxins aspartate and glutamate) are being tested without conclusive results so far.
    2) Selegiline (an anti-Parkinson drug) and hydergine (a vasodilator and metabolic enhancer) may slow the rate of functional decline in some patients with AD, but are of unproved benefit; they have few side effects and are well tolerated.
    3) Propentofylline inhibits glutamate release and increases cerebral blood flow; studies have demonstrated cognitive improvements, awaiting approval for use in the US.
    4) There is evidence that antiinflammatory agents (e.g., nonsteroidal antiinflammatories) may slow disease progression, however results with prednisone have not been positive so far.
    5) Antioxidants such as vitamin E (α-tocopherol) and idebenone have shown some promise in slowing functional decline in AD.
    6) Newer estrogen-based compounds are being tested (estrogen promotes neuronal function and cerebral blood flow, but has not been effective in treating AD).
    7) Nerve growth factors prevent cholinergic cell loss and are being intensively studied.
  - Controlling behavior
    1) Neuroleptics may be needed to control behavior, but most are anticholinergic and may worsen cognitive function with many side effects; newer drugs, such as clozapine and risperidone, decrease agitation and psychosis with fewer side effects.
    2) Anxiolytics may help with anxiety and insomnia but often result in confusion and ataxia.
    3) Antidepressants may be indicated for associated depression, but also often have anticholinergic effects. Serotonin uptake inhibitors (fluoxetime, citalopram) are undergoing testing.

Pathophysiology → Clinical Link

What is going on in the disease process that influences how the patient presents and how he or she should be managed?

What should you do now that you understand the underlying pathophysiology?

Genetics of AD are very complicated and polygenic, except in the case of early-onset familial inheritance; the genetic links are still being defined.	Population screening for AD is not possible nor desirable at this time; a family history of early-onset AD (50s or younger) should be investigated.
Decreased acetylcholine is a primary feature of AD pathophysiology.	Tacrine and donepezil probably improve cognition by increasing ACH, but more effective drugs with fewer side effects are needed.
Two protein gene products, Abeta-amyloid protein and ApoE, have been identified as being key components of the structural abnormalities characteristic of AD; there are inflammatory, metabolic, and excitotoxic components to the pathophysiology of AD.	Further understanding of these processes, and identification of others, may lead to more specific AD therapies; numerous trials are underway.
The clinical manifestations of AD, especially in the late stages, can be easily confused with delirium, which is an acute state that requires rapid intervention.	Evaluation for the rapidity of onset of symptoms, amount of agitation, and severity or disorientation and reduced consciousness must be done quickly and carefully to rule out a treatable and potentially life-threatening cause of delirium.
Numerous other causes for dementia exist including vascular disease, depression, chronic infection, endocrine or metabolic disease, and drugs.	The diagnosis of AD is one of exclusion; careful exam and lab analysis is necessary to rule out treatable causes of dementia.
AD occurs in the elderly and is associated with low levels of ACH.	Although caregiver burden is very significant in AD, treatment with neuroleptics, anxiolytics, or antidepressants is associated with considerable toxicity.

Suggested Reading

Adams, T., & Page, S. (2000). New pharmacological treatments for Alzheimer's disease: Implications for dementia care nursing. *Journal of Advanced Nursing, 31,* 1183-1188.

Almkvist, O., Jelic, V., Amberla, K., Lindahl, E., Meurling, L., & Nordberg, A. (2001). Responder characteristics to a single oral dose of cholinesterase inhibitor: A double-blind placebo-controlled study with tacrine in Alzheimer patients. *Dementia & Geriatric Cognitive Disorders, 12,* 22-32.

Askanas, V., & Engel, W. K. (2001). Inclusion-body myositis: Newest concepts of pathogenesis and relation to aging and Alzheimer disease. *Journal of Neuropathology & Experimental Neurology, 60,* 1-14.

Backman, L., Small, B. J., & Fratiglioni, L. (2001). Stability of the preclinical episodic memory deficit in Alzheimer's disease. *Brain, 124*(Pt 1), 96-102.

Behl, C. (1999). Alzheimer's disease and oxidative stress: Implications for novel therapeutic approaches. *Progress in Neurobiology, 57*(3), 301-323.

Birks, J., & Flicker, L. (2000). Selegiline for Alzheimer's disease. *Cochrane Database of Systematic Reviews [computer file],* CD000442.

Birks, J., Iakovidou, V., & Tsolaki, M. (2000). Rivastigmine for Alzheimer's disease. *Cochrane Database of Systematic Reviews [computer file],* CD001191.

Birks, J. S., & Melzer, D. (2000). Donepezil for mild and moderate Alzheimer's disease. *Cochrane Database of Systematic Reviews [computer file],* CD001190.

Blass, J. P., Sheu, R. K., & Gibson, G. E. (2000). Inherent abnormalities in energy metabolism in Alzheimer disease. Interaction with cerebrovascular compromise. *Annals of the New York Academy of Sciences, 903,* 204-221.

Bonilla, E., Tanji, K., Hirano, M., Vu, T. H., DiMauro, S., & Schon, E. A. (1999). Mitochondrial involvement in Alzheimer's disease. *Biochimica et Biophysica Acta, 1410*(2), 171-182.

Cappa, A., Calcagni, M. L., Villa, G., Giordano, A., Marra, C., De Rossi, G., Puopolo, M., & Gainotti, G. (2001). Brain perfusion abnormalities in Alzheimer's disease: Comparison between patients with focal temporal lobe dysfunction and patients with diffuse cognitive impairment. *Journal of Neurology, Neurosurgery & Psychiatry, 70,* 22-27.

Celsis, P. (2000). Age-related cognitive decline, mild cognitive impairment or preclinical Alzheimer's disease? *Annals of Medicine, 32,* 6-14.

Chemerinski, E., Petracca, G., Sabe, L., Kremer, J., & Starkstein, S. E. (2001). The specificity of depressive symptoms in patients with Alzheimer's disease. *American Journal of Psychiatry, 158,* 68-72.

Christen, Y. (2000). Oxidative stress and Alzheimer disease. *American Journal of Clinical Nutrition, 71,* 621S-629S.

Collie, A., & Maruff, P. (2000). The neuropsychology of preclinical Alzheimer's disease and mild cognitive impairment. *Neuroscience & Biobehavioral Reviews, 24,* 365-374.

Cotter, R. L., Burke, W. J., Thomas, V. S., Potter, J. F., Zheng, J., & Gendelman, H. E. (1999). Insights into the neurodegenerative process of Alzheimer's disease: A role for mononuclear phagocyte-associated inflammation and neurotoxicity. *Journal of Leukocyte Biology, 65*(4), 416-427.

Coughlan, C. M., & Breen, K. C. (2000). Factors influencing the processing and function of the amyloid beta precursor protein—A potential therapeutic target in Alzheimer's disease? *Pharmacology & Therapeutics, 86,* 111-145.

Czech, C., Tremp, G., & Pradier, L. (2000). Presenilins and Alzheimer's disease: Biological functions and pathogenic mechanisms. *Progress in Neurobiology, 60,* 363-384.

de la Monte, S. M., Lu, B. X., Sohn, Y. K., Etienne, D., Kraft, J., Ganju, N., & Wands, J. R. (2000). Aberrant expression of nitric oxide synthase III in Alzheimer's disease: Relevance to cerebral vasculopathy and neurodegeneration. *Neurobiology of Aging, 21,* 309-319.

de la Torre, J. C. (2000). Critically attained threshold of cerebral hypoperfusion: The CATCH hypothesis of Alzheimer's pathogenesis. *Neurobiology of Aging, 21,* 331-342.

Doody, R. S. (1999). Clinical profile of donepezil in the treatment of Alzheimer's disease. *Gerontology, 45*(Suppl 1), 23-32.

Dooley, M., & Lamb, H. M. (2000). Donepezil: A review of its use in Alzheimer's disease. *Drugs & Aging, 16,* 199-226.

Drouet, B., Pincon-Raymond, M., Chambaz, J., & Pillot, T. (2000). Molecular basis of Alzheimer's disease. *Cellular & Molecular Life Sciences, 57,* 705-715.

Emilien, G., Beyreuther, K., Masters, C. L., & Maloteaux, J. M. (2000). Prospects for pharmacological intervention in Alzheimer disease. *Archives of Neurology, 57,* 454-459.

Felician, O., & Sandson, T. A. (1999). The neurobiology and pharmacotherapy of Alzheimer's disease. *Journal of Neuropsychiatry & Clinical Neurosciences, 11*(1), 19-31.

Flicker, L., & Grimley, E. J. (2000). Piracetam for dementia or cognitive impairment. *Cochrane Database of Systematic Reviews [computer file],* CD001011.

Flynn, B. L. (1999). Pharmacologic management of Alzheimer disease, part I: Hormonal and emerging investigational drug therapies. *Annals of Pharmacotherapy, 33*(2), 178-187.

Flynn, B. L., & Ranno, A. E. (1999). Pharmacologic management of Alzheimer disease, part II: Antioxidants, antihypertensives, and ergoloid derivatives. *Annals of Pharmacotherapy, 33*(2), 188-197.

George-Hyslop, P. H. (2000). Molecular genetics of Alzheimer's disease. *Biological Psychiatry, 47,* 183-199.

Growdon, J. H. (1999). Biomarkers of Alzheimer disease. *Archives of Neurology, 56*(3), 281-283.

Grundman, M. (2000). Vitamin E and Alzheimer disease: The basis for additional clinical trials. *American Journal of Clinical Nutrition, 71,* 630S-636S.

Halliday, G., Robinson, S. R., Shepherd, C., & Kril, J. (2000). Alzheimer's disease and inflammation: A review of cellular and therapeutic mechanisms. *Clinical & Experimental Pharmacology & Physiology, 27,* 1-8.

Hebert, L. E., Scherr, P. A., McCann, J. J., Beckett, L. A., & Evans, D. A. (2001). Is the risk of developing Alzheimer's disease greater for women than for men? *American Journal of Epidemiology, 153,* 132-136.

Hellstrom-Lindahl, E. (2000). Modulation of beta-amyloid precursor protein processing and tau phosphorylation by acetylcholine receptors. *European Journal of Pharmacology, 393,* 255-263.

Higgins, J. P., & Flicker, L. (2000). Lecithin for dementia and cognitive impairment. *Cochrane Database of Systematic Reviews [computer file],* CD001015.

Huang, X., Cuajungco, M. P., Atwood, C. S., Moir, R. D., Tanzi, R. E., & Bush, A. I. (2000). Alzheimer's disease, beta-amyloid protein and zinc. *Journal of Nutrition, 130,* 1488S-1492S.

Hyman, B. T., Strickland, D., & Rebeck, G. W. (2000). Role of the low-density lipoprotein receptor-related protein in beta-amyloid metabolism and Alzheimer disease. *Archives of Neurology, 57,* 646-650.

Jann, M. W. (2000). Rivastigmine, a new-generation cholinesterase inhibitor for the treatment of Alzheimer's disease. *Pharmacotherapy, 20,* 1-12.

Kalaria, R. N. (2000). The role of cerebral ischemia in Alzheimer's disease. *Neurobiology of Aging, 21,* 321-330.

Kudo, T., Imaizumi, K., Tanimukai, H., Katayama, T., Sato, N., Nakamura, Y., Tanaka, T., Kashiwagi, Y., Jinno, Y., Tohyama, M., & Takeda, M. (2000). Are cerebrovascular factors involved in Alzheimer's disease? *Neurobiology of Aging, 21,* 215-224.

Lehtovirta, M., Laakso, M. P., Frisoni, G. B., & Soininen, H. (2000). How does the apolipoprotein E genotype modulate the brain in aging and in Alzheimer's disease? A review of neuroimaging studies. *Neurobiology of Aging, 21,* 293-300.

Lerner, A. J. (1999). Women and Alzheimer's disease. *Journal of Clinical Endocrinology & Metabolism, 84*(6), 1830-1834.

Levy, E., Sastre, M., Kumar, A., Gallo, G., Piccardo, P., Ghetti, B., & Tagliavini, F. (2001). Codeposition of cystatin C with amyloid-beta protein in the brain of Alzheimer disease patients. *Journal of Neuropathology & Experimental Neurology, 60,* 94-104.

Liddell, M. B., Lovestone, S., & Owen, M. J. (2001). Genetic risk of Alzheimer's disease: Advising relatives. *British Journal of Psychiatry, 178,* 7-11.

Lovestone, S. (1999). Early diagnosis and the clinical genetics of Alzheimer's disease. *Journal of Neurology, 246*(2), 69-72.

McGeer, P. L., & McGeer, E. G. (2000). Autotoxicity and Alzheimer disease. *Archives of Neurology, 57,* 789-790.

Monk, D., & Brodaty, H. (2000). Use of estrogens for the prevention and treatment of Alzheimer's disease. *Dementia & Geriatric Cognitive Disorders, 11,* 1-10.

Mrak, R. E., & Griffin, W. S. (2000). Interleukin-1 and the immunogenetics of Alzheimer disease. *Journal of Neuropathology & Experimental Neurology, 59,* 471-476.

Murer, M. G., Yan, Q., & Raisman-Vozari, R. (2001). Brain-derived neurotrophic factor in the control human brain, and in Alzheimer's disease and Parkinson's disease. *Progress in Neurobiology, 63,* 71-124.

Nishimura, M., Yu, G., & St. George-Hyslop, P.H. (1999). Biology of presenilins as causative molecules for Alzheimer disease. *Clinical Genetics, 55*(4), 219-225.

Nourhashemi, F., Gillette-Guyonnet, S., Andrieu, S., Ghisolfi, A., Ousset, P. J., Grandjean, H., Grand, A., Pous, J., Vellas, B., & Albarede, J. L. (2000). Alzheimer disease: Protective factors. *American Journal of Clinical Nutrition, 71,* 643S-649S.

Olin, J., Schneider, L., Novit, A., & Luczak, S. (2000). Hydergine for dementia. *Cochrane Database of Systematic Reviews [computer file],* CD000359.

Palacios, S., Cifuentes, I., Menendez, C., & von Helde, S. (2000). The central nervous system and HRT. *International Journal of Fertility & Womens Medicine, 45,* 13-21.

Poehlman, E. T., & Dvorak, R. V. (2000). Energy expenditure, energy intake, and weight loss in Alzheimer disease. *American Journal of Clinical Nutrition, 71,* 650S-655S.

Prasad, K. N., Hovland, A. R., Cole, W. C., Prasad, K. C., Nahreini, P., Edwards-Prasad, J., & Andreatta, C. P. (2000). Multiple antioxidants in the prevention and treatment of Alzheimer disease: Analysis of biologic rationale. *Clinical Neuropharmacology, 23,* 2-13.

Prior, R., Wihl, G., & Urmoneit, B. (2000). Apolipoprotein E, smooth muscle cells and the pathogenesis of cerebral amyloid angiopathy: The potential role of impaired cerebrovascular A beta clearance. *Annals of the New York Academy of Sciences, 903,* 180-186.

Qizilbash, N., Birks, J., Lopez-Arrieta, J., Lewington, S., & Szeto, S. (2000). Tacrine for Alzheimer's disease. *Cochrane Database of Systematic Reviews [computer file],* CD000202.

Richards, S. S., & Hendrie, H. C. (1999). Diagnosis, management, and treatment of Alzheimer disease: A guide for the internist. *Archives of Internal Medicine, 159*(8), 789-798.

Rohn, T. T., Head, E., Su, J. H., Anderson, A. J., Bahr, B. A., Cotman, C. W., & Cribbs, D. H. (2001). Correlation between caspase activation and neurofibrillary tangle formation in Alzheimer's disease. *American Journal of Pathology, 158,* 189-198.

Sasaki, N., Toki, S., Chowei, H., Saito, T., Nakano, N., Hayashi, Y., Takeuchi, M., & Makita, Z. (2001). Immunohistochemical distribution of the receptor for advanced glycation end products in neurons and astrocytes in Alzheimer's disease. *Brain Research, 888,* 256-262.

Schmidt, R., Schmidt, H., & Fazekas, F. (2000). Vascular risk factors in dementia. *Journal of Neurology, 247,* 81-87.

Thomas, T. (2000). Monoamine oxidase-B inhibitors in the treatment of Alzheimer's disease. *Neurobiology of Aging, 21,* 343-348.

Thompson, C. & Briggs, M. (2000). Support for carers of people with Alzheimer's type dementia. *Cochrane Database of Systematic Reviews [computer file],* CD000454.

VanDenBerg, C. M., Kazmi, Y., & Jann, M. W. (2000). Cholinesterase inhibitors for the treatment of Alzheimer's disease in the elderly. *Drugs & Aging, 16,* 123-138.

Vickers, J. C., Dickson, T. C., Adlard, P. A., Saunders, H. L., King, C. E., & McCormack, G. (2000). The cause of neuronal degeneration in Alzheimer's disease. *Progress in Neurobiology, 60,* 139-165.

Yanagisawa, K. (2000). Neuronal death in Alzheimer's disease. *Internal Medicine, 39,* 328-330.

Case Study*

Alzheimer Disease

INITIAL HISTORY

- 76-year-old woman.
- Told daughter she had not been feeling well.
- Shopping for groceries with daughter.
- Became separated in the aisles.
- Became confused and angry when store employees and others tried to assist her.
- Now 30 minutes later.

Question 1   What is your differential diagnosis based on the information you now have?

Question 2   What other questions would you like to ask now? (These questions should be asked of the patient first, and then of a reliable historian separately.)

_____

*Gail L. Kongable contributed this case study.

ADDITIONAL HISTORY
- The daughter has noticed increased anxiety and confusion in her mother on several occasions.
- No personal or family history of psychological illness.
- Daughter describes language problems, such as trouble finding words.
- Problems with abstract thinking.
- Poor or decreased judgment.
- Disorientation in place and time.
- Changes in mood and behavior.
- Changes in personality.

FURTHER HISTORY
- No history of trauma or recent infection.
- Family history: father and brother have died from stroke and heart disease; mother had Alzheimer disease.
- Current medications: aspirin, 325 mg daily; hydrochlorothiazide, 25 mg BID.
- No other medical history.
- No known allergies.

Question 3 Now what do you think about her history?

PHYSICAL EXAMINATION
- Alert elderly woman in no acute distress.
- T = 37 orally; P = 85 and regular; RR = 15 and unlabored; BP 158/88 right arm sitting.

HEENT, Skin, Neck
- Pupils are small and react to light sluggishly.
- Ocular fundus is pale; vessels are narrow and attenuated.
- Dentures present, buccal and pharyngeal membranes are moist without lesions or exudate.
- Pale, dry with senile lentigines.
- Transparent with decreased turgor.
- Minor multiple ecchymosis noted on forearms.
- No other lesions or abrasions.
- No lymphadenopathy, no thyromegaly.
- Trachea is midline.
- Carotid pulses full and equal bilaterally without bruit.
- No jugular venous distension.

Lungs
- Increased anterior/posterior diameter, with mild kyphosis.
- No shortness of breath.
- Lungs clear to auscultation throughout, bilaterally.

Cardiac
- Apical pulse at 5th ICS, L MCL.
- Regular rate and rhythm.
- Normal S_1, S_2; no murmurs, clicks, or rubs.

Abdomen, Extremities, Neurological
- Round, symmetric with no apparent masses or hernias.
- No scars or lesions.
- Bowel sounds present; no bruits.
- Tympany to percussion in all quadrants; no masses or organomegaly.
- No redness, cyanosis, skin lesions.
- Symmetric with no swelling or atrophy.
- Warm bilaterally.
- All pulses present and equal bilaterally.
- No lymphadenopathy.
- Orientation to person, time, and place inconsistent.
- Pinprick, light touch, vibration intact; able to identify a key.
- Motor: no atrophy, weakness or tremor; rapid alternating movements smooth.
- DTRs all 2+.
- No Babinski.

Musculoskeletal
- Gait slightly wide based; unable to tandem walk.
- No Romberg.
- Joints and muscles symmetric; no swelling, masses, deformities, tenderness.
- Mild kyphosis of the spine.
- Joints: full, smooth range of motion; no crepitance, tenderness.
- Extremities: able to maintain flexion and extension against resistance without tenderness.

Question 4   What studies would you initiate now while preparing your interventions?

Question 5 What therapies would you initiate immediately while awaiting result of the lab studies?

LABORATORY RESULTS

- Head CT scan showed one small capsular infarction, no mass lesion or edema, no hydrocephalus.
- No significant abnormal results of chemistry, hematology, and metabolic screens.
- MMSE findings of impairment of memory and three other cognitive areas.
- Geriatric Depression Scale (GDS) is positive for memory difficulty, disrupted sleep-wake cycle, apathy, increased dependence (classic for Alzheimer disease).

Question 6 What does Alzheimer dementia look like on CT scan?

EMERGENCY ROOM COURSE

- Patient is cooperative, in no apparent distress.
- Becomes less confused with repeated explanation of circumstances.
- Physical exam now unchanged.
- No repeat lab studies.

Question 7 What do you think is happening?

Question 8   Now what should be done and what can the patient expect?

HOSPITAL COURSE

- Response to therapy: stable condition.
- Discharged to home in the care of daughter after 24 hours.

Question 9   What instructions and medications should this patient go home with?

Question 10   What steps can she take to prevent future problems?

21

Epilepsy*

DEFINITION

- Epilepsy, as defined by the Commission on Epidemiology and Prognosis of Epilepsy, is the occurrence of at least two unprovoked seizures with at least a 24-hour separation between those seizures.

- Neither seizures nor epilepsy is a diagnosis or disease entity itself; it is a symptom of other processes that affect the brain in a variety of ways, but has the final common clinical expression of a seizure.

- Seizures are the cardinal manifestation of epilepsy, though not all patients with seizures have epilepsy.

- A seizure is an excessive or abnormal sudden, high frequency discharge of the brain's neurons.

- Status epilepticus is defined as continuous or repeating seizures that occur so rapidly that the patient does not recover consciousness between them.

CLASSIFICATION

- The diagnosis, treatment, and prognosis of seizure disorders depend on the correct identification of types of seizures and epilepsy. There are two currently accepted classification schemes, the International Classification of Epileptic Seizures [ICES] and the International Classification of Epilepsies and Epileptic Syndromes [ICEES].

- **Overview of ICES**
    - Partial seizures begin in a focal or restricted part of the cortex.
        1) Simple partial seizures: consciousness is not impaired. They are further subdivided into various categories based on signs and symptoms produced by the seizure.
        2) Complex partial seizures: consciousness is impaired. Complex partial seizures can arise from any cortical area, yet they are frequently considered equivalent to temporal lobe seizures; they are frequently preceded by an aura.
        3) Partial seizures may evolve into secondarily generalized seizures. The secondarily generalized seizures are usually tonic-clonic.
    - Generalized seizures begin with epileptiform activity over the entire cortex.
        1) Absence seizures are brief generalized seizures without prominent motor manifestations and are typically associated with a generalized 3-Hz spike-and-wave pattern on the electroencephalogram (EEG).
        2) Myoclonic seizures appear as singular or successive shock-like body jerks; the EEG would show generalized discharges.

---

*Lucy R. Paskus and Valentina L. Brashers contributed this chapter.

4) Tonic seizures cause sudden, sustained tone, and are frequently manifested as flexor or extensor posturing. They may be accompanied by a guttural cry as air is forced out of closed vocal cords.

5) Tonic-clonic seizures often evolve from tonic to clonic movements and may be preceded by brief myoclonic or clonic activity.

6) Atonic seizures, also know as "drop attacks," result from a sudden brief loss of tone.

- Unclassified epileptic seizures may not always fall clearly into one category in practice, although it is important to remember that a single patient may present with several different seizure types.

- **Overview of ICEES**
  - Like ICES, ICEES divides seizure types into partial, generalized, and undetermined. While ICES categorizes seizure type, ICEES expands this classification scheme to include more information about the cause and clinical manifestations of the seizure. Subcategories of the epilepsies and epileptic syndromes include the following:
    1) Idiopathic: most common; no obvious underlying cause or pathological alteration other than a presumed genetic predisposition.
    2) Symptomatic: occur as a result of a defined cerebral disorder.
    3) Cryptogenic: suspected to be symptomatic despite absence of definitive proof of the underlying cause.

- Both the ICES and ICEES are useful but they also they have their limitations. Both are so detailed as to be impractical for most nonneurologists; new classification schemes are being proposed.

EPIDEMIOLOGY

- Epilepsy is one of the most common chronic neurological disorders in the United States, with a prevalence of approximately 0.5%.

- The cumulative lifetime risk of having a seizure is 8%.

- Half the lifetime risk of developing epilepsy occurs during childhood or adolescence.

- During childhood, rates are highest during the first year of life and then drop sharply; rates drop off again during adolescence; over age 50, the rate of epilepsy begins to increase again, secondary to cerebrovascular disease and cerebral vascular accidents.

- The mortality rate of a patient with epilepsy is 2 to 4 times the nonepileptic population, with the mortality being highest in the 10 years after diagnosis.

- 10% of deaths in patients with epilepsy are directly related to a seizure or status epilepticus, while 5% of deaths are secondary to a fatal accident during a seizure.

- The suicide risk in people with epilepsy is 25 times that of the general population.

PATHOPHYSIOLOGY

- A few of the familial epilepsies have been found to have a genetic basis, with mutations in the ion channels that modulate neuronal firing; however, for the vast majority of the epilepsies a genetic link has yet to be discovered.

- One or more of the following mechanisms are postulated to be involved in the genesis and spread of epileptic discharges.
  - Disturbances in the excitation/inhibition balance in the hypothalamus is thought to be a major factor in the etiology of epilepsy.

1) Excitatory amino acids (EAAs) are in a physiologic balance with the inhibitory neurotransmitters.

2) Glutamate, an EAA, is the primary excitatory neurotransmitter in the central nervous system and acts primarily through activation of the N-methyl-D-aspartate (NMDA) receptors.

3) Gamma-amniobutyric acid (GABA) is the primary inhibitory neurotransmitter.

4) Both decreased GABAergic inhibition and an increase in glutamatergic excitation are thought to be critically involved in the cellular mechanisms underlying the initiation and spread of epileptic seizures and the processes that lead to epileptogenesis and, as a consequence, chronic epilepsy.

5) Many new antiepileptic drugs (AEDs) are targeted at enhancing GABA activity. While currently available NMDA antagonists are excessively neurotoxic, studies are ongoing to evaluate newer drugs aimed at inhibiting glutamate activity.

- Changes in voltage-regulated ion channels in neuronal membranes that lead to excessive depolarization or excessive action potential firing. Potential ion channel defects include voltage sensitive calcium-, potassium-, or sodium-channels and sodium/hydrogen exchangers.

- Changes in gap junctions result in altered interneuronal communication and changes in neural synchrony. These gap junctions are influenced by serum pH (alkalosis tends to stimulate epileptogenic communication, while acidosis inhibits it) but there are no current pharmacologic therapies that target the gap junction. A ketogenic diet may affect the gap junction by altering pH.

PATIENT PRESENTATION

History

Positive family history of seizures; febrile seizures as a child; head injury; CNS infection; stroke; heart disease; reported lapses of consciousness; episodes of incontinence; seizure activity witnessed by others; history of motor vehicle accidents or other unexplained injuries; alcohol or drug abuse or toxicity.

Symptoms

Localized seizure-like movements on one part of the body; episodic loss of consciousness; focal neurologic deficits; visual changes; headache; confusion; incontinence, tongue-biting; fatigue; tearfulness; incontinence; symptoms from injuries.

Examination

Between seizures, the exam may be completely normal; witnessed seizures allow for confirmation of the diagnosis; focal neurologic findings; evidence of injury; evidence of drug or alcohol abuse.

DIFFERENTIAL DIAGNOSIS

- Not seizures
  - Syncope: cardiac disease, orthostatic blood pressure changes, vasovagal episodes.
  - Psychogenic "seizures;" parasomnias; somatoform disorder; malingering; factitious disorder (eg. Munchausen's syndrome).
  - Migraines.
- Not epilepsy
  - Alcohol abuse/withdrawal.
  - Vascular pathology (transient ischemic attacks, stroke).
  - Tumor.

- Drug induced: antipsychotics, theophylline, tricyclic antidepressants, meperidine, cyclosporin, cisplatin, and beta-lactam antibiotics can cause seizures at therapeutic doses.

- Drug withdrawal: anticonvulsants, benzodiazepines, barbiturates, and baclofen.

- Metabolic disarray: hypoglycemia, hypo-/hypernatremia, hypo-/hypercalcemia

- Anoxia: cardiac arrest, carbon monoxide poisoning, asphyxiation.

- Fever: more common in young children.

- Infections.

- Cranial trauma.

- Eclampsia.

KEYS TO ASSESSMENT

- Goals of evaluation are as follows:

  - Verify that a seizure has occurred.

    1) Epilepsy is essentially a clinical diagnosis and more than one witnessed classical generalized tonic-clonic convulsion or many absences can be diagnostic of epilepsy.

    2) Obtain a detailed patient interview and, if possible, an interview of those who witnessed the seizure; these subjective accounts can assist in differential diagnosis, as well as establishing seizure type.

  - Rapidly identify potential life-threatening causes (trauma, myocardial infarction, stroke, metabolic disarray, drug toxicity).

    1) When a seizure occurs within well-defined circumstances, such as a stroke or head injury, the focus should be on treating the underlying cause and preventing seizure recurrence.

    2) An urgent metabolic and toxic screening is necessary for every patient presenting with a first generalized seizure, with particular attention paid to natremia and glycemia.

  - When the patient is known to have epilepsy and is under treatment, a seizure should not be managed in the atmosphere of an emergency; priority should be placed understanding what triggered the seizure (e.g., improper medication use, alcohol, skipped meals, sleep deprivation, stress, fever).

  - Physical examination should include a thorough neurological exam to look for focal deficits.

    1) When the neuro exam is abnormal, magnetic resonance imaging (MRI) becomes urgent.

    2) Following a normal neuro exam, patients should have an EEG and magnetic resonance imaging (MRI) on an outpatient basis; the MRI scheduled as soon as possible if the EEG shows abnormal activity.

  - EEG:

    1) EEG is essential to appropriately categorize and manage epilepsy.

    2) In an isolated first seizure, EEG findings may be of little value in predicting risk of recurrence, but may be used in deciding when to initiate treatment with AEDs.

    3) Incidence of epileptiform activity in people without seizures is 0% to 3.8%.

    4) Many patients with epilepsy have a normal EEG on one or more occasion.

    5) Repetition of EEGs and the use of different activations (hyperventilation, photic stimulation, sleep) increase the chances of finding paroxysmal activity in epileptic patients.

    6) The interictal EEG recording is an important localizing and prognostic tool in epilepsy surgery evaluation.

- MRI:

  1) Demonstrates structural lesions, though not necessarily epileptogenic focus.

  2) Crucial in presurgical evaluation.

  3) Experimental fMRI (functional MRI) and MRSI (MR spectroscopic imaging).

- Positron emission tomography (PET) identifies the foci of epileptogenesis as an area of interictal hypometabolism.

- Single photon emission computed tomography (SPECT) measures distribution of blood flow; can be applied during seizures since tracers can be mixed at the bedside.

KEYS TO MANAGEMENT

- **Pharmacologic**

  - In a patient with one seizure and without risk factors for recurrence (prior neurologic injury or lesions, history of epilepsy in a sibling, or an EEG with generalized epileptiform discharges), it is reasonable to withhold anti-epileptic drugs (AEDs) if the patient is willing and informed.

  - After a second seizure, the risk for recurrence is 80% to 90% and the patient must be treated with AEDs.

  - The common link among older and new AEDs is their ability to moderate excitatory and inhibitory neurotransmission by affecting several different sites, such as ion channels, neurotransmitter receptors, and neurotransmitter metabolism. Some of the more commonly used older and new AEDs are:

OLDER AEDs	NEW AEDs
Phenytoin	Felbamate
Carbamazepine	Gabapentin
Phenobarbital	Lamotrigine
Valproic acid	Tiagabine
Benzodiazepines	Topiramate
	Vigabatin
	Zonisamide

  - Initial therapy for epilepsy is monotherapy.

  - Approximately 70% of patients can achieve seizure control with AEDs.

  - Dosing of medications:

    1) A very low dose is used for the first few days, then a gradual increase.

    2) Generalized tonic-clonic seizures typically require a lower dose than partial seizures.

    3) There are increased adverse drug reactions with an increased dose.

    4) The final decision about which dose is appropriate will take into account the individual characteristics of the patient; a complete and detailed medical and social history is helpful in choosing the appropriate AED.

    5) The best AED is the one that controls seizures without causing unacceptable side effects.

    6) The nature of the seizure that the patient is experiencing, as well as the specific epileptic syndrome, may influence the choice of AED.

- Use of AEDs in women:

  1) Cosmetic consequences of epilepsy therapy include weight gain or weight loss, hair growth on face and arms or hair loss, facial acne, and gingival hypertrophy.

  2) There is the potential for catamenial epilepsy (seizures associated with menstrual cycle) related to relative lack of progesterone during luteal phase of cycle (estrogen is proconvulsant, and progesterone is anti-convulsant).

  3) There is often a decreased effectiveness of oral contraceptives (oral contraceptives should contain at least 50 micrograms of estrogen).

  4) Seizure frequency may be increased during pregnancy.

  5) In children born to women with epilepsy, there is an increased risk for infant mortality, congenital malformation, low birth weight, developmental delays and neonatal hemorrhage (important to supplement with vitamin K during last month of pregnancy).

- The role of plasma drug concentrations:

  1) Routine drug monitoring is not recommended at this time, however, drug levels may provide important references in adjusting dosages, ruling out noncompliance, and toxicity.

  2) Many of the new AEDs demonstrate marked inter- and intra-individual pharmacodynamic variability and the role of therapeutic drug monitoring is being explored.

- Polypharmacy in drug-resistant epilepsy:

  1) Polypharmacy is generally utilized after failure of successive monotherapy.

  2) Combine drugs with different mechanisms of action.

  3) Avoid drugs with similar adverse effects.

- Deciding when to stop drug therapy in the seizure-free patient:

  1) A patient on monotherapy who has been seizure free more than 2 years may be a candidate for drug withdrawal.

  2) An abnormal EEG suggests a poor prognosis of successful medication withdrawal.

  3) Implications of drug withdrawal should be discussed with the patient, especially the probability of relapse.

  4) If withdrawal is indicated and agreed upon, it should take place gradually over no less than 6 months.

- **Surgical**

  - Surgery is typically reserved for those patients who fail medical management but is probably underused in the management of refractory epilepsy.

  - There must be a well-localized epileptogenic focus and the focus must be located such that the surgery would not result in severe speech or memory deficits.

  - The prototype of surgically remediable epilepsy syndromes is temporal lobe epilepsy; one of the most common forms of epilepsy and also one of the most refractory.

  - Pediatric epilepsy surgery is increasing secondary to the delineation of certain catastrophic epileptic disorders of infants and young children, and the greater understanding of the plasticity of the developing brain.

Pathophysiology → Clinical Link

What is going on in the disease process that influences how the patient presents and how he or she should be managed?

What should you do now that you understand the underlying pathophysiology?

Seizures are categorized by their clinical appearance and EEG pattern; these categories are correlated with prognosis and response to medication.	A careful history of a seizure from observers, as well as an EEG, is essential to the appropriate identification of the seizure type and selection of the proper drug.
Seizures are most likely the result of an imbalance of excitatory (glutamate) and inhibitory (GABA) neurotransmitters and/or abnormal ionic exchange at the neuronal membrane.	The older AEDs work primarily by stabilizing neuronal membrane ionic activity; the newer drugs are aimed at modulating glutamate and/or GABA activity.
Seizures can result from many causes, including anoxia, space-occupying lesions, infarctions, toxins, metabolic disarray, trauma, and infections.	A thorough evaluation with special emphasis on the neurologic exam and laboratories is essential in the new-onset seizure patient, and a MRI should be done quickly if there is any evidence of localized neurologic disease.
An EEG can be abnormal in people without epilepsy and can be normal in patients with epilepsy.	The EEG is most useful in the evaluation of new-onset seizures if it can be correlated by observed epileptic activity; thus, activators, such as sleep deprivation, hyperventilation, and photic stimulation with observation of the patient, may be indicated to confirm the diagnosis.
The efficacy and side effects of the AEDs varies significantly between individual patients.	The selection of appropriate pharmacologic management must also be based on psychosocial information obtained from the patient and family.
Hormone changes in women through the menstrual cycle, with the use of oral contraceptives, and with pregnancy are associated with an increased risk of seizures. In addition, epilepsy and the use of AEDs during pregnancy is associated with many potential complications for the infant.	Women with epilepsy require a high level of vigilance for potential complications, and expert management of especially during pregnancy.

Suggested Reading

Adab, N., Jacoby, A., Smith, D., & Chadwick, D. (2001). Additional educational needs in children born to mothers with epilepsy. *Journal of Neurology, Neurosurgery & Psychiatry, 70,* 15-21.

Arunkumar, G., & Morris H. (1998). Epilepsy update: New medical and surgical treatment options. *Cleveland Clinic Journal of Medicine, 65*(10), 527-32, 534-537.

Austin, J. K., Harezlak, J., Dunn, D. W., Huster, G. A., Rose, D. F., & Ambrosius, W. T. (2001). Behavior problems in children before first recognized seizures. *Pediatrics, 107,* 115-122.

Beaumont, A., & Whittle, I. R. (2000). The pathogenesis of tumour associated epilepsy. *Acta Neurochirurgica, 142*(1), 1-15.

Berg, A. T., Shinnar, S., Levy, S. R., Testa, F. M., Smith-Rapaport, S., Beckerman, B., & Ebrahimi, N. (2001). Defining early seizure outcomes in pediatric epilepsy: The good, the bad and the in-between. *Epilepsy Research, 43,* 75-84.

Bernard, C., Cossart, R., Hirsch, J. C., Esclapez, M., & Ben Ari, Y. (2000). What is GABAergic inhibition? How is it modified in epilepsy? *Epilepsia, 41*(Suppl 6), S90-S95.

Binnie, C. D. (2000). Vagus nerve stimulation for epilepsy: A review. *Seizure, 9*(3), 161-169.

Bowman, E. S., & Coons, P. M. (2000). The differential diagnosis of epilepsy, pseudoseizures, dissociative identity disorder, and dissociative disorder not otherwise specified. *Bulletin of the Menninger Clinic, 64*(2), 164-180.

Boylan, L. S. (2001). Postictal psychosis related regional cerebral hyperfusion. *Journal of Neurology, Neurosurgery & Psychiatry, 70,* 137-138.

Briellmann, R. S., Jackson, G. D., Torn-Broers, Y., & Berkovic, S. F. (2001). Causes of epilepsies: Insights from discordant monozygous twins. *Annals of Neurology, 49,* 45-52.

Burgess, D. L., & Noebels, J. L. (2000). Calcium channel defects in models of inherited generalized epilepsy. *Epilepsia, 41*(8), 1074-1075.

Carlen, P. L., Skinner, F., Zhang, L., Naus, C., Kushnir, M., & Perez Velazquez, I. J. (2000). The role of gap junctions in seizures. *Brain Research–Brain Research Reviews, 32*(1), 235-241.

Chapman, A. G. (2000). Glutamate and epilepsy. *Journal of Nutrition, 130*(4S), 1043S-1045S.

Coulter, D. A. (2001). Epilepsy-associated plasticity in gamma-aminobutyric acid receptor expression, function, and inhibitory synaptic properties. *International Review of Neurobiology, 45,* 237-252.

Cramer, J. A., Fisher, R., Ben Menachem, E., French, J., & Mattson, R. H. (1999). New antiepileptic drugs: Comparison of key clinical trials. *Epilepsia, 40*(5), 590-600.

Devinsky, O. (1999). Patients with refractory seizures. *New England Journal of Medicine, 340*(20), 1565-1570.

Dubeau, F., & McLachlan, R. S. (2000). Invasive electrographic recording techniques in temporal lobe epilepsy. *Canadian Journal of Neurological Sciences, 27*(Suppl 1), S29-S34.

Engel, J., Jr. (1999). The timing of surgical intervention for mesial temporal lobe epilepsy: A plan for a randomized clinical trial. *Archives of Neurology, 56*(11), 1338-1341.

Ensom, M. H. (2000). Gender-based differences and menstrual cycle-related changes in specific diseases: Implications for pharmacotherapy. *Pharmacotherapy, 20*(5), 523-539.

Feely, M. (1999). Fortnightly review: Drug treatment of epilepsy. *British Medical Journal, 318*(7176), 106-109.

Fowle, A. J., & Binnie, C. D. (2000). Uses and abuses of the EEG in epilepsy. *Epilepsia, 41*(Suppl 3), S10-S8l.

Gordon, N. (2000). Cognitive functions and epileptic activity. *Seizure, 9*(3), 184-188.

Greenwood, R. S. (2000). Adverse effects of antiepileptic drugs. *Epilepsia, 41*(Suppl 2), S42-S52.

Greenwood, R. S., & Tennison, M. B. (1999). When to start and stop anticonvulsant therapy in children. *Archives of Neurology, 56*(9), 1073-1077.

Hirose, S., Okada, M., Kaneko, S., & Mitsudome, A. (2000). Are some idiopathic epilepsies disorders of ion channels? A working hypothesis. *Epilepsy Research, 41*(3), 191-204.

Jones, M. W., & Anderman, F. (2000). Temporal lobe epilepsy surgery: Definition of candidacy. *Canadian Journal of Neurological Sciences, 27*(Suppl 1), S11-S13.

Juhasz, C., Chugani, D. C., Muzik, O., Watson, C., Shah, J., Shah, A., & Chugani, H. T. (2000). Relationship between EEG and positron emission tomography abnormalities in clinical epilepsy. *Journal of Clinical Neurophysiology, 17*(1), 29-42.

Krumholz, A. (1999). Nonepileptic seizures: Diagnosis and management. *Neurology, 53*(5 Suppl 2), S76-S83.

Lester, H. A., & Karschin, A. (2000). Gain of function mutants: Ion channels and G protein-coupled receptors. *Annual Review of Neuroscience, 23,* 89-125.

Logsdon-Pokorny, V. K. (2000). Epilepsy in adolescents: Hormonal considerations. *Journal of Pediatric & Adolescent Gynecology, 13*(1), 9-13.

Loscher, W. (1998). Pharmacology of glutamate receptor antagonists in the kindling model of epilepsy. *Progress in Neurobiology, 54*(6), 721-741.

Mattson, R. H. (1998). Medical management of epilepsy in adults. *Neurology, 51*(5 Suppl 4), S15-S20.

McAbee, G. N., & Wark, J. E. (2000). A practical approach to uncomplicated seizures in children. *American Family Physician, 62*(5), 1109-1116.

Morrell, M. J. (1999). Epilepsy in women: The science of why it is special. *Neurology, 53*(4 Suppl 1), S42-S48.

Moshe, S. L. (2000). Mechanisms of action of anticonvulsant agents. *Neurology, 55*(5 Suppl 1), S32-S40.

Nsour, W. M., Lau, C. B. S., & Wong, I. C. (2000). Review on phytotherapy in epilepsy. *Seizure, 9*(2), 96-107.

Owens, D. F. & Kriegstein, A. R. (2001). Maturation of channels and receptors: Consequences for excitability. *International Review of Neurobiology, 45,* 43-87.

Pachlatko, C. (1999). The relevance of health economics to epilepsy care. *Epilepsia, 40*(Suppl 8), S3-S7.

Parrent, A. G., & Lozano, A. M. (2000). Stereotactic surgery for temporal lobe epilepsy. *Canadian Journal of Neurological Sciences, 27*(Suppl 1), S79-S84.

Pellock, J. M. (1999). Managing pediatric epilepsy syndromes with new antiepileptic drugs. *Pediatrics, 104*(5 Pt 1), 1106-1116.

Perucca, E. (2000). Is there a role for therapeutic drug monitoring of new anticonvulsants? *Clinical Pharmacokinetics, 38*(3), 191-204.

Pimentel, J. (2000). Current issues on epileptic women. *Current Pharmaceutical Design, 6*(8), 865-872.

Prasad, A. N., Prasad, C., & Stafstrom, C. E. (1999). Recent advances in the genetics of epilepsy: Insights from human and animal studies. *Epilepsia, 40*(10), 1329-1352.

Rho, J. M., & Sankar, R. (1999). The pharmacologic basis of antiepileptic drug action. *Epilepsia, 40*(11), 1471-1483.

Rogawski, M. A. (2000). KCNQ2/KCNQ3 K+ channels and the molecular pathogenesis of epilepsy: Implications for therapy. *Trends in Neurosciences, 23*(9), 393-398.

Schramm, J., Kral, T., Grunwald, T., & Blumcke, I. (2001). Surgical treatment for neocortical temporal lobe epilepsy: Clinical and surgical aspects and seizure outcome. *Journal of Neurosurgery, 94,* 33-42.

Silfvenius, H. (1999). Cost and cost-effectiveness of epilepsy surgery. *Epilepsia, 40*(Suppl 8), S32-S39.

Sloviter, R. S. (1999). Status epilepticus-induced neuronal injury and network reorganization. *Epilepsia, 40*(Suppl 1), S34-S39.

So, E. L. (2000). Integration of EEG, MRI, and SPECT in localizing the seizure focus for epilepsy surgery *Epilepsia, 40*(Suppl 1), S34-39.

So, E. L., O'Brien, T. J., Brinkmann, B. H., & Mullan, B. P. (2000). The EEG evaluation of single photon emission computed tomography abnormalities in epilepsy. *Journal of Clinical Neurophysiology, 17*(1), 10-28.

Stephen, L. J., & Brodie, M. J. (2000). Epilepsy in elderly people. *Lancet, 355*(9213), 1441-1446.

Swann, J. W., Lee, C. L., Smith, K. L., & Hrachovy, R. A. (2000). Developmental neuroplasticity and epilepsy. *Epilepsia, 41*(8), 1078-1079.

Swann, J. W., Smith, K. L., & Lee, C. L. (2001). Neuronal activity and the establishment of normal and epileptic circuits during brain development. *International Review of Neurobiology, 45,* 89-118.

Teyler, T. J., Morgan, S. L., Russell, R. N., & Woodside, B. L. (2001). Synaptic plasticity and secondary epileptogenesis. *International Review of Neurobiology, 45,* 253-267.

Tomson, T. (2000). Mortality in epilepsy. *Journal of Neurology, 247*(1), 15-21.

Tomson, T., & Johannessen, S. I. (2000). Therapeutic monitoring of the new antiepileptic drugs. *European Journal of Clinical Pharmacology, 55*(10), 697-705.

Tuxhorn, I., Moch, A., & Holthausen, H. (2000). Pediatric epilepsy surgery: State of the art, recent developments and future perspectives. *Epileptic Disorders, 2*(1), 53-55.

Waagepetersen, H. S., Sonnewald, U., & Schousboe, A. (1999). The GABA paradox: Multiple roles as metabolite, neurotransmitter, and neurodifferentiative agent. *Journal of Neurochemistry, 73*(4), 1335-1342.

Wada, J. A. (2001). Epilepsy as a progressive (or nonprogressive "benign") disorder. *International Review of Neurobiology, 45,* 481-504.

Wiebe, S. (2000). Epidemiology of temporal lobe epilepsy. *Canadian Journal of Neurological Sciences, 27*(Suppl 1), S6-S10.

Willmore, L.J. (1998). Epilepsy emergencies: The first seizure and status epilepticus. *Neurology, 51*(5 Suppl 4), S34-38.

Yerby, M. S. (2000). Quality of life, epilepsy advances, and the evolving role of anticonvulsants in women with epilepsy. *Neurology, 55*(5 Suppl 1), S54-58.

Case Study*

Epilepsy

INITIAL HISTORY

- 15-year-old boy.
- Playing touch football when symptoms developed.
- Was tackled and became unreasonably angry at his friend.
- Fell to the ground with sudden onset of unconsciousness.
- Body stiffened with arms and legs extended.
- Did not breathe for about 10 seconds.
- Began violent, rhythmic, muscular contractions accompanied by strenuous hyperventilation which lasted 2 to 3 minutes.
- Incontinent of urine.
- Lay limp, breathing quietly, and woke up confused.
- Now 1 hour later in the emergency room.

Question 1   What is your differential diagnosis based on the information you now have?

Question 2   What other questions would you like to ask now?

---

*Gail L. Kongable contributed this case study.**

ADDITIONAL HISTORY

- No memory of the event; first memory was of finding himself on the ground.
- No history of seizures.
- Denies taking any drugs or alcohol.
- No recent upper respiratory or other infections.
- History of minor head injury as a child with loss of consciousness.
- Had complained of headache to his mother earlier in the day.
- No nausea or vomiting.
- Had been having a stressful time in school.
- Older sister had a seizure with high fever at age 3, none since.

Question 3   What do you think about his history?

PHYSICAL EXAMINATION

- Alert but tired teenager in no apparent distress.
- BP = 115/72 mmHg, sitting; T = 37 orally; P = 72, regular; RR = 14, regular and unlabored.

Skin, HEENT

- Pink, warm, dry; no lesions or abrasions.
- .Conjunctiva pink, moist.
- Visual acuity 20/20 without glasses.
- Fundi without lesions or hemorrhages.
- Nasal mucosa pink, moist without lesions, no exudate.
- Bite wound left lateral tongue, no exudate.
- Pharynx pink without exudate.

Neck

- Supple.
- No adenopathy, no thyromegaly.
- No bruits.

Lungs

- Chest expansion full, symmetrical.
- Normal diaphragmatic position and excursion.
- Lung sounds clear to auscultation throughout all lobes bilaterally.

Cardiac
- Apical pulse palpated at 4th intercostal space, midclavicular line.
- Heart rate and rhythm regular.
- No murmurs, clicks, gallops, extrasystoles.

Abdomen, Extremities
- Nondistended.
- Bowel sounds present and not hyperactive.
- Liver percusses 2 cm below right costal margin (RCM), overall size is 8 cm.
- No tenderness, masses, organomegaly.
- Brisk capillary refill at 3 seconds, no edema, no clubbing.

Neurological
- Alert, oriented, somewhat sleepy.
- Cranial nerves II-XII intact.
- Strength 5/5 throughout.
- DTRs 2+ and symmetrical.
- Sensory intact to touch.
- No Romberg.
- Able to perform rapid alternating movements (RAM) smoothly without error.

Question 4 What studies would you initiate now while preparing your interventions?

Question 5 What therapies would you initiate immediately while awaiting results of the lab studies?

LABORATORY
- CBC, chemistries, liver function studies, and urinalysis are all within normal ranges.
- Head CT and MRI normal.

EMERGENCY ROOM COURSE
- Patient becomes increasingly irritable and anxious.
- He experiences a second seizure with sudden loss of consciousness, generalized tonic convulsion is closely followed by alternating clonic convulsions.
- The event lasts about 3 minutes.
- The patient appears to sleep for about 5 minutes (postictal).
- The patient awakens confused.

PHYSICAL EXAMINATION NOW
- P = 110, regular; RR = 20; BP = 130/76.
- Lungs are clear to auscultation, no aspiration.
- Skin diaphoretic, warm.
- Patient sleepy, oriented to name only.
- Neurologic exam remains normal.

Question 6 What interventions should be initiated now?

RESPONSE TO THERAPY
- No further seizure activity over the next 4 hours.
- Patient is drowsy and oriented when awakened from sleep.
- RR = 12

Question 7 Now what should be done and what can the patient expect?

HOSPITAL COURSE

- The patient does well with no further seizures.
- He continues to be tired but has no other adverse effects.
- He is discharged home on the second day.

Question 8   What instructions and medications should the patient go home with?

22

Acute Bacterial Meningitis

DEFINITION

- Infection of the meninges by bacteria, usually with an underlying encephalitis.

EPIDEMIOLOGY

- There are 3 cases per 100,00 persons per year in the United States; median age is 25 years.
- Risk factors include extremes of age, splenectomy, sickle-cell disease, alcoholism, liver disease, otitis media, sinusitis, pneumonia, diabetes, immunosuppression, ventricular shunt, cerebrospinal fluid (CSF) leak, and recent neurosurgical procedures.
- Community-acquired meningitis is preceded by nasopharyngeal colonization.
- Since the use of the *Haemophilus influenzae* (*H. influenza*) vaccine became widespread, the incidence of bacterial meningitis has declined and there has been a shift in the most likely etiologic microorganisms.
  - <1 month old: Group B streptococci.
  - >1 month and older: *Streptococcus pneumoniae* (pneumococcus).
  - *Neisseria meningitidis* (meningococcus): common in ages 2 to 18 years.
- Penicillin resistance of streptococcal infections is now estimated at 25% to 35% (>40% in children 6 years old) and resistance to cefotaxime is 15%.
- Staphylococcus and gram-negative microorganisms are more common in older patients and in infections due to trauma and nosocomial exposure.
- Listeria monocytogenes causes up to 10% of infections, especially in newborns (probable GI source).
- Acute bacterial meningitis is nearly always fatal without treatment; there is a 10% mortality even with therapy.

PATHOPHYSIOLOGY

- Bacteria invade the central nervous system (CNS) due to the combination of aggressive microorganism ± host immunosuppression ± repetitive seeding.
- Bacteria invade the CNS (Fig. 22-1, top of next page).
  - Hematogenous: mucosal colonization of the nasopharynx or infections of the lung and skin result in seeding of the blood and transport to the meninges.
  - Contiguous: spreads directly to the meninges from otitis media or sinusitis.
  - Direct entry: trauma, lumbar puncture, or surgery can lead to direct inoculation of the CSF.
- Encapsulated microorganisms are the most common: pneumococcus, meningococcus, and *H. influenza* usually from a respiratory or cranial source and multiply rapidly in the CSF.
- Once in the CSF, bacterial products (especially lipopolysaccharide [LPS] and peptidoglycan) stimulate the production of inflammatory cytokines from endothelial cells and astrocytes including TNFα, IL-1, IL-8, and nitrous oxide (NO).

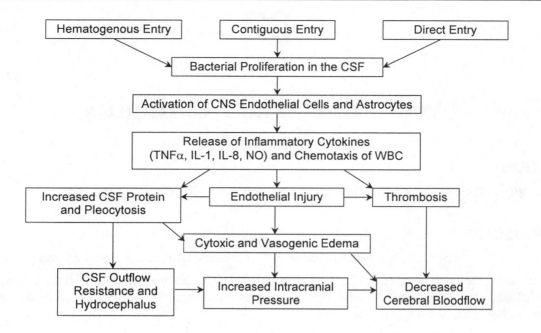

Fig. 22-1 Pathogenesis of Bacterial Meningitis

- These cytokines are chemotactic for neutrophils and lymphocytes resulting in the adhesion of the leukocytes to the endothelium, and endothelial injury and disruption of the blood-brain barrier leading to protein and cellular accumulation in the CSF.

- Endothelial injury also causes initiation of the coagulation cascade and vasogenic edema.

- Increased intracranial pressure (ICP), due to edema and CSF outflow obstruction, leads to reduced cerebral blood flow (CBF) when then leads to brain ischemia and, eventually, death.

PATIENT PRESENTATION

There are two types of onset:

- Rapid (25%): hospitalized within 24-hours of the onset of symptoms; high mortality rate.

- Slow (75%): days to weeks of preceding prodromal symptoms.

History

Recent upper respiratory symptoms; exposure to other ill individuals; sinusitis or otitis media; recent neurosurgery; immunosuppression; sickle-cell disease.

Symptoms

Headache; fever; stiff neck; rash; somnolence or irritability; photophobia; vomiting; seizures; blurred vision; numbness or weakness.

Examination

Fever; decreased level of consciousness; nuchal rigidity; Brudzinski and Kernig signs; cranial nerve palsies; focal neurologic deficits; rashes.

DIFFERENTIAL DIAGNOSIS

- Viral meningitis
- Subarachnoid hemorrhage

- Migraine
- Influenza
- Carcinomatous meningitis
- Parameningeal foci of infection

KEYS TO ASSESSMENT

- Lumbar puncture: CSF results in bacterial meningitis.
    - Pressure increased (mean pressure = 30 cm H_2O)
    - Protein increased (>150 mg/dl)
    - Leukocytes: polymorphonuclear neutrophils (PMNs) (>1000/μl)
    - Glucose decreased (<40 mg/dl); lactate increased
    - Lactic dehydrogenase (LDH): increased
    - Gram stain 60% to 80% sensitive, >90% specific
    - Culture 70% to 85% sensitive
    - India ink: look for cryptococcus
    - Counter immunoelectrophoresis (CIE), latex agglutination, polymerase chain reactions (PCR) for *S. pneumoniae, N. meningitidis, H. influenza, S. agalactiae,* HSV, enterovirus, and Listeria.
- Other CSF studies are being used in experimental trials.
    - C-reactive protein is elevated in over 97% of bacterial meningitis but is nonspecific.
    - CSF procalcitonin is highly specific for bacterial meningitis but not highly sensitive.
    - TNFα, IL-1, IL-6, complement, and endothelins are all being evaluated.
- Serum reveals increased white blood cells (WBC) and possible electrolyte disturbances, especially if the patient develops the syndrome of inappropriate antidiuretic hormone (SIADH) resulting in hyponatremia.
- Computed tomography (CT) or magnetic resonance imaging (MRI) should be obtained if there is evidence of increased intracranial pressure, equivocal CSF results, or focal neurologic findings on the physical examination.

KEYS TO MANAGEMENT

- Early recognition, early identification, and rapid initiation are crucial to patient survival.
- The delay of antibiotics is a serious problem in all hospitals; cultures will not be decreased in diagnostic sensitivity if antibiotics are begin 1 to 2 hours before lumbar puncture.
- Isolation of the patient is indicated until the microorganism has been identified.
- Antibiotics: empiric often necessary.
    - They should cover likely microorganisms: use gram stain results or broad empiric coverage.
    - They must penetrate the blood-brain barrier and be bactericidal: leukocyte phagocytosis is inefficient in CSF due to deficiency of complement and specific antibodies.
    - The choice of empiric antibiotics includes combinations of broad spectrum cephalosporins (ceftriaxone, cefotaxime, ceftazidime) or meropenem plus vancomycin (some regimens include ampicillin especially in young children).

- – If possible, it is best to later tailor therapy to the gram stain, polymerase chain reaction (PCR), or culture results.

- Dexamethasone
  - – Used in children over 6 weeks of age with the first dose of antibiotics; it reduces the risk of complications such as hearing loss.
  - – It is still debated in adults; it may be useful if there is clear evidence of increased intracranial pressure.

- Monitoring and managing sequelae.
  - – ICP pressure bolt and management of increased ICP.
  - – Anticonvulsants for recurrent seizures.
  - – Support for sepsis.
  - – Shunt for refractory hydrocephalus.
  - – Support for disseminated intravascular coagulation (DIC) or syndrome of inappropriate antidiuretic hormone (SIADH).

- Reassess for long-term sequela: up to 25% of children have prolonged complications such as deafness, mental retardation, seizure disorder, spasticity, or paresis.

- Prevention:
  - – Vaccination
    1) *H. influenza*: vaccinate all children >2 months of age.
    2) *N. meningitidis*: vaccinate asplenic, immunocompromised, travelers to endemic areas, community and college outbreaks, and household contacts.
    3) *S. pneumoniae*: vaccinate adults >65 years of age; those with chronic cardiovascular, pulmonary, hepatic, or renal disease; diabetics; alcoholism; CSF leak; immunocompromised; asplenia; lymphoma; HIV; nephrotic syndrome; or multiple myeloma; administer booster every 6 years.
  - – Chemoprophylaxis
    1) Contacts of cases of meningococcal disease: rifampin, minocycline, ciprofloxacin.
    2) Contacts of cases of *H. influenza* meningitis: rifampin.

Pathophysiology $\rightarrow$	**Clinical Link**
What is going on in the disease process that influences how the patient presents and how he or she should be managed?	*What should you do now that you understand the underlying pathophysiology?*

Encapsulated microorganisms are common pathogens in bacterial meningitis, and the immune defenses in the CSF are relatively weak, so these microorganisms can multiply quickly.	Meningitis can progress rapidly to significant neurologic injury and must be treated with antibiotics that are bactericidal, not just bacteristatic, and for which the microorganism is not resistant.
The first step in host response to CSF bacterial invasion is via the production of inflammatory cytokines from endothelial cells and astrocytes (TNFα, IL-1, NO).	Meningitis is characterized by intense inflammation of the meninges and underlying brain tissue; drugs that block the various cytokines are being tested and steroids are used in children (still controversial in adults).
Increased intracranial pressure is the most ominous sequelae of meningitis and can result in decreased cerebral blood flow, brain ischemia, and herniation.	Patients must be monitored for deteriorating mental status, changes in vital signs, and papilledema; pressure monitoring and treatment with hyperventilation and osmotic agents may be necessary.
Meningitis and subarachnoid hemorrhage can occur in otherwise young and healthy people, and both present with headache, change in mental status, meningismus, and focal neurological deficits, particularly cranial nerve palsies.	Subarachnoid hemorrhage must be ruled out in a patient who does not describe the usual infectious prodromal symptoms and who has clinical evidence of increased intracranial pressure with MRI or (CT) scanning.
Bacteria in the CSF cause changes in the blood-brain barrier that allow cells (usually neutrophils) and protein into the CSF, use up the glucose, and produce lactate with their metabolism, and can often be seen on gram stain or cultured and be tested for with polymerase chain reaction (PCR).	Diagnosis of meningitis is usually made by lumbar puncture with CSF analysis indicating increased protein, neutrophils, and lactate, decreased glucose, and positive stains, cultures, and PCR testing.
The CSF has limited immunologic protection and microorganisms can multiply quickly with rapid deterioration of the patient and risk for long-term sequelae and death.	Rapid institution of broad-spectrum empiric antibiotics is crucial to patient outcomes and should not be delayed because performing diagnostic tests including the lumbar puncture.

Suggested Reading

Bartt, R. (2000). Listeria and atypical presentations of Listeria in the central nervous system. *Seminars in Neurology, 20*(3), 361-373.

Bracco, D., & Ravussin, P. (2000). Neuroinflammation and infection. *Current Opinion in Anaesthesiology. 13*(5), 523-528.

Chowdhury, M. H., & Tunkel, A. R. (2000). Antibacterial agents in infections of the central nervous system. *Infectious Disease Clinics of North America, 14,* 391-408.

Dichgans, M., Jager, L., Mayer, T., Schorn, K., & Pfister, H. W. (1999). Bacterial meningitis in adults: Demonstration of inner ear involvement using high-resolution MRI. *Neurology, 52*(5), 1003-1009.

Drake, R., Dravutski, J., & Voss, L. (2000). Hearing in children after meningococcal meningitis. *Journal of Paediatrics & Child Health, 36*(3), 240-243.

Fassbender, K., Eschenfelder, C., & Hennerici, M. (1999). Fas (APO-1/CD95) in inflammatory CNS diseases: Intrathecal release in bacterial meningitis. *Journal of Neuroimmunology, 93*(1-2), 122-125.

Gendrel, D., & Bohuon, C. (2000). Procalcitonin as a marker of bacterial infection. *Pediatric Infectious Disease Journal. 19*(8), 679-688.

Grimwood, K., Anderson, P., Anderson, V., Tan, L., & Nolan, T. (2000). Twelve year outcomes following bacterial meningitis: Further evidence for persisting effects. *Archives of Disease in Childhood, 83*(2), 111-116.

Hardy, S. J., Christodoulides, M., Weller, R. O., & Heckels, J. E. (2000). Interactions of *Neisseria meningitidis* with cells of the human meninges. *Molecular Microbiology, 36*(4), 817-829.

Hasbun, R., Aronin, S. I., & Quagliarello, V. J. (1999). Treatment of bacterial meningitis. *Comprehensive Therapy, 25*(2), 73-81.

Hatala, R., & Attia, J. (2000). Computed tomography for predicting complications of lumbar puncture. *Journal of the American Medical Association, 283*(8), 1004.

Heyderman, R., & Klein, N. (2000). Emergency management of meningitis. *Journal of the Royal Society of Medicine, 93*(5), 225-229.

Hussein, A. S., & Shafran, S. D. (200). Acute bacterial meningitis in adults: A 12-year review. *Medicine, 79*(6), 360-368.

Klinger, G., Chin, C., Beyene, J., & Perlman, M. (2000). Predicting the outcome of neonatal bacterial meningitis. *Pediatrics, 106*(3), 477-482.

Koedel, U., & Pfister, H. W. (1999). Oxidative stress in bacterial meningitis. *Brain Pathology, 9*(1), 57-67.

Lopez-Cortes, L. F., Marquez-Arbizu, R., Jimenez-Jimenez, L. M., Jimenez-Mejias, E., Caballero-Granado, F. J., Rey-Romero, C., Polaina, M., & Pachon, J. (2000). Cerebrospinal fluid tumor necrosis factor-alpha, interleukin-1beta, interleukin-6, and interleukin-8 as diagnostic markers of cerebrospinal fluid infection in neurosurgical patients. *Critical Care Medicine, 28*(1), 215-219.

Lortholary, O., Dromer, F., Mathoulin, P., Fitting, C., Improvisi, L., Cavaillon, J. M., Dupont, B., & French Cryptococcosis Study Group. (2001). Immune mediators in cerebrospinal fluid during cryptococcosis are influenced by meningeal involvement and human immunodeficiency virus serostatus. *Journal of Infectious Diseases, 183,* 294-302.

MacLennan, J., Obaro, S., Deeks, J., Lake, D., Elie, C., Carlone, G., Moxon, E. R., & Greenwood, B. (2001). Immunologic memory 5 years after meningococcal A/C conjugate vaccination in infancy. *Journal of Infectious Diseases, 183,* 97-104.

Marion, D. (2000). Aseptic versus bacterial postoperative meningitis: Cytokines as a distinguishing marker. *Critical Care Medicine, 28*(1), 281-282.

Moller, K., Larsen ,F. S., Qvist, J., Wandall, J. H., Knudsen, G. M., Gjorup, I. E., & Skinhoj, P. (2000). Dependency of cerebral blood flow on mean arterial pressure in patients with acute bacterial meningitis. *Critical Care Medicine, 28*(4), 1027-1032.

Moller, K., & Skinhoj P. (2000). Guidelines for managing acute bacterial meningitis. *British Medical Journal, 320*(7245), 1290.

Moller, K., Skinhoj, P., Knudsen, G. M., & Larsen, F. S. (2000). Effect of short-term hyperventilation on cerebral blood flow autoregulation in patients with acute bacterial meningitis. *Stroke, 31*(5), 1116-1122.

Moller, K., Strauss, G., Thomsen, G., Larsen, F., Skinhoj, P., & Knudsen, G. (2000). Cerebral blood flow, oxidative metabolism, and cerebrovascular carbon dioxide reactivity in patients with acute bacterial meningitis. *European Journal of Anaesthesiology—Supplement 17,* (Suppl 19), 88.

Nahab, F. B., Worrell, G. A., & Weinshenker, B. G. (2001). 25-year-old man with recurring headache and confusion. *Mayo Clinic Proceedings, 76,* 75-78.

Narchi, H. (2001). Aseptic meningitis. *Pediatrics, 107*(2), 451.

Negrini, B., Kelleher, K. J., & Wald, E. R. (2000). Cerebrospinal fluid findings in aseptic versus bacterial meningitis. *Pediatrics, 105*(2), 316-319.

Perkins, B. A. (2000). New opportunities for prevention of Meningococcal disease. *Journal of the American Medical Association, 283*(21), 2842-2844.

Pfister, L., Tureen, J., Shaw, S., Christen, S., Ferriero, D., Tauber, M., & Leib, S. (2000). Endothelin inhibition improves cerebral blood flow and is neuroprotective in pneumococcal meningitis. *Annals of Neurology, 47*(3), 329-335.

Rajnik, M., & Ottolini, M. G. (2000). Serious infections of the central nervous system: Encephalitis, meningitis, and brain abscess. *Adolescent Medicine, 11*(2), 401-425.

Ramers, C., Billman, G., Hartin, M., Ho, S., & Sawyer, M. (2000). Impact of a diagnostic cerebrospinal fluid enterovirus polymerase chain reaction test on patient management. *Journal of the American Medical Association, 283*(20), 2680-2685.

Roos, K. L. (2000). Acute bacterial meningitis. *Seminars n Neurology, 20*(3), 293-306.

Rosenstein, N. E., & Perkins, B. A. (2000). Update on Haemophilus influenzae serotype b and meningococcal vaccines. *Pediatric Clinics of North America, 47*(2), 337-352, vi.

Schwarz, S., Bertram, M., Schwab, S., Andrassy, K., & Hacke, W. (2000). Serum procalcitonin levels in bacterial and abacterial meningitis. *Critical Care Medicine, 28*(6), 1828-1832.

Sherwood, E., & Prough, D. (200). Interleukin-8, neuroinflammation, and secondary brain injury. *Critical Care Medicine, 28(4),* 1221-1223.

Silber, E., Sonnenberg, P., Ho, K. C., Koornhof, H. J., Eintracht, S., Morris, L., & Saffer, D. (1999). Meningitis in a community with a high prevalence of tuberculosis and HIV infection. *Journal of the Neurological Sciences, 162*(1), 20-26.

Sormunen, P., Kallio, M. J., Kilpi, T., & Peltola, H. (1999). C-reactive protein is useful in distinguishing Gram stain-negative bacterial meningitis from viral meningitis in children. *Journal of Pediatrics, 134*(6), 725-729.

Teach, S. J., & Geil, P. A. (1999). Incidence of bacteremia, urinary tract infections, and unsuspected bacterial meningitis in children with febrile seizures. *Pediatric Emergency Care, 15*(1), 9-12.

van der, F. M., Stockhammer, G., Vonk, G. J., Nikkels, P. G., Diemen-Steenvoorde, R. A., van der Vlist, G. J., Rupert, S. W., Schmutzhard, E., Gunsilius, E., Gastl, G., Hoepelman, A. I., Kimpen, J. L., & Geelen, S. P. (2001). Vascular endothelial growth factor in bacterial meningitis: Detection in cerebrospinal fluid and localization in postmortem brain. *Journal of Infectious Diseases, 183,* 149-153.

Woolley, A. L., Kirk, K. A., Neumann, A. M. J., McWilliams, S. M., Murray, J., Freind, D., & Wiatrak, B. J. (1999). Risk factors for hearing loss from meningitis in children: The Children's Hospital experience. *Archives of Otolaryngology—Head & Neck Surgery, 125(5),* 509-514.

Case Study

Acute Bacterial Meningitis

INITIAL HISTORY

- 22-year-old female college student who just completed winter exams.
- Felt well until about 1 week ago when she developed an upper respiratory infection.
- Improved slowly but over the past 2 days has developed increasing cough production of rusty sputum, fever, myalgias, and now a bitemporal headache.

Question 1   What other questions about her symptoms would you like to ask this patient?

ADDITIONAL HISTORY

- She states that her neck feels stiff and sore.
- She feels tired and is having trouble concentrating.
- Bright lights make her eyes hurt and her vision is slightly blurry; she denies double vision.
- She has had no rashes, vomiting, or diarrhea.
- She has had some shaking chills.
- She does not recall any of her recent contacts being ill.
- She denies dyspnea or chest pain.

Question 2   What other questions about her history would you like to ask?

PAST MEDICAL HISTORY
- She denies any past history of meningitis, head trauma, or neurological disease; or pneumonia, immunodeficiency, or severe infections.
- She has never been hospitalized.
- She was tested for HIV last year and was negative; she has not been sexually active in 13 months.
- She is on no medications and has no allergies.
- She has a 10-pack/year smoking history.
- She had the usual childhood immunizations but has received none in recent years.

PHYSICAL EXAMINATION
- Well-built, well-nourished female appearing tired but in no acute distress; coughing occasionally.
- T = 38E orally; P = 85 and regular; RR = 20; BP = 95/75 right arm sitting.

Skin
- Warm and moist.
- No rashes on careful inspection.
- No cyanosis.

HEENT, Neck
- PERRLA, difficult to visualize fundi due to photophobia but no papilledema seen.
- Ears and throat clear without lesions or exudates.
- Neck stiff and painful with flexion.
- Positive Kernig and Brudzinski signs.

Lungs
- No chest deformity; chest expansion symmetrical.
- Dullness to percussion over the right posterior inferior lung field.
- Inspiratory crackles with egophony in the right posterior lung field.

Cardiac, Extremities
- Apical impulse at the 5th intercostal space at the midclavicular line.
- Regular rate and rhythm without murmurs or gallops.
- Pulses full and symmetrical in all extremities.
- No cyanosis, clubbing, rashes, or edema.

Abdomen, Neurological
- Nondistended; no tenderness; no masses or organomegaly.
- Bowel sounds heard in all four quadrants.
- Oriented x 4 but mildly lethargic.
- Cranial nerves all intact including ocular movements.
- Strength 5/5 and symmetrical throughout.
- Sensory intact and symmetrical.
- DTR 2+ and symmetrical.
- Gait steady.

Question 3   What are the pertinent positive and negative findings on exam and what might they mean?

Question 4   What is your differential diagnosis at this time?

Question 5   What laboratory tests and therapeutic interventions would be indicated at this time?

LABORATORY
- Serum chemistries normal.
- WBC = $12,000/mm^3$ (90% PMNs); HCT = 40%; platelets = $280,000/mm^3$.
- Sputum gram stain = numerous PMNs with numerous gram-positive diplococci.
- Chest x-ray = dense right lower lobe infiltrate with air bronchograms.

LUMBAR PUNCTURE/CEREBROSPINAL FLUID RESULTS
- Opening pressure = 30 cm water.
- Increased protein; decreased glucose; increased lactate.
- 120 WBC/mm^3, all PMNs.
- Gram stain positive for gram-positive diplococci.
- India ink negative for fungi.

Question 6   How would you interpret these lab findings?

Question 7   What antibiotics would be indicated?

HOSPITAL COURSE
- Patient is admitted.
- Her fever gradually resolves.
- She experiences decreasing headache and lethargy.

Question 8   For what complications should this patient be monitored?

23

Menopausal Osteoporosis

DEFINITION

- A value of bone mineral density 2.5 standard deviations or more below the young adult mean.
- The disease is characterized by low bone mass and microarchitectural deterioration of bone tissue, leading to enhanced bone fragility and a consequent increase in fracture risk. It is age-related, and it is associated with decreases in stature and kyphosis. Type I = menopausal osteoporosis, type II = senile osteoporosis.

EPIDEMIOLOGY

- In the U.S., 15% of postmenopausal Caucasian women and 35% of women older than 65 have osteoporosis.
- One in every two Caucasian women will suffer an osteoporotic fracture in her lifetime.
- 25% of women over age 60 have spinal compression, 40% of women will develop vertebral fractures by age 75, and 20% of women will develop hip fractures by age 90.
- After hip fracture, less than 50% of people are able to return to fully independent functioning and 12-24% will die within a year.
- 15% of young adults in the United States have osteopenia.
- 40% to 80% of the risk for osteoporosis is due to heredity; genes that have been implicated include vitamin D receptor, estrogen receptor, androgen receptor, collagen type 1 alpha 1, and IL-6 gene polymorphisms.
- Risk factors:
    - History of fracture as an adult or history of fracture in a first degree relative
    - Caucasian race
    - Advanced age
    - Low body weight (<127 lbs)
    - Smoking, heavy caffeine intake
    - Low calcium or high phosphate intake
    - Sedentary lifestyle
    - Dementia and/or depression
    - Medications (steroids, phenytoin, heparin, warfarin)

PATHOPHYSIOLOGY

- Maximum bone mass is achieved at age 25 to 35 and is determined by genetics, amount of mechanical loading (exercise), nutrition (ex. calcium intake), and hormone use.

- Bone remodeling occurs constantly in the healthy adult at maturity with no net change in bone mass. Osteoclasts excavate erosion cavities on bone surfaces and osteoblasts fill in the cavities with new bone giving it greater strength and repairing microfractures.

- Hormonal and cytokine factors that influence bone remodeling include estrogen, testosterone, calcitonin, parathyroid hormone (PTH), 1,25 dihydroxyvitamin D, interleukins-1 and -6 (IL-1, IL-6), transforming growth factor, and tumor necrosis factor (TNF).

- Women lose 30% to 50% of their trabecular bone with aging. The amount of bone loss is dependent on the peak bone mass and the rate of bone loss.

- Estrogen accelerates osteoclast apoptosis and prolongs the life of the osteoblasts, thus limiting the activity of the osteoclasts such that infilling of the erosion sites by osteoblasts is relatively preserved until menopause. In addition, estrogen increases intestinal and renal absorption of calcium and increases vitamin D receptor activity.

- Gonadal insufficiency (estrogen loss) accelerates bone turnover with increasing osteoclast activity, progressively greater surface of the bone being occupied by remodeling events, and less effective filling of erosion cavities by osteoblasts leading to osteopenia and osteoporosis. The most rapid loss of bone occurs in the first year after menopause.

- Dietary calcium insufficiency or vitamin D deficiency increase bone resorption and the risk for osteoporosis.

- Turnover is more rapid in trabecular (cancellous) bone (vertebral column, distal radius, proximal femur) than in cortical bone with a loss of bone mineral density and disconnectivity of the trabecular elements leading to increased likelihood of fracture.

- Osteoporosis of trabecular bone increases the risk of vertebral compression fracture, fractures of the distal forearm, and hip fracture.

PATIENT PRESENTATION

History

Postmenopausal or surgical oophorectomy, elderly, housebound, late menarche, family history, thin, Caucasian or Asian, poor diet (low in calcium, high in phosphates), smoking, caffeine, history of fractures, family history of fractures, dementia or depression, medications.

Symptoms

Loss of height, back pain, pain at fracture sites; more than 65% of individuals with compression fracture are asymptomatic.

Examination

Reduced height for weight, thin, "dowager hump," evidence of fracture.

DIFFERENTIAL DIAGNOSIS

- Senile osteoporosis
- Iatrogenic osteoporosis (drugs)
- Multiple myeloma
- Hyperthyroidism
- Hyperparathyroidism
- Cushing disease
- Type I diabetes

- Osteomalacia (low calcium, vitamin D deficiency)
- Rheumatic disease

KEYS TO ASSESSMENT

- Identify at-risk patients.
- Yearly heights.
- Consider measuring follicle-stimulating hormone (FSH) levels if perimenopausal.
- Laboratory evaluation to rule out other causes of osteopenia:
  - Glucose (diabetes)
  - Blood urea nitrogen (BUN) and creatinine (Cr) (renal disease)
  - Calcium, phosphorous (hyperparathyroidism)
  - T_3, T_4 (hyperthyroidism), parathyroid hormone (PTH)
  - Alkaline phosphatase (high in malignancy, multiple myeloma, Paget)
  - Serum protein electrophoresis (multiple myeloma)
  - Others as indicated by physical examination
- Laboratory to confirm osteoporosis:
  - Urinary type I collagen
  - Cross-linked N-telopeptide (NTX)
- Diagnostics:
  - X-rays are useful in evaluating for compression fractures but osteopenia is evident only after 30% of the bone is lost. Phalangeal bone density can be done to predict hip fracture risk.
  - Dual energy x-ray absorptiometry (DEXA) is the diagnostic modality of choice and is indicated in post menopausal women who are of low body weight and not on estrogen. It can also be used to monitor the effectiveness of therapy in women with known osteoporosis.
    1) Healthy: one standard deviation of peak bone mass
    2) Osteopenia: 1.0-2.4 standard deviations below peak bone mass
    3) Osteoporosis: ≥2.5 standard deviations below peak bone mass
  - Others:
    1) Quantitative ultrasound
    2) Quantitative computed tomography (CT) scanning

KEYS TO MANAGEMENT

- **Prevention**
  - Maintain adequate calcium intake.
    1) Important to begin in the prepubertal period and continue throughout life.
    2) Calcium citrate is the most easily absorbed, however dairy products are even more effective due to improved absorption with milk-based protein (MBP).
    3) When combined with exercise, can reduce hip fracture risk but will not prevent spinal bone loss.

- Reduce phosphorous intake (soft drinks, prepared foods).
- Supplement vitamin D if not getting adequate sun exposure or dietary insufficiency.
- Exercise both pre- and postmenopausally.
    1) Exercise should be begun in youth to maximize bone density.
    2) Weight-bearing and exercise increases total body calcium as well as vertebral bone density in postmenopausal women.
- Smoking cessation, avoid excessive caffeine intake.
- Avoid osteopenic medications (steroids, thyroxine) if possible.
- Oral contraceptives for anorexia or extreme exercise resulting in secondary amenorrhea.

- **Pharmacologic treatment**
    - **Estrogen**
        1) Prevents bone loss, increases bone density, decreases fracture risk.
        2) 0.625 mg orally or 0.3 mg combined with calcium replacement is the minimal effective dose; must be combined with progestins in women with an intact uterus to prevent endometrial cancer.
        3) Treatment should be begun soon after menopause to maximize bone density.
        4) Nonosseous benefits are numerous (see Chapter 25).
        5) The benefits must be weighed against the increase in breast cancer risk (see Chapter 9) and thrombophlebitis.
    - **Selective estrogen receptor modulators (SERMS)**
        1) Raloxifene is approved for use in osteoporosis and has been shown to significantly increase bone mineral density and reduce the risk of fractures without increased risk for endometrial or breast cancer (see Chapters 9 and 25).
        2) Tibolone is a steroid receptor modulator that has been shown to be effective in some studies at reducing fracture risk.
    - **Bisphosphonates**
        1) Alendronate reduces hip and spinal fractures by about 50% and increases bone mineral density significantly within 2 to 3 years; other bisphosphonates include etidronate and risedronate.
        2) Work by suppressing bone turnover by blocking osteoclasts action on the bone; sometimes described as functioning as a bone "shield."
        3) Well tolerated with few side effects except for esophageal and GI irritation; alendronate can be given weekly.
        4) Should be considered in place of estrogen in women with risks for breast cancer or thrombophlebitis; some studies are finding them even more effective when used in combination with estrogen or SERMS.
    - **Calcitonin**
        1) Can be given SQ or via nasal spray.
        2) Increases bone mass and decreases fracture rate (less than HRT or bisphosphonates).
        3) Can be used for its analgesic effect on painful osteoporotic bone fractures.

- **Fluorides**
    1) Reduces fracture risk, but less so than estrogen.
    2) A low dose has tolerable side effects but can cause significant toxicity in some patients.
- **Parathyroid hormone (teriparatide)**
    1) Preliminary results show dramatic increases in bone mineral density in women with severe osteoporosis.
    2) Requires daily injections.
    3) Expected to be approved in the US in 2002.
- **Others/experimental**
    1) Anticytokines
    2) Osteoprotegerin
    3) Ipriflavon
    4) HMG CoA reductase inhibitors (statins)
    5) Strontium
    6) Nonsteroidal antiinflammatory drugs and COX 2 inhibitors

- **Monitoring therapy**
    - Follow heights
    - Follow serum calcium
    - Consider monitoring urinary type I collagen and cross-linked N-telopeptide (NTX) as measures of bone turnover (should decrease with treatment).
    - If on estrogen, obtain careful breast, pelvic, pap, and maturation index annually

Pathophysiology → Clinical Link

What is going on in the disease process that influences how the patient presents and how he or she should be managed?

What should you do now that you understand the underlying pathophysiology?

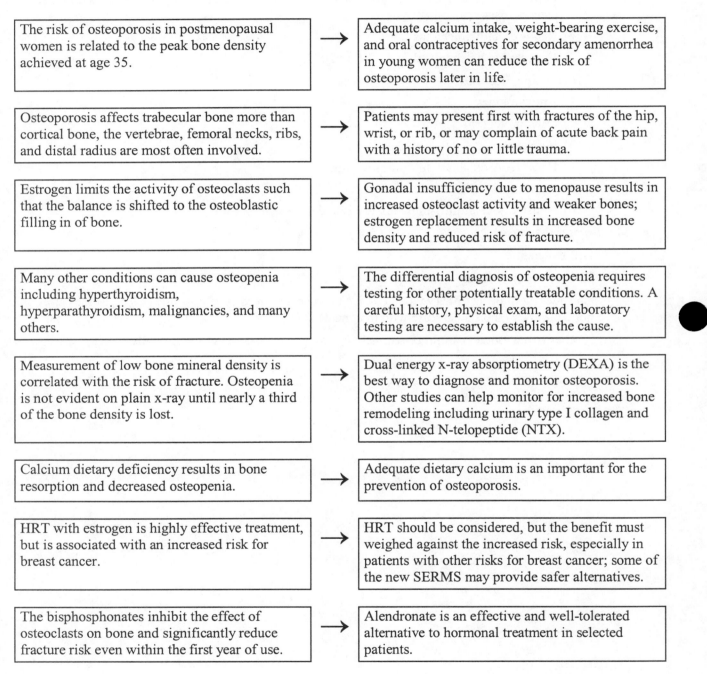

Pathophysiology	Clinical Link
The risk of osteoporosis in postmenopausal women is related to the peak bone density achieved at age 35.	Adequate calcium intake, weight-bearing exercise, and oral contraceptives for secondary amenorrhea in young women can reduce the risk of osteoporosis later in life.
Osteoporosis affects trabecular bone more than cortical bone, the vertebrae, femoral necks, ribs, and distal radius are most often involved.	Patients may present first with fractures of the hip, wrist, or rib, or may complain of acute back pain with a history of no or little trauma.
Estrogen limits the activity of osteoclasts such that the balance is shifted to the osteoblastic filling in of bone.	Gonadal insufficiency due to menopause results in increased osteoclast activity and weaker bones; estrogen replacement results in increased bone density and reduced risk of fracture.
Many other conditions can cause osteopenia including hyperthyroidism, hyperparathyroidism, malignancies, and many others.	The differential diagnosis of osteopenia requires testing for other potentially treatable conditions. A careful history, physical exam, and laboratory testing are necessary to establish the cause.
Measurement of low bone mineral density is correlated with the risk of fracture. Osteopenia is not evident on plain x-ray until nearly a third of the bone density is lost.	Dual energy x-ray absorptiometry (DEXA) is the best way to diagnose and monitor osteoporosis. Other studies can help monitor for increased bone remodeling including urinary type I collagen and cross-linked N-telopeptide (NTX).
Calcium dietary deficiency results in bone resorption and decreased osteopenia.	Adequate dietary calcium is an important for the prevention of osteoporosis.
HRT with estrogen is highly effective treatment, but is associated with an increased risk for breast cancer.	HRT should be considered, but the benefit must weighed against the increased risk, especially in patients with other risks for breast cancer; some of the new SERMS may provide safer alternatives.
The bisphosphonates inhibit the effect of osteoclasts on bone and significantly reduce fracture risk even within the first year of use.	Alendronate is an effective and well-tolerated alternative to hormonal treatment in selected patients.

Suggested Reading

Adami, S., Bruni, V., Bianchini, D., Becorpi, A., Lombardi, P., Campagnoli, C., Ferrari, A., Marchesoni, T., & Balena, R. (2000). Prevention of early postmenopausal bone loss with cyclical etidronate. *Journal of Endocrinological Investigation, 23*(5), 310-316.

Alekel, D. L., Germain, A. S., Peterson, C. T., Hanson, K. B., Stewart, J. W., & Toda, T. (2000). Isoflavone-rich soy protein isolate attenuates bone loss in the lumbar spine of perimenopausal women. *American Journal of Clinical Nutrition, 72*(3), 844-852.

Anonymous. (2001). Once-a-week alendronate for postmenopausal osteoporosis is as effective as once-daily dosing. *Geriatrics, 56,* 19.

Beardsworth, S. A., Kearney, C. E., & Purdie, D. W. (1999). Prevention of postmenopausal bone loss at lumbar spine and upper femur with tibolone: A two-year randomised controlled trial. *British Journal of Obstetrics & Gynaecology, 106*(7), 678-683.

Beauchesne, M. F., & Miller, P. F. (1999). Etidronate and alendronate in the treatment of postmenopausal osteoporosis. *Annals of Pharmacotherapy, 33*(5), 587-599.

Bjarnason, N. H., Byrjalsen, I., Hassager, C., Haarbo, J., & Christiansen, C. (2000). Low doses of estradiol in combination with gestodene to prevent early postmenopausal bone loss. *American Journal of Obstetrics & Gynecology, 183*(3), 550-560.

Bjarnason, N. H., & Christiansen, C. (2000). The influence of thinness and smoking on bone loss and response to hormone replacement therapy in early postmenopausal women. *Journal of Clinical Endocrinology & Metabolism, 85*(2), 590-596.

Compston, J. E. (2001). Sex steroids and bone. *Physiological Reviews, 81,* 419-447.

De, L. V., Ditto, A., la Marca, A., Lanzetta, D., Massafra, C., & Morgante, G. (2000). Bone mineral density and biochemical markers of bone turnover in peri- and postmenopausal women. *Calcified Tissue International, 66*(4), 263-267.

Downs, R. W., Jr., Bell, N. H., Ettinger, M. P., Walsh, B. W., Favus, M. J., Mako, B., Wang, L., Smith, M. E., Gormley, G. J., & Melton, M. E. (2000). Comparison of alendronate and intranasal calcitonin for treatment of osteoporosis in postmenopausal women. *Journal of Clinical Endocrinology & Metabolism, 85*(5), 1783-1788.

Feltrin, G. P., Nardin, M., Marangon, A., Khadivi, Y., Calderone, M., & De Conti, G. (2000). Quantitative ultrasound at the hand phalanges: Comparison with quantitative computed tomography of the lumbar spine in postmenopausal women. *European Radiology, 10*(5), 826-831.

Fogelman, I., Ribot, C., Smith, R., Ethgen, D., Sod, E., & Reginster, J. Y. (2000). Risedronate reverses bone loss in postmenopausal women with low bone mass: Results from a multinational, double-blind, placebo-controlled trial. BMD-MN Study Group. *Journal of Clinical Endocrinology & Metabolism, 85*(5), 1895-1900.

Freedman, M., San Martin, J., O'Gorman, J., Eckert, S., Lippman, M. E., Lo, S. C., Walls, E. L., & Zeng, J. (2001). Digitized mammography: A clinical trial of postmenopausal women randomly assigned to receive raloxifene, estrogen, or placebo. *Journal of the National Cancer Institute, 93,* 51-56.

Ganry, O., Baudoin, C., & Fardellone, P. (2000). Effect of alcohol intake on bone mineral density in elderly women: The EPIDOS Study. Epidemiologie de l'Osteoporose. *American Journal of Epidemiology, 151*(8), 773-780.

Greenspan, S. L., Harris, S. T., Bone, H., Miller, P. D., Orwoll, E. S., Watts, N. B., & Rosen, C. J. (2000). Bisphosphonates: Safety and efficacy in the treatment and prevention of osteoporosis. *American Family Physician, 61*(9), 2731-2736.

Gulam, M., Thornton, M. M., Hodsman, A. B., & Holdsworth, D. W. (2000). Bone mineral measurement of phalanges: Comparison of radiographic absorptiometry and area dual x-ray absorptiometry. *Radiology, 216*(2), 586-591.

Halbekath, J., Becker-Bruser, W., & Wille, H. (2000). Raloxifene and risk of vertebral fracture in postmenopausal women. *Journal of the American Medical Association, 283*(17), 2236-2237.

Heaney, R. P. (2001). Protein intake and bone health: The influence of belief systems on the conduct of nutritional science. *American Journal of Clinical Nutrition, 73,* 5-6.

Heinemann, D. F. (2000). Osteoporosis. An overview of the National Osteoporosis Foundation clinical practice guide. *Geriatrics, 55*(5), 31-36.

Iqbal, M. M. (2000).Osteoporosis: Epidemiology, diagnosis, and treatment. *Southern Medical Journal, 93*(1), 2-18.

Kado, D. M., Browner, W. S., Palermo, L., Nevitt, M. C., Genant, H. K., & Cummings, S. R. (1999). Vertebral fractures and mortality in older women: A prospective study. Study of Osteoporotic Fractures Research Group. *Archives of Internal Medicine, 159*(11), 1215-1220.

Kato, I., Toniolo, P., Zeleniuch-Jacquotte, A., Shore, R. E., Koenig, K. L., Akhmedkhanov, A., & Riboli, E. (2000). Diet, smoking and anthropometric indices and postmenopausal bone fractures: A prospective study. *International Journal of Epidemiology, 29*(1), 85-92.

Keen, R. W., Woodford-Richens, K. L., Grant, S. F., Ralston, S. H., Lanchbury, J. S., & Spector, T. D. (1999). Association of polymorphism at the type I collagen (COL1A1) locus with reduced bone mineral density, increased fracture risk, and increased collagen turnover. *Arthritis & Rheumatism, 42*(2), 285-290.

Lane, J. M., Russell, L., & Khan, S. N. (2000). Osteoporosis. *Clinical Orthopaedics & Related Research,* (372), 139-150.

LeBoff, M. S., Kohlmeier, L., Hurwitz, S., Franklin, J., Wright, J., & Glowacki, J. (1999). Occult vitamin D deficiency in postmenopausal US women with acute hip fracture. *Journal of the American Medical Association, 281*(16), 1505-1511.

Masahashi, T., Negoro, Y., Kuroki, T., Asai, M., Noguchi, M., & Nakanishi, M. (1999). Biochemical markers of bone turnover during hormone replacement therapy. *International Journal of Gynaecology & Obstetrics, 64*(2), 163-166.

Mather, K. J., Meddings, J. B., Beck, P. L., Scott, R. B., & Hanley, D. A. (2001). Prevalence of IgA-antiendomysial antibody in asymptomatic low bone mineral density. *American Journal of Gastroenterology, 96,* 120-125.

Melton, L. J., III. (2000). Excess mortality following vertebral fracture. *Journal of the American Geriatrics Society, 48*(3), 338-339.

Meunier, P. J., Delmas, P. D., Eastell, R., McClung, M. R., Papapoulos, S., Rizzoli, R., Seeman, E., & Wasnich, R. D. (1999). Diagnosis and management of osteoporosis in postmenopausal women: Clinical guidelines. International Committee for Osteoporosis Clinical Guidelines. *Clinical Therapeutics, 21*(6), 1025-1044.

Miller, P. D. (1999). Management of osteoporosis. *Advances in Internal Medicine, 44,* 175-207.

Mincey, B. A., Moraghan, T. J., & Perez, E. A. (2000). Prevention and treatment of osteoporosis in women with breast cancer. *Mayo Clinic Proceedings, 75*(8), 821-829.

Ongphiphadhanakul, B., Chanprasertyothin, S., Payatikul, P., Tung, S. S., Piaseu, N., Chailurkit, L., Chansirikarn, S., Puavilai, G., & Rajatanavin, R. (2000). Oestrogen-receptor-alpha gene polymorphism affects response in bone mineral density to oestrogen in post-menopausal women. *Clinical Endocrinology, 52*(5), 581-585.

Raisz, L. G., & Weicker, L. P., Jr. (2000). Screening for osteoporosis: A clinical, social, and economic dilemma. *Mayo Clinic Proceedings, 75*(9), 885-887.

Ravn, P., Weiss, S. R., Rodriguez-Portales, J. A., McClung, M. R., Wasnich, R. D., Gilchrist, N. L., Sambrook, P., Fogelman, I., Krupa, D., Yates, A. J., Daifotis, A., & Fuleihan, G. E. (2000). Alendronate in early postmenopausal women: Effects on bone mass during long-term treatment and after withdrawal. Alendronate Osteoporosis Prevention Study Group. *Journal of Clinical Endocrinology & Metabolism, 85*(4), 1492-1497.

Recker, R. R., Davies, K. M., Dowd, R. M., & Heaney, R. P. (1999). The effect of low-dose continuous estrogen and progesterone therapy with calcium and vitamin D on bone in elderly women. A randomized, controlled trial. *Annals of Internal Medicine, 130*(11), 897-904.

Roe, E. B., Chiu, K. M., & Arnaud, C. D. (2000). Selective estrogen receptor modulators and postmenopausal health. *Advances in Internal Medicine, 45,* 259-278.

Sairanen, S., Karkkainen, M., Tahtela, R., Laitinen, K., Makela, P., Lamberg-Allardt, C., & Valimaki, M. J. (2000). Bone mass and markers of bone and calcium metabolism in postmenopausal women treated with 1,25-dihydroxyvitamin D (Calcitriol) for four years. *Calcified Tissue International, 67*(2), 122-127.

Sellmeyer, D. E., Stone, K. L., Sebastian, A., & Cummings, S. R. (2001). A high ratio of dietary animal to vegetable protein increases the rate of bone loss and the risk of fracture in postmenopausal women. Study of Osteoporotic Fractures Research Group. *American Journal of Clinical Nutrition, 73,* 118-122.

Sheth, P. (1999). Osteoporosis and exercise: A review. *Mount Sinai Journal of Medicine, 66*(3), 197-200.

Simonelli, C. (2000). Practical issues in bone mineral density testing. *Journal of the American Medical Womens Association, 55*(4), 228-233.

Siris, E. (2000). Alendronate in the treatment of osteoporosis: A review of the clinical trials. *Journal of Womens Health & Gender-Based Medicine, 9*(6), 599-606.

Sunyer, T., Lewis, J., Collin-Osdoby, P., & Osdoby, P. (1999). Estrogen's bone-protective effects may involve differential IL-1 receptor regulation in human osteoclast-like cells. *Journal of Clinical Investigation, 103*(10), 1409-1418.

Tobias, J. H., & Compston, J. E. (1999). Does estrogen stimulate osteoblast function in postmenopausal women? *Bone, 24*(2), 121-124.

Tonino, R. P., Meunier, P. J., Emkey, R., Rodriguez-Portales, J. A., Menkes, C. J., Wasnich, R. D., Bone, H. G., Santora, A. C., Wu, M., Desai, R., & Ross, P. D. (2000). Skeletal benefits of alendronate: 7-year treatment of postmenopausal osteoporotic women. Phase III Osteoporosis Treatment Study Group. *Journal of Clinical Endocrinology & Metabolism, 85*(9), 3109-3115.

Ullom-Minnich, P. (1999). Prevention of osteoporosis and fractures. *American Family Physician, 60*(1), 194-202.

Vogt, T. M., Ross, P. D., Palermo, L., Musliner, T., Genant, H. K., Black, D., & Thompson, D. E. (2000). Vertebral fracture prevalence among women screened for the Fracture Intervention Trial and a simple clinical tool to screen for undiagnosed vertebral fractures. Fracture Intervention Trial Research Group. *Mayo Clinic Proceedings, 75*(9), 888-896.

Watts, N. B. (1999). Postmenopausal osteoporosis. *Obstetrical & Gynecological Survey, 54*(8), 532-538.

Weaver, C. M., Peacock, M., & Johnston, C. C. J. (1999). Adolescent nutrition in the prevention of postmenopausal osteoporosis. *Journal of Clinical Endocrinology & Metabolism, 84*(6), 1839-1843.

Wong, J. C., Lewindon, P., Mortimer, R., & Shepherd, R. (2001). Bone mineral density in adolescent females with recently diagnosed anorexia nervosa. *International Journal of Eating Disorders, 29,* 11-16.

Case Study*

Menopausal Osteoporosis

INITIAL HISTORY
- 66-year-old female.
- Back pain for 6 to 8 weeks.
- Pain is constant and aggravated by activity.
- Ibuprofen provides temporary relief.

Question 1   What is the differential diagnosis at this time?

Question 2   What additional questions would you like to ask her about her symptoms?

ADDITIONAL HISTORY
- Patient denies any acute or previous injury to her back.
- She states she has had a slight reduction in height.
- She denies change in weight.
- She denies any unusual bleeding.
- She denies fever or chills.
- She denies heat or cold intolerance or changes in her hair, skin, or nails.

*****Leslie Buchanan contributed this case study.**

Question 3   What would you like to ask her about her past medical history and family history?

PAST MEDICAL HISTORY

- Patient has a history of mild hypertension for which she takes an ACE inhibitor.
- She has never taken any other medications long-term.
- She has been postmenopausal since age 48 but does not take hormones at the advice of her nurse practitioner.
- She denies endocrine or renal disease.
- She denies a personal history of breast cancer but has a family history in both her mother and sister.
- Her mammogram last year was negative.
- Her mother had a fractured hip from a fall 10 years ago.

Question 4   What would you like to ask her about her lifestyle?

LIFESTYLE HISTORY

- Gets very little exercise, mostly light housework.
- Rarely gets outdoors.
- 20 pack/year smoking history.
- Drinks an occasional glass of wine.
- Drinks 4 to 5 caffeinated beverages per day.
- Does not take calcium or vitamin D supplements.

PHYSICAL EXAMINATION

- 66-year-old white female of slight stature, walking with normal gait in no acute distress.
- Height = 5' 3.5"; weight = 120 lbs.
- T = 37 orally; P = 84 regular; RR = 20 and unlabored; BP = 154/88 sitting.

Skin, HEENT

- Dry skin; nails cracking.
- No areas of tenderness, slight hair thinning.
- Tympanic membranes pearly without bulging or retraction.
- Conjunctiva clear, PERRL, funduscopic without lesions.
- Clear without drainage or erythema.

Neck

- Moderate cervical lordosis.
- No bony tenderness.
- Full range of motion without pain elicited.
- Thyroid nontender without thyromegaly, no masses palpable.
- No adenopathy.

Chest

- Normal chest excursion, clear to auscultation and percussion.
- Cardiac exam with regular rate and rhythm without murmurs or gallops.

Abdomen, Neurologic

- Bowel sounds present throughout.
- No tenderness; no organomegaly; no masses.
- Alert and oriented x3, recent and remote memory intact.
- Cranial nerves intact.
- No focal motor deficits; no gross sensory deficits.
- DTRs 1+ and symmetrical throughout.
- Negative Kernig and Brudzinski signs.

Musculoskeletal

- Tenderness with palpation of the bony prominences of L1 and L2.
- Limited flexion and extension of the back.
- Lateral bending unlimited and nonpainful.
- No dorsal kyphosis (dowager hump).
- No deformity or swelling of joints.

Question 5   What are the pertinent positive and negative findings on physical exam?

Question 6   What initial diagnostic testing is indicated?

LUMBOSACRAL SPINE X-RAY RESULTS

- Osteopenia
- Compression fracture of L2

Question 7   Based on these results, what further diagnostic testing is now indicated?

LABORATORY RESULTS

- Serum chemistries, including phosphate, and calcium normal.
- CBC normal.
- Thyroid function tests normal.
- Rheumatoid factor negative.
- Serum and 24-hour urine alkaline phosphates normal.
- Erythrocyte sedimentation rate and serum protein electrophoresis normal.
- Dual energy x-ray densitometry consistent with significant osteopenia.

Question 8   Now what is your diagnosis?

Question 9 What is your treatment plan?

Question 10 What further care would you recommend?

24

Osteoarthritis

DEFINITION

- Osteoarthritis (OA) is defined as a heterogeneous group of conditions that leads to joint symptoms and signs which are associated with defective integrity of articular cartilage in addition to related changes in the underlying bone.
- Primary osteoarthritis is idiopathic and can be generalized or localized.
- Secondary osteoarthritis occurs due to an identifiable risk factor or cause such as joint trauma, anatomic abnormalities, infection, neuropathy, hemophilia, metabolic alterations in cartilage (hemochromatosis), or subchondral bone alteration (acromegaly, Paget disease).

EPIDEMIOLOGY

- OA is the most common form of joint disease in the world.
- It affects approximately 7% of the United States population; it affects 60% to 70% of people over age 65.
- There is an increasing risk with increasing age; prevalence is rising rapidly as the population ages.
- Autosomal dominant hereditary patterns have been identified in certain subgroups of osteoarthritis.
  - Primary generalized OA associated with human lymphocyte antigen (HLA) A1 B8 haplotype.
  - Familial chondrocalcinosis (crystal deposition in joints).
  - Chondrodysplasias.
- Several genes have been linked to various changes in cartilage components (e.g., mutation on chromosome 12 [COL2A1] linked to abnormal type II collagen).
- The risk factors for primary OA include increasing age, obesity, repetitive joint overuse, immobilization, and increased bone density (less "shock absorption;" see below).

PATHOPHYSIOLOGY

- Cartilage components become disorganized and degraded in OA.
  - Mechanical factors result in the release of enzymes (collagenase and stromelysin) resulting in proteoglycan depletion and type II collagen disordering.
  - There is a loss of the cartilage matrix, especially at the medial cartilage surface.
  - Inflammatory cytokines (interleukin-1 [IL-1], prostaglandin E2 [PGE 2], tumor necrosis factor α [TNF α], interleukin-6 [IL-6], nitric oxide) promote joint inflammation and cartilage degradation.
  - Chondrocytes become unresponsive to growth factors, such as transforming growth factor-β and insulin-like growth factor, and cannot fully compensate for matrix loss. An imbalance of cartilage synthesis and degradation develops with abrasions, pitting, and fissuring of the articular surface.
  - The articular cartilage becomes overhydrated and swollen.

- Matrix degradation and overhydration lead to a loss in compressive stiffness and elasticity with transmission of greater mechanical stress to the subchondral bone.

- The subchondral trabecular bone is damaged and loses its normal hydraulic "shock absorption;" bone cysts may form from this excess subchondral bone stress.

- Repair mechanisms at the edge of the articular surface (cartilage-bone interface) result in increased synthesis of cartilage and bone forming overgrowths called osteophytes.

- Some patients are found to have various forms of calcium crystals concentrated in the damaged articular cartilage. The pathogenesis of this crystal deposition is unclear but is correlated with a more rapid disease progression in these patients.

- Articular cartilage requires physiologic weight loading and motion to allow adequate penetration of nutrients from the synovial fluid into the cartilage; nonphysiologic loads (either in excess or insufficient) result in poor cartilage nutrition.

- Human joints require maximal mobility while avoiding articular tissue injury. One hypothesis is that there is a "protective muscular reflex" that prevents the joint from exceeding its normal range of excursion. It has been postulated that disordered neuromuscular activity may play a role in the pathogenesis of OA.

- Joint instability is correlated with a high risk of OA. Increasing the strength of the "bridging" muscles across a joint can improve joint stability, decrease joint loading, and reduce mechanical stress. Thus, exercise can improve symptoms and joint function, even though there may be little radiologic improvement.

- The pain of OA is believed to be due to three major causes: pain with movement from mechanical factors, pain at rest from synovial inflammation, and night pain from intraosseous hypertension.

PATIENT PRESENTATION

History

Family history of OA; history of joint trauma; weight gain; occupation that includes repetitive movements, especially of the knees (squatting), elbows and back (heavy lifting), and hands (assembly line and mill work).

Symptoms

Nagging pain that has been present for years in one or more joints and waxes, wanes in intensity according to the weather and exertion; stiffness after prolonged inactivity that "loosens up" with activity (may become permanent in late stages); swelling and deformity, especially of the knees and fingers, with development of "knobby" joints at the distal and proximal interphalangeal joints (DIP and PIP); inability to grip with the hands or comb the hair; restricted walking and fatigue.

Examination

Limping gait; Heberden's nodes (DIP osteophytes) and Bouchard nodes (PIP osteophytes); flexor and lateral deviations of the distal phalanx; decreased range of motion and crepitus with passive motion; swelling, warmth, and tenderness (inflammation) during "flares."

DIFFERENTIAL DIAGNOSIS

- Secondary osteoarthritis
- Rheumatoid arthritis
- Gout

- Systemic lupus erythematosus
- Rheumatic fever
- Septic arthritis

KEYS TO ASSESSMENT

- Carefully assess all joints for deformity, creptitus, and decreasing range of motion.
- Examine the eyes, skin, and organs for evidence of systemic rheumatic disease.
- In a patient with (1) a classic history for OA, (2) a joint exam revealing Heberdens nodes and decreased range of motion without evidence of significant joint deformity or inflammation, and (3) a general physical exam without evidence of systemic disease, consideration should be given for empiric treatment without further diagnostic testing.
- Specific joint involvement is frequently assessed with x-ray (weight bearing for the knee), look for joint space narrowing, subchondral bone cysts, and sclerosis, and osteophytes.
- Serum markers for evidence of articular cartilage destruction are being used experimentally as a means of detecting OA before there is radiologic evidence. These include keratin sulfate and cartilage oligomeric matrix protein; these are not yet indicated for routine evaluation.
- Technetium 99 m scintigraphy and magnetic resonance imaging (MRI) are sensitive indicators of OA but they contribute little to the general clinical evaluation of OA.
- In a patient with severe disease or suspicious aspects to the history and physical, further diagnostic testing is indicated.
    - Chemistries, including blood urea nitrogen (BUN) and creatinine (Cr).
    - Erythrocyte sedimentation rate (ESR) and rheumatoid factors.
    - Other specific tests for rheumatologic disease, such as anti-deoxyribonucleic acid (anti-DNA), HLA-B27, and uric acid.
    - Arthrocentesis with chemistries, cell counts, cultures and stain, and rheumatoid factor.

KEYS TO MANAGEMENT

- The American College of Rheumatology Guidelines for OA management suggest beginning therapy with nonpharmacologic modalities, adding acetaminophen (up to 1 gram four times per day) and proceeding to low dose and then high dose nonsteroidal antiinflammatory drugs if symptoms remain refractory.
- Nonpharmacologic
    - Exercise improves symptoms and quality of life in patients with mild to moderate OA.
    - Physical therapy, including passive range of motion and water exercises, can improve function.
    - Occupational therapy can help with assistive devices for activities of daily living.
    - Heat application, transcutaneous electric nerve stimulation (TENS), and acupuncture can be considered.
    - Diet for weight loss if appropriate.
    - Increased intake of vitamin C has been correlated with decreased OA progression and pain.
    - Ultrasound (diathermy) facilitates tendon extensibility, relaxes muscles, and decreases pain.

- Pharmacologic
    - Use of capsaicin as a topical analgesic (decreases neuronal substance P, a neurotransmitter implicated in arthritis pain).
    - Acetaminophen has been shown in many studies to be as effective in reducing pain for mild to moderate OA as nonsteroidal antiinflammatory drugs (NSAIDs).
    - Although OA is now known to have an inflammatory component, NSAIDS use is associated with some risk and they should be used only when simple analgesics fail to control symptoms.
        1) The risk of side effects (upper gastrointestinal [GI] ulceration and bleeding) are of particular risk in the elderly.
        2) There is evidence that NSAIDs may inhibit cartilage synthesis and repair, and have even been associated with acceleration of disease progression.
        3) Some patients will have greater analgesia with NSAIDs than acetaminophen. They usually they will respond at low doses thus reducing the risk of side effects.
        4) New nonsteroidal antiinflammatory drugs block only the cyclooxygenase 2 enzyme (COX-2 inhibitors), thus, maximizing the antiinflammatory and analgesic effects while minimizing GI side effects (celecoxib, rofecoxib).
    - Chondroprotective drugs are undergoing extensive research include glucosamine polysulfate, chondroitin sulfate, sodium pentosan polysulfate, and glycosaminoglycan peptide complex orally. These have been found to improve symptoms in most patients with few side effects.
    - Intraarticular injection of steroids or hyaluronic acid during acute inflammatory "flares" can provide rapid symptom relief. Frequency of steroid injections greater than 3 to 4 times per year may be associated with decreased cartilage repair.
    - Oral tetracycline derivatives have been found to be chondroprotective and are undergoing extensive investigation.
- Other
    - Orthopedic surgery (including arthroscopic procedures), such as joint debridement, abrasion arthroplasty, chondral shaving, and joint replacement, can be used with selected patients.
    - Autologous chondrocyte implantation has been used in some patients with severe disease. Early studies are encouraging.
    - Gene therapy with introduction of chondroprotective genes in to chondrocytes is being explored.

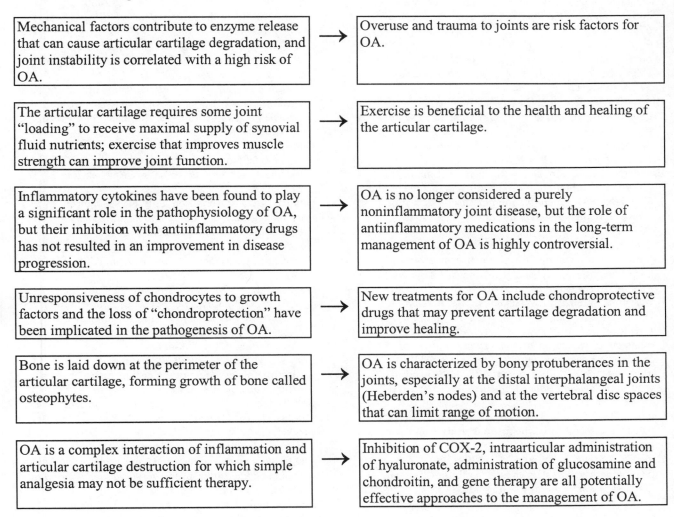

Pathophysiology → Clinical Link

What is going on in the disease process that influences how the patient presents and how he or she should be managed?

What should you do now that you understand the underlying pathophysiology?

Pathophysiology	Clinical Link
Mechanical factors contribute to enzyme release that can cause articular cartilage degradation, and joint instability is correlated with a high risk of OA.	→ Overuse and trauma to joints are risk factors for OA.
The articular cartilage requires some joint "loading" to receive maximal supply of synovial fluid nutrients; exercise that improves muscle strength can improve joint function.	→ Exercise is beneficial to the health and healing of the articular cartilage.
Inflammatory cytokines have been found to play a significant role in the pathophysiology of OA, but their inhibition with antiinflammatory drugs has not resulted in an improvement in disease progression.	→ OA is no longer considered a purely noninflammatory joint disease, but the role of antiinflammatory medications in the long-term management of OA is highly controversial.
Unresponsiveness of chondrocytes to growth factors and the loss of "chondroprotection" have been implicated in the pathogenesis of OA.	→ New treatments for OA include chondroprotective drugs that may prevent cartilage degradation and improve healing.
Bone is laid down at the perimeter of the articular cartilage, forming growth of bone called osteophytes.	→ OA is characterized by bony protuberances in the joints, especially at the distal interphalangeal joints (Heberden's nodes) and at the vertebral disc spaces that can limit range of motion.
OA is a complex interaction of inflammation and articular cartilage destruction for which simple analgesia may not be sufficient therapy.	→ Inhibition of COX-2, intraarticular administration of hyaluronate, administration of glucosamine and chondroitin, and gene therapy are all potentially effective approaches to the management of OA.

Suggested Reading

Abramson, S. B. (1999). The role of COX-2 produced by cartilage in arthritis. *Osteoarthritis & Cartilage, 7*(4), 380-381.

Alexander, C. J. (1999). Heberden's and Bouchard's nodes. *Annals of the Rheumatic Diseases, 58*(11), 675-678.

Bailey, A. J., & Knott, L. (1999). Molecular changes in bone collagen in osteoporosis and osteoarthritis in the elderly [review, 61 refs]. *Experimental Gerontology, 34*(3), 337-351.

Blumenfeld, I., & Livne, E. (1999). The role of transforming growth factor (TGF)-beta, insulin-like growth factor (IGF)-1, and interleukin (IL)-1 in osteoarthritis and aging of joints. *Experimental Gerontology, 34*(7), 821-829.

Brander, V. A., Kaelin, D. L., Oh, T. H., & Lim, P. A. (2000). Rehabilitation of orthopedic and rheumatologic disorders. 3. Degenerative joint disease. *Archives of Physical Medicine & Rehabilitation, 81*(3 Suppl 1), S67-S72

Brandt, K. D., Smith, G. N., Jr., & Simon, L. S. (2000). Intraarticular injection of hyaluronan as treatment for knee osteoarthritis: What is the evidence? *Arthritis & Rheumatism, 43*(6), 1192-1203.

Brosseau, L., Welch, V., Wells, G., deBie, R., Gam, A., Harman, K., Morin, M., Shea, B., & Tugwell, P. (2000). Low level laser therapy (classes I, II and III) for the treatment of osteoarthritis. *Cochrane Database of Systematic Reviews [computer file], (2),* CD002046.

Burkholder, J. F. (2000). Osteoarthritis of the hand: A modifiable disease. *Journal of Hand Therapy, 13*(2), 79-89.

Clemett, D., & Goa, K. L. (2000). Celecoxib: A review of its use in osteoarthritis, rheumatoid arthritis and acute pain. *Drugs, 59*(4), 957-980.

Concoff, A. L., & Kalunian, K. C. (1999). What is the relation between crystals and osteoarthritis? *Current Opinion in Rheumatology, 11*(5), 436-440.

Creamer, P. (1999). Intra-articular corticosteroid treatment in osteoarthritis. *Current Opinion in Rheumatology, 11*(5), 417-421.

Crowther, C. L. (1999). COX-2 inhibitors. *Lippincott's Primary Care Practice, 3*(4), 394-396.

Day, R., Morrison, B., Luza, A., Castaneda, O., Strusberg, A., Nahir, M., Helgetveit, K. B., Kress, B., Daniels, B., Bolognese, J., Krupa, D., Seidenberg, B., & Ehrich, E. (2000). A randomized trial of the efficacy and tolerability of the COX-2 inhibitor rofecoxib vs ibuprofen in patients with osteoarthritis. Rofecoxib/Ibuprofen Comparator Study Group. *Archives of Internal Medicine, 160*(12), 1781-1787.

Delafuente, J. C. (2000). Glucosamine in the treatment of osteoarthritis. *Rheumatic Diseases Clinics of North America, 26*(1), 1-11.

Dequeker, J. (1999). The inverse relationship between osteoporosis and osteoarthritis. *Advances in Experimental Medicine & Biology, 455,* 419-422.

Estes, J. P., Bochenek, C., & Fasler, P. (2000). Osteoarthritis of the fingers. *Journal of Hand Therapy, 13*(2), 108-123.

Evans, C. H., & Robbins, P. D. (1999). Potential treatment of osteoarthritis by gene therapy. *Rheumatic Diseases Clinics of North America, 25*(2), 333-344.

Freemantle, N. (2000). Cost-effectiveness of non-steroidal anti-inflammatory drugs (NSAIDs)—What makes a NSAID good value for money? *Rheumatology (Oxford), 39*(3), 232-234.

Ghosh, P. (1999). The pathobiology of osteoarthritis and the rationale for the use of pentosan polysulfate for its treatment. *Seminars in Arthritis & Rheumatism, 28*(4), 211-267.

Golden, B. D., & Abramson, S. B. (1999). Selective cyclooxygenase-2 inhibitors. *Rheumatic Diseases Clinics of North America, 25*(2), 359-378.

Goldring, M. B. (2000). The role of the chondrocyte in osteoarthritis. *Arthritis & Rheumatism, 43*(9), 1916-1926.

Goldstein, D. J., Wang, O., Todd, L. E., Gitter, B. D., DeBrota, D. J., & Iyengar, S. (2000). Study of the analgesic effect of lanepitant in patients with osteoarthritis pain. *Clinical Pharmacology & Therapeutics, 67*(4), 419-426.

Gomes, J. L., Marczyk, L. R., & Ruthner, R. P. (2001). Arthroscopic exposure of the patellar articular surface. *Arthroscopy, 17,* 98-100.

Gotzsche, P. C. (2000). Non-steroidal anti-inflammatory drugs. *British Medical Journal, 320*(7241), 1058-1061.

Hawker, G. A., Wright, J. G., Coyte, P. C., Williams, J. I., Harvey, B., Glazier, R., & Badley, E. M. (2000). Differences between men and women in the rate of use of hip and knee arthroplasty. *New England Journal of Medicine, 342*(14), 1016-1022.

Hawkey, C. J., Jackson, L., Harper, S. E., Simon, T. J., Mortensen, E., & Lines, C. R. (2001). Review article: The gastrointestinal safety profile of rofecoxib, a highly selective inhibitor of cyclooxygenase-2, in humans. *Alimentary Pharmacology & Therapeutics, 15,* 1-9.

Holderbaum, D., Haqqi, T. M., & Moskowitz, R. W. (1999). Genetics and osteoarthritis: Exposing the iceberg. *Arthritis & Rheumatism, 42*(3), 397-405.

Hurwitz, D. E., Sharma, L., & Andriacchi, T. P. (1999). Effect of knee pain on joint loading in patients with osteoarthritis. *Current Opinion in Rheumatology, 11*(5), 422-426.

Kang, R., Ghivizzani, S. C., Muzzonigro, T. S., Herndon, J. H., Robbins, P. D., & Evans, C. H. (2000). Orthopaedic applications of The Marshall R. Urist Young Investor Award. Orthopaedic applications of gene therapy. From concept to clinic. *Clinical Orthopaedics & Related Research, 375,* 324-337.

Kee, C. C. (2000). Osteoarthritis: Manageable scourge of aging. *Nursing Clinics of North America, 35*(1), 199-208.

Kent, H. (2000). Pinpointing the genes at work in osteoarthritis and cardiovascular disease. *Canadian Medical Association Journal, 162*(11), 1604.

Kirwan, J., & Quilty, B. (878). The patient with osteoarthritis. *Practitioner, 243*(1605), 873-876.

Krane, S. M. (2001). Petulant cellular acts: Destroying the ECM rather than creating it [letter; comment]. *Journal of Clinical Investigation, 107,* 31-32.

Ladislas, R. (2000). Cellular and molecular mechanisms of aging and age related diseases. *Pathology Oncology Research, 6*(1), 3-9.

Lane, N. E., & Buckwalter, J. A. (1999). Exercise and osteoarthritis. *Current Opinion in Rheumatology, 11*(5), 413-416.

Lane, S. R., Trindade, M. C., Ikenoue, T., Mohtai, M., Das, P., Carter, D. R., Goodman, S. B., & Schurman, D. J. (2000). Effects of shear stress on articular chondrocyte metabolism. *Biorheology, 37*(1-2), 95-107.

Lockard, M. A. (2000). Exercise for the patient with upper quadrant osteoarthritis. *Journal of Hand Therapy, 13*(2), 175-183.

Loeser, R. F. (2000). Chondrocyte integrin expression and function. *Biorheology, 37*(1-2), 109-116.

Lotz, M., Hashimoto, S., & Kuhn, K. (1999). Mechanisms of chondrocyte apoptosis. *Osteoarthritis & Cartilage, 7*(4), 389-391.

Mandell, B. F. (1999). COX 2-selective NSAIDs: Biology, promises, and concerns. *Cleveland Clinic Journal of Medicine, 66*(5), 285-292.

Manek, N. J., & Lane, N. E. (2000). Osteoarthritis: Current concepts in diagnosis and management. *American Family Physician, 61*(6), 1795-1804.

McAlindon, T. (2001). Glusoamine for osteoarthritis: Dawn of a new era? *Lancet, 357,* 247-248.

McAlindon, T. E., LaValley, M. P., Gulin, J. P., & Felson, D. T. (2000). Glucosamine and chondroitin for treatment of osteoarthritis: A systematic quality assessment and meta-analysis. *Journal of the American Medical Association, 283*(11), 1469-1475.

Mckinney, R. H., & Ling, S. M. (2000). Osteoarthritis: No cure, but many options for symptom relief. *Cleveland Clinic Journal of Medicine, 67*(9), 665-671.

Myers, S. L. (2000). Synovial fluid markers in osteoarthritis. *Rheumatic Diseases Clinics of North America, 25*(2), 433-449.

O'Connor, W. J., Botti, T., Khan, S. N., & Lane, J. M. (2000). The use of growth factors in cartilage repair. *Orthopedic Clinics of North America, 31*(3), 399-410.

Peat, G., McCarney, R., & Croft, P. (2001). Knee pain and osteoarthritis in older adults: A review of community burden and current use of primary health care. *Annals of the Rheumatic Diseases, 60,* 91-97.

Puppione, A. A. (1999). Management strategies for older adults with osteoarthritis: How to promote and maintain function. *Journal of the American Academy of Nurse Practitioners, 11*(4), 167-171.

Reginster, J. Y., Deroisy, R., Rovati, L. C., Lee, R. L., Lejeune, E., Bruyere, O., Giacovelli, G., Henrotin, Y., Dacre, J. E., & Gossett, C. (2001). Long-term effects of glucosamine sulphate on osteoarthritis progression: A randomised, placebo-controlled clinical trial. *Lancet, 357,* 251-256.

Rovati, L. C., Annefeld, M., Giacovelli, G., Schmid, K., & Setnikar, I. (1999). Glucosamine in osteoarthritis. *Lancet, 354*(9190), 1640-1642.

Ryan, L. M., & Cheung, H. S. (1999). The role of crystals in osteoarthritis. *Rheumatic Diseases Clinics of North America, 25*(2), 257-267.

Saxon, L., Finch, C., & Bass, S. (1999). Sports participation, sports injuries and osteoarthritis: Implications for prevention [review, 80 refs]. *Sports Medicine, 28*(2), 123-135.

Sharkey, N. A., Williams, N. I., & Guerin, J. B. (2000). The role of exercise in the prevention and treatment of osteoporosis and osteoarthritis. *Nursing Clinics of North America, 35*(1), 209-221.

Sowers, M., & Lachance, L. (1999). Vitamins and arthritis. The roles of vitamins A, C, D, and E [review, 79 refs]. *Rheumatic Diseases Clinics of North America, 25*(2), 315-332.

Studer, R., Jaffurs, D., Stefanovic-Racic, M., Robbins, P. D., & Evans, C. H. (1999). Nitric oxide in osteoarthritis. *Osteoarthritis & Cartilage, 7*(4), 377-379.

Uebelhart, D., & Williams, J. M. (1999). Effects of hyaluronic acid on cartilage degradation. *Current Opinion in Rheumatology, 11*(5), 427-435.

Verhagen, A. P., de Vet, H. C., de Bie, R. A., Kessels, A. G., Boers, M., & Knipschild, P. G. (2000). Balneotherapy for rheumatoid arthritis and osteoarthritis. *Cochrane Database of Systematic Reviews* (2) *[computer file],* CD000518.

Weale, A. E., Halabi, O. A., Jones, P. W., & White, S. H. (2001). Perceptions of outcomes after unicompartmental and total knee replacements. *Clinical Orthopaedics & Related Research, 382,* 143-153.

Wen, D. Y. (2000). Intra-articular hyaluronic acid injections for knee osteoarthritis. *American Family Physician, 62*(3), 565-570.

Wollheim, F. A. (2000). Serum markers of articular cartilage damage and repair. *Rheumatic Diseases Clinics of North America, 25*(2), 417-432.

Wright, K. E., Maurer, S. G., & Di Cesare, P. E. (2000). Viscosupplementation for osteoarthritis. *American Journal of Orthopedics (Chatham, NJ), 29*(2), 80-88.

Case Study

Osteoarthritis

INITIAL HISTORY

- 74-year-old woman complaining of a several-year history of aching in her knees, right greater than left, that is worse when it rains.
- Now she is having difficulty going up the stairs in her home.
- She has also had low back pain for many years.
- Suffered a broken right hip 3 years ago when she fell on an icy sidewalk.

Question 1   What questions would you like to ask this patient about her symptoms?

ADDITIONAL HISTORY

- Her knees started to get significantly more painful after she gained 15 pounds over the past 6 months.
- She denies any swollen, red, hot, or deformed joints.
- She played field hockey in college and had a right knee injury at that time, but never needed surgery.
- Her joints are the most stiff after she has been sitting or lying still, they "loosen up" with activity.
- Her back pain doesn't seem to be getting any worse and her hip seems to have healed well.
- She denies any numbness, weakness, or shooting pains in her legs.
- She takes ibuprofen 400 mg QID with some relief, but it gives her indigestion.

Question 2   What would you like to ask this patient about her medical history?

YET MORE HISTORY

- She denies ever having been told she has arthritis.
- She has been worried about osteoporosis, but has never been diagnosed as having it.
- She has had mild hypertension for many years and was once hospitalized for diverticulitis.
- She denies cardiac, lung, or renal diseases, and has never had blood in her stool or an ulcer.
- She had a hysterectomy without oophorectomy 20 years ago and has never taken hormones.
- She is taking no prescribed medications and has no allergies.

Question 3   Are there any important things to ask her about her lifestyle and social history?

LIFESTYLE AND SOCIAL HISTORY

- She exercises regularly in the pool but can no longer walk daily as she has in the past.
- She has a well-balanced diet but it is high in prepared foods and soft drinks and low in calcium.
- She does not smoke and drinks 1 to 2 mixed drinks each evening.
- She lives with her 80-year-old sister in a 2-story home on the outskirts of town.

Question 4   Based on the history alone, what is the differential diagnosis of this patient's musculoskeletal complaints?

PHYSICAL EXAMINATION

- Alert, obese white female in no distress.
- T = 37 orally; P = 70 and regular; RR = 12 and unlabored; BP = 155/88 right arm, sitting.

HEENT, Skin, Neck

- PERRL, fundi without vascular changes, pharynx clear.
- Skin without rashes or ecchymoses.
- No thyromegaly, adenopathy, or bruits.

Lungs, Cardiac
- Good chest excursion; lungs clear to auscultation and percussion.
- RRR without murmurs or gallops.

Abdomen, Neurological
- Abdomen without tenderness or organomegaly; stool heme negative.
- Cranial nerves intact; sensory exam normal and symmetrical.
- Strength 5/5 in both upper extremities; 4/5 in lower extremities.
- Gait slow but without specific deficits.

Musculoskeletal
- Full passive and active range of motion at shoulders and elbows.
- Decreased range of motion and Bouchard's and Heberden's nodes in bilateral hand exam.
- Back with decreased flexion and extension with mild scoliosis.
- Both knees enlarged with decreased range of motion and crepitus, right greater than left.
- Right hip with decreased external and internal rotation but without pain.
- No joint heat, tenderness, or erythema.

Question 5   What are the pertinent positives and negatives in this patient's exam?

Question 6   What laboratory studies are indicated now?

LABORATORY RESULTS

- Chemistries, including BUN, Cr, calcium, and phosphate, normal.
- CBC, including HCT, normal.
- Thyroid functions normal.
- X-ray of right knee reveals joint space narrowing, subchondral sclerosis, and bone cysts; no radiographic evidence of osteoporosis.
- X-ray of lumbosacral spine reveals disc space narrowing and osteophyte formation, especially at L3-L4 and L4-L5 without evidence of compression fracture.

Question 7   What is the diagnosis?

Question 8   How should this patient be managed?

25

Alterations During Menopause

DEFINITION

- Menopause is defined by the World Health Organization as the permanent cessation of menstruation resulting from the loss of ovarian follicular activity. After 12 consecutive months of amenorrhea, the final menstrual period is retrospectively designated as the time of menopause.

- Postmenopause is defined as commencing from the time of the final menstrual period.

- Perimenopause (climacteric) or menopause transition is defined as the physiologic antecedents associated with the transition from premenopausal to postmenopausal follicular function and comprises the period of time (2 to 8 years) preceding the menopause and one year following the final menses. Thus, the last year of the perimenopause coincides with the first year of the postmenopause.

EPIDEMIOLOGY

- Women in the United States can now expect to spend a third of their lives postmenopausal.

- The average age of menopause is between 48 and 52 years (age 51 is most often quoted) but anytime between age 40 and 60 is normal.

- The factors associated with early menopause include smoking (average 1 to 2 years younger), menstrual cycles shorter than 26 days, gynecologic surgery (without oophorectomy), and cancer chemotherapy or radiotherapy (ovarian failure in 40% to 85%, especially if age over 40 during treatment).

- The factors associated with late menopause include early menarche and high parity.

- Although this is a natural process of aging, 90% of women are symptomatic and there are clear health implications.

  - The type and number of climacteric symptoms are related to race, ethnicity, education, perceived life stressors, and amount of exercise and leisure interests.

  - The onset of symptoms often occurs during the perimenopause before cessation of menses.

PATHOPHYSIOLOGY

- The transition to menopause occurs due to an interaction of central nervous system, endocrine, and ovarian events leading to an increase in the rate of loss of ovarian follicles resulting in irregular reproductive cycles. Although the loss of ovarian estrogen release is key to the symptoms of the climacteric, several discoveries suggest that there is a more complex interaction of events.

  - FSH begins to rise in an intermittent and unpredictable way beginning at age 40, even when estradiol and progesterone levels remain normal and menstrual cycles are regular.

  - Hot flashes and sleep disturbances (felt to be more directly related to hypothalamic dysfunction than to pure estrogen deficiency) can occur beginning age 40, even when estradiol and cycles remain normal.

  - Desynchronization of neural signals with changes in the daily and monthly rhythmicity of hormone levels has been documented before measurable primary ovarian dysfunction occurs.

- Inhibin A and inhibin B are ovarian and pituitary compounds that form a secondary negative feedback loop on the hypothalamic/pituitary axis that is independent of hormone levels. The neuroendocrine changes seen prior to ovarian failure (ex. ↑ FSH) are seen when inhibin B levels decline beginning in the early 40s.

- Early perimenopause

  - There are fewer oocytes by the time of the perimenopause (ovary contains 380,000 oocytes at menarche but there is significant oocyte atresia and one is used per cycle).

  - The cycle length is slightly shortened because of a shortened follicular phase (first clinical indication of the perimenopause).

  - Follicle-stimulating hormone (FSH) levels begin to rise (first laboratory indication of the perimenopause).

  - Ovarian gonadotropin receptors diminish.

- Middle perimenopause

  - There are changes in the menstrual pattern with unpredictable variations in cycle length; women often experience long intermenstrual intervals interspersed with short cycles.

  - The unpredictable variations are probably due to erratic maturation of the remaining ovarian follicles with some ovulatory cycles (estrogen rise followed by leuteinizing hormone [LH] and progesterone secretion) mixed with anovulatory cycles (no LH and progesterone surge).

  - Follicle-stimulating hormone (FSH) levels rise significantly (>25 mIU/mL).

  - Early symptoms include hot flashes, breast tenderness, and dysfunctional uterine bleeding.

- Late perimenopause and postmenopause

  - There is no ovulation, estradiol levels fall.

  - Ovarian stroma continues to produce androgens (androstenedione and testosterone).

  - Androstenedione is converted to estrone and estradiol in peripheral fat cells so that there is some protective estrogen effect until late in life, especially in obese women.

  - A small amount of progesterone is made by the adrenal gland.

- Effects of estrogen deficiency

  - Atherosclerotic cardiovascular disease: increased risk of coronary and cerebrovascular disease (proposed mechanisms include decreased ability to heal vascular injury, decreased endogenous vasodilators [ex. nitric oxide], decreased insulin sensitivity, decreased high density lipoprotein and increased low density lipoprotein [especially small dense LDL; downregulates hepatic LDL receptors], increased Lp[a]).

  - Cognitive defects, dementia, and central nervous system injury: proposed mechanisms include dysregulation of numerous neurotransmitters, decrease in neuronal growth factors, decreases in cerebral blood flow, increased silent cerebral ischemic events, and altered sleep patterns (ex. sleep related disordered breathing, insomnia).

  - Osteoporosis: increased osteoclast activity (see Chapter 23).

  - Genitourinary atrophy and dysfunction: atrophic vaginitis, urethritis, incontinence, uterovaginal prolapse (proposed mechanisms include vaginal wall atrophy, increases in vaginal pH, thinning of the urethral mucosa, decreased sensitivity of the alpha-adrenergic receptors at the bladder neck, atrophy of the bladder trigone).

- Vasomotor instability (hot flash): affects 80% to 85% of U.S. women and begins in the perimenopause.

    1) A specific thermoregulatory disorder triggered by a neuroendocrine imbalance from the hypothalamus that is believed to be initiated by estrogen deficiency.

    2) Characterized by low level surges in LH occurring several times every hour; LH centers in the hypothalamus are near areas that regulate body temperature.

    3) 70% of these LH surges result in an increase in skin temperature of up to 4° C with associated symptoms.

    4) Increased frequency of symptomatic episodes has been associated with stress. It may be mediated in part by the lack of estrogen regulation of catecholamines; exercise appears to help this aspect.

    5) Peripheral vasodilation is followed by vasoconstriction and shiver.

    6) Episodes of flushing of the skin, perspiration, palpitations, nausea, and dizziness.

    7) May disrupt sleep cycles.

    8) Presence of hot flashes may be associated with an increased risk for osteoporosis and other metabolic abnormalities, such as hyperglycemia, but this is controversial.

- Other: increases in intraabdominal fat, decreases in skeletal muscle contractility, alterations in integument structure.

PATIENT PRESENTATION

History

Woman in her late 40s or early 50s; menstrual cycle changes with shortened cycles followed by erratic cycles; smoking; chemotherapy; surgery; hormone use.

Symptoms

- Perimenopausal symptomatology involves three interacting factors:
    - Loss of estrogen
    - Sociologic changes in aging
    - Psychologic changes in aging
- Perimenopausal and menopausal symptomatology:
    - Hot flashes/perspiration
    - Atrophic vaginitis/vaginal discharge/dyspareunia
    - Uterovaginal prolapse/urethritis/stress incontinence
    - Decreased cognitive ability/memory loss
    - Fatigue/insomnia/anxiety/mood lability
    - Decreased muscle strength
    - Osteoporosis/fractures
    - Alopecia/hirsutism
    - Skin dryness/pruritus/wrinkles

Examination

Dry skin, alopecia; hirsutism; loss of height; vaginal dryness and discharge; uterine prolapse; evidence of atherosclerotic disease.

KEYS TO ASSESSMENT

- If patient is younger than 40 years of age, evaluate for possible causes of premature menopause (gynecologic surgery especially with oophorectomy, chemotherapy, congenital abnormalities [Turner syndrome]).

- Obtain a careful menstrual history including menarche, premenopause, perimenopause, and any postmenopausal bleeding.

- Carefully review symptoms: ask about sleep, fatigue, and mood; and about exercise, smoking, and diet.

- Assess for medical contraindications for hormone replacement (breast or endometrial cancer, active thrombotic disease, undiagnosed uterine bleeding, hepatic failure).

- Perform a careful physical exam with special attention to cardiovascular and gynecologic exams.

- Consider possible laboratory evaluation for osteoporosis (see Chapter 23).

- Measure serum FSH levels.

- Assess the patient's symptoms and risk for cardiovascular disease and osteoporosis.

- Assess the patient's understanding and perceptions of hormone replacement therapy.

KEYS TO MANAGEMENT

- Nonpharmacologic

    - Exercise has been shown to result in improvement in hot flashes, mood, muscle strength, bone mineral density, and overall quality of life while decreasing postmenopausal cardiac risk.

    - Smoking cessation can result in improved estrogen effects and decreased cardiovascular risk.

    - Help the patient identify and avoid stimuli that trigger vasomotor flashes, including alcohol, caffeine, and hot spicy foods; layered clothing may help with temperature control.

    - Modify diet to include soy; vitamins B, C, and E; and milk (contains calcium and L-tryptophan to promote sleep).

    - Educate the patient about using vaginal lubricants.

    - Create a safe and caring environment for patients so that open discussion can occur about symptoms, aging, and relationship concerns, and provide reassurance that all women experience some difficulties in making the transition to older life can be very helpful.

- Hormone replacement therapy (HRT)

    - There remains considerable controversy over the risks and benefits of HRT.

    - Risks:

        1) Increased risk for breast cancer (see Chapter 9).

        2) Increased risk for endometrial cancer if HRT is given without progesterone ("unopposed estrogen") in patients who have not undergone hysterectomy.

        3) Increased risk of thromboembolic disease.

        4) In patients with known atherosclerotic cardiovascular disease, may increase the risk of ischemic events in the short run when administered for secondary prevention (increases C-reactive protein and promotes thombosis).

        5) Increased risk for gallbladder symptoms.

        6) May increase frequency and severity of headache in patients with migraines.

        7) It may worsen hepatic failure in patients with underlying hepatic disease.

- Benefits of HRT are numerous.
  1) Prevention and treatment of osteoporosis (see Chapter 23).
  2) Improvement in cardiovascular risk factors, including an improved lipid profile (decreases low density lipoprotein [LDL] and lipoprotein [a] [Lp(a)] and increases high density lipoprotein [HDL]).
  3) Possible reduction in risk for atherosclerosis (decreases LDL oxidation and its incorporation into vessel walls and may promote endothelial repair). Although estrogens have been shown to have multiple beneficial effects on vascular function, results from recently published prospective studies on HRT for the primary prevention of coronary artery disease have not shown significant reductions in ischemic events.
  4) Reduction in the incidence of restenosis and recurrent MI after coronary stenting.
  5) Reduction in clinically unsuspected cerebral ischemic events.
  6) Improved carbohydrate metabolism (improves insulin sensitivity and diabetic control).
  7) Reduced risk of Alzheimer's disease and improved cognitive function and memory (improves synaptogenesis and cerebral blood flow).
  8) Improved self-image and mood, and improves sleep.
  9) Increased muscle strength.
  10) Reduction in hot flashes.
  11) Prevention and treatment of urogenital atrophy (vaginitis, urethritis, uterine prolapse).
- Decisions about HRT or alternatives should be collaborative with the patient and should be made after careful assessment of the risks versus the benefits for each individual. Several authors have suggested decision-trees to decide which patients will likely benefit from HRT.
- The type of hormone replacement should be tailored to the individual patient.
  1) Oral estrogen comes as conjugated (Premarin), esterified (Ogen) or micronized (Estrace). Dose is controversial but evidence suggests that 0.3 mg is adequate.
  2) Transdermal estrogen is also effective, avoids first pass through liver in patients with compromised liver function; it may cause localized bruising.
  3) Estrogen should be given daily. The common dose of Premarin is 0.625 mg/day but new studies suggest that 0.3 mg/day results in positive bone and lipid changes without inducing endometrial hyperplasia (more study is needed).
  4) Progesterone should be given to all women who receive estrogen and have a uterus.
  5) The duration of HRT remains highly controversial. Bone mineralization will reverse rapidly with cessation of estrogen, and cardiovascular risk also rises, however, the risk of breast cancer is greatest in those taking estrogens for 10 years or more.
- Alternatives to HRT:
  1) The selective estrogen receptor modulators (SERMS) are an expanding group of drugs that have estrogenic effects on some tissues and antiestrogenic effects on others. Raloxifene has been approved for the treatment of osteoporosis and improves the lipid profile, but does not increase the risk of breast or endometrial cancer. The cardiovascular effects of raloxifene are less than those seen with estrogens, however, so the search for better SERMS continues.
  2) Progestins alone can help reduce hot flashes but they are associated with dysfunctional uterine bleeding, mood changes, and worsening of vaginal atrophy.
  3) Androgens are used with estrogen in some women to increase libido, decrease breast tenderness, and decrease migraines; there is no indication for androgens alone.

4) Phytoestrogens are estrogen-like compounds created by the intestinal bacterial conversion of iso flavonoids (found in soybean products) and lignins (found in cereals, seeds, and nuts); they may have an antiestrogenic (and possibly anticancer) effect on breast tissue while reducing hot flashes.

5) A variety of other drugs have been used for vasomotor symptoms with variable effectiveness, including clonidine, methyldopa, and paroxetine hydrochloride.

6) For patients with significant risks for breast cancer or preexisting coronary disease, other approaches to cardiovascular risk reduction should be considered, such as statins.

Pathophysiology $\rightarrow$ Clinical Link

What is going on in the disease process that influences how the patient presents and how he or she should be managed?

What should you do now that you understand the underlying pathophysiology?

Perimenopause is characterized by fewer oocytes with decreased follicular estradiol production.	Premenopausal causes of increased oocyte loss (e.g., chemotherapy) can result in early onset menopause.
Decreased estradiol levels, increased FSH, erratic ovulation, and decreased ovarian gonadotropin receptors are associated with perimenopause.	The perimenopausal period can be diagnosed by increasing FSH levels and changes in the menstrual cycle such as shortened intermenstrual periods.
Estrogen is important to maintaining normal functioning of the skin, neurons, blood vessels, bones, muscles, and the urogenital epithelium.	Perimenopausal estrogen deficiency is characterized by thin, dry skin, decreased cognitive ability, increased cardiovascular risk, osteoporosis, decreased muscle strength, and atrophic vaginitis.
In the last perimenopause, LH levels demonstrate low-level frequent, episodic surges associated with hypothalamic-induced changes in body temperature. These LH surges are inhibited by exogenous estrogen replacement.	Vasomotor instability (hot flashes) occurs frequently in perimenopausal women and is associated with a feeling of heat and sweating that can be effectively treated with HRT.
Hot flashes cause sleep cycle disturbance.	HRT improves sleep.
Estrogen decreases LDL and Lp(a), increases HDL, improves vascular dilation, and decreases LDL oxidation and its incorporation into the vessel.	HRT reduces cardiovascular risk profiles, however a reduction in actual ischemic events has not been documented. The search for a better form of hormone replacement continues.
Estrogen causes an increase in breast cancer risk, an increase in endometrial hyperplasia and endometrial cancer risk, and an increase in the risk of thromboembolism.	Patients should be well-educated about their individual risk-benefit profile for HRT, and treatment discussions should be made collaboratively with the patient and tailored to her individual needs.
New selective estrogen receptor modulators have antiestrogen effects in the breast, and have variable effects on estrogen receptors in bone, heart, liver, and endometrium.	New options for HRT may reduce the risk of breast and improve osteoporosis and cardiovascular risk, however better drugs are needed.

Suggested Reading

Anonymous. (1999). Hormone replacement therapy. Clinical Synthesis Panel on HRT. *Lancet, 354*(9173), 152-155.

Anonymous. (2000). A decision tree for the use of estrogen replacement therapy or hormone replacement therapy in postmenopausal women: Consensus opinion of The North American Menopause Society. *Menopause, 7*(2), 76-86.

Anonymous. (2000). Phytoestrogens. *Medical Letter on Drugs & Therapeutics, 42*(1072), 17-18.

Appling, S. E., Allen, J. K., Van Zandt, S., Olsen, S., Brager, R., & Hallerdin, J. (2000). Knowledge of menopause and hormone replacement therapy use in low-income urban women. *Journal of Womens Health & Gender-Based Medicine, 9*(1), 57-64.

Armstrong, A. L., Oborne, J., Coupland, C. A., Macpherson, M. B., Bassey, E. J., & Wallace, W. A. (1996). Effects of hormone replacement therapy on muscle performance and balance in post-menopausal women. *Clinical Science, 91*(6), 685-690.

Arpels, J. C. (1996). The female brain hypoestrogenic continuum from the premenstrual syndrome to menopause. A hypothesis and review of supporting data. *Journal of Reproductive Medicine, 41*(9), 633-639.

Bartlik, B., & Goldstein, M. Z. (2000). Maintaining sexual health after menopause. *Psychiatric Services, 51*(6), 751-753.

Benazzi, F. (2000). Female depression before and after menopause. *Psychotherapy & Psychosomatics, 69*(5), 280-283.

Berstein, L. M., Tsyrlina, E. V., Kolesnik, O. S., Gamajunova, V. B., & Adlercreutz, H. (2000). Catecholestrogens excretion in smoking and non-smoking postmenopausal women receiving estrogen replacement therapy. *Journal of Steroid Biochemistry & Molecular Biology, 72*(3-4), 143-147.

Boggs, P. P., & Rosenthal, M. B. (2000). Helping women help themselves: Developing a menopause discussion group. *Clinical Obstetrics & Gynecology, 43*(1), 207

Brzezinski, A., & Benshushan, A. (2000). Neuropeptides, neurotransmitters, body weight, and menopause *Menopause, 7*(3), 137-139.

Burger, H. G. (1999). The endocrinology of the menopause [Review, 21 refs]. *Journal of Steroid Biochemistry & Molecular Biology, 69*(1-6), 31-35.

Burger, H. G., Dudley, E. C., Cui, J., Dennerstein, L., & Hopper, J. L. (2000). A prospective longitudinal study of serum testosterone, dehydroepiandrosterone sulfate, and sex hormone-binding globulin levels through the menopause transition. *Journal of Clinical Endocrinology & Metabolism, 85*(8), 2832-2838.

Burstein, H. J., & Winer, E. P. (2000). Primary care for survivors of breast cancer. *New England Journal of Medicine, 343*(15), 1086-1094.

Bush, T. L. (2000). Preserving cardiovascular benefits of hormone replacement therapy. *Journal of Reproductive Medicine, 45*(3 Suppl), 259-273.

Carr, M. C., Kim, K. H., Zambon, A., Mitchell, E. S., Woods, N. F., Casazza, C. P., Purnell, J. Q., Hokanson, J. E., Brunzell, J. D., & Schwartz, R. S. (2000). Changes in LDL density across the menopausal transition. *Journal of Investigative Medicine, 48*(4), 245-250.

Cutson, T. M., & Meuleman, E. (2000). Managing menopause. *American Family Physician, 61*(5), 1391-1400.

D'Agostino, R. B., Russell, M. W., Huse, D. M., Ellison, R. C., Silbershatz, H., Wilson, P. W., & Hartz, S. C. (2000). Primary and subsequent coronary risk appraisal: New results from the Framingham study. *American Heart Journal, 139*(2 Pt 1), 272-281.

Falkeborn, M., Schairer, C., Naessen, T., & Persson, I. (2000). Risk of myocardial infarction after oophorectomy and hysterectomy. *Journal of Clinical Epidemiology, 53*(8), 832-837.

Fillenbaum, G. G., Hanlon, J. T., Landerman, L. R., & Schmader, K. E. (2001). Impact of estrogen use on decline in cognitive function in a representative sample of older community-resident women. *American Journal of Epidemiology, 153,* 137-144.

Franceschi, S., Gallus, S., Talamini, R., Tavani, A., Negri, E., & La Vecchia, C. (2000). Menopause and colorectal cancer. *British Journal of Cancer, 82*(11), 1860-1862.

Ganz, P. A., Greendale, G. A., Petersen, L., Zibecchi, L., Kahn, B., & Belin, T. R. (2000). Managing menopausal symptoms in breast cancer survivors: Results of a randomized controlled trial. *Journal of the National Cancer Institute, 92*(13), 1054-1064.

Gold, E. B., Sternfeld, B., Kelsey, J. L., Brown, C., Mouton, C., Reame, N., Salamone, L., & Stellato, R. (2000). Relation of demographic and lifestyle factors to symptoms in a multi-racial/ethnic population of women 40-55 years of age. *American Journal of Epidemiology, 152*(5), 463-473.

Gorodeski, G. I. (2000). Effects of menopause and estrogen on cervical epithelial permeability. *Journal of Clinical Endocrinology & Metabolism, 85*(7), 2584-2595.

Grady, D., Brown, J. S., Vittinghoff, E., Applegate, W., Varner, E., Snyder, T., & The HERS Research Group. (2001). Postmenopausal hormones and incontinence: The Heart and Estrogen/Progestin Replacement Study. *Obstetrics & Gynecology, 97,* 116-120.

Greendale, G. A., Lee, N. P., & Arriola, E. R. (1999). The menopause. *Lancet, 353*(9152), 571-580.

Greendale, G. A., & Sowers, M. (1997). The menopause transition. *Endocrinology & Metabolism Clinics of North America, 26*(2), 261-277.

Grodstein, F., Stampfer, M. J., Manson, J. E., Colditz, G. A., Willett, W. C., Rosner, B., Speizer, F. E., & Hennekens, C. H. (1996). Postmenopausal estrogen and progestin use and the risk of cardiovascular disease. *New England Journal of Medicine, 335*(7), 453-461.

Hadji, P., Hars, O., Bock, K., Sturm, G., Bauer, T., Emons, G., & Schulz, K. D. (2000). The influence of menopause and body mass index on serum leptin concentrations. *European Journal of Endocrinology, 143*(1), 55-60.

Hayward, C. S., Kelly, R. P., & Collins, P. (2000). The roles of gender, the menopause and hormone replacement on cardiovascular function. *Cardiovascular Research, 46*(1), 28-49.

Igarashi, M., Saito, H., Morioka, Y., Oiji, A., Nadaoka, T., & Kashiwakura, M. (2000). Stress vulnerability and climacteric symptoms: Life events, coping behavior, and severity of symptoms. *Gynecologic & Obstetric Investigation, 49*(3), 170-178.

Jacobsen, B. K., Heuch, I., & Kvale, G. (2000). On mortality from ischemic heart disease in women with very late menopause. *Journal of Clinical Epidemiology, 53*(4), 435-436.

Joakimsen, O., Bonaa, K. H., Stensland-Bugge, E., & Jacobsen, B. K. (2000). Population-based study of age at menopause and ultrasound assessed carotid atherosclerosis: The Tromso Study. *Journal of Clinical Epidemiology, 53*(5), 525-530.

Jones, C. R., & Czajkowski, L. (2000). Evaluation and management of insomnia in menopause. *Clinical Obstetrics & Gynecology, 43*(1), 184-197.

Jones, K. P. (2000). Hormone replacement therapy: Making a 45-year plan. *Clinical Obstetrics & Gynecology, 43*(1), 213-218.

Jones, K. P. (2000). Menopause and cognitive function: Estrogens and alternative therapies. *Clinical Obstetrics & Gynecology, 43*(1), 198-206.

Kamali, P., Muller, T., Lang, U., & Clapp, J. F., III. (2000). Cardiovascular responses of perimenopausal women to hormonal replacement therapy. *American Journal of Obstetrics & Gynecology, 182*(1 Pt 1), 17-22.

Kass-Annese, B. (2000). Alternative therapies for menopause. *Clinical Obstetrics & Gynecology, 43*(1), 162-183.

Kawano, H., Motoyama, T., Hirai, N., Yoshimura, T., Kugiyama, K., Ogawa, H., Okamura, H., & Yasue, H. (2001). Effect of medroxyprogesterone acetate plus estradiol on endothelium-dependent vasodilation in postmenopausal women. *American Journal of Cardiology, 87,* 238-240.

Kuller, L. H., Simkin-Silverman, L. R., Wing, R. R., Meilahn, E. N., & Ives, D. G. (2001). Women's Healthy Lifestyle Project. A randomized clinical trial: Results at 54 months [online]. *Circulation, 103,* 32-37.

Lewis-Barned, N. J., Sutherland, W. H., Walker, R. J., de Jong, S. A., Walker, H. L., Edwards, E. A., Markham, V., & Goulding, A. (2000). Plasma cholesteryl ester fatty acid composition, insulin sensitivity, the menopause and hormone replacement therapy. *Journal of Endocrinology, 165*(3), 649-655.

Luciano, A. A., Miller, B. E., Schoenenfeld, M. J., Schaser, R. J., & Ogen/Provera Study Group. (2001). Effects of estrone sulfate alone or with medroxyprogesterone acetate on serum lipoprotein levels in postmenopausal women. *Obstetrics & Gynecology, 97,* 101-108.

Luoto, R., Sharrett, A. R., Schreiner, P., Sorlie, P. D., Arnett, D., & Ephross, S. (2000). Blood pressure and menopausal transition: The Atherosclerosis Risk in Communities Study (1987-95). *Journal of Hypertension, 18*(1), 27-33.

Mahon, S. M., & Williams, M. (2000). Information needs regarding menopause. Results from a survey of women receiving cancer prevention and detection services. *Cancer Nursing, 23*(3), 176-185.

Majmudar, N. G., Robson, S. C., & Ford, G. A. (2000). Effects of the menopause, gender, and estrogen replacement therapy on vascular nitric oxide. *Journal of Clinical Endocrinology & Metabolism, 85*(4), 1577-1583.

Maroulis, G. B. (2000). Alternatives to estrogen replacement therapy. *Annals of the New York Academy of Sciences, 900,* 413-415.

Mattsson, L. A., Bohnet, H. G., Gredmark, T., Torhorst, J., Hornig, F., & Huls, G. (1999). Continuous, combined hormone replacement: Randomized comparison of transdermal and oral preparations. *Obstetrics & Gynecology, 94*(1), 61-65.

Mingo, C., Herman, C. J., & Jasperse, M. (2000). Women's stories: Ethnic variations in women's attitudes and experiences of menopause, hysterectomy, and hormone replacement therapy. *Journal of Womens Health & Gender-Based Medicine, 9*(Suppl 2), S27-S38.

Mix, C., Bergmann, S., Kocis, K., Richter, P., & Jaross, W. (2000). Lipids and stability of menopausal status in middle-aged women within two years. *Clinica y Laboratorio, 46*(3-4), 153-156.

Murray, J. L. (2000). Options and issues in managing menopause. *American Family Physician, 61*(5), 1285.

Rodriguez, C., Calle, E. E., Patel, A. V., Tatham, L. M., Jacobs, E. J., & Thun, M. J. (2001). Effect of body mass on the association between estrogen replacement therapy and mortality among elderly US women. *American Journal of Epidemiology, 153,* 145-152.

Schairer, C., Lubin, J., Troisi, R., Sturgeon, S., Brinton, L., & Hoover, R. (2000). Menopausal estrogen and estrogen-progestin replacement therapy and breast cancer risk. *Journal of the American Medical Association, 283*(4), 485-491.

Shaver, J. L., & Zenk, S. N. (2000). Sleep disturbance in menopause. *Journal of Womens Health & Gender-Based Medicine, 9*(2), 109-118.

Shaw, C. R. (1997). The perimenopausal hot flash: Epidemiology, physiology, and treatment. *Nurse Practitioner, 22*(3), 55-56.

Sherwin, B. B. (1997). Estrogen effects on cognition in menopausal women. *Neurology, 48*(Suppl 7), S21-S26.

Shifren, J. L., & Schiff, I. (2000). The aging ovary. *Journal of Womens Health & Gender-Based Medicine, 9*(Suppl 1), S3-S7.

Somekawa, Y., Chiguchi, M., Ishibashi, T., & Aso, T. (2001). Soy intake related to menopausal symptoms, serum lipids, and bone mineral density in postmenopausal Japanese women. *Obstetrics & Gynecology, 97,* 109-115.

Stearns, V., Isaacs, C., Rowland, J., Crawford, J., Ellis, M. J., Kramer, R., Lawrence, W., Hanfelt, J. J., & Hayes, D. F. (2000). A pilot trial assessing the efficacy of paroxetine hydrochloride (Paxil) in controlling hot flashes in breast cancer survivors. *Annals of Oncology, 11*(1), 17-22.

Tchernof, A., Poehlman, E. T., & Despres, J. P. (2000). Body fat distribution, the menopause transition, and hormone replacement therapy. *Diabetes & Metabolism, 26*(1), 12-20.

Toth, M. J., Tchernof, A., Sites, C. K., & Poehlman, E. T. (2000). Menopause-related changes in body fat distribution. *Annals of the New York Academy of Sciences, 904*, 502-506.

Wise, P. M., Smith, M. J., Dubal, D. B., Wilson, M. E., Krajnak, K. M., & Rosewell, K. L. (1999). Neuroendocrine influences and repercussions of the menopause [review, 60 refs]. *Endocrine Reviews, 20*(3), 243-248.

Zhang, Y., Felson, D. T., Ellison, R. C., Kreger, B. E., Schatzkin, A., Dorgan, J. F., Cupples, L. A., Levy, D., & Kiel, D. P. (2001). Bone mass and the risk of colon cancer among postmenopausal women: The Framingham Study. *American Journal of Epidemiology, 153*, 31-37.

Case Study

Alterations During Menopause

INITIAL HISTORY

- 54-year old white female.
- Complaining of fatigue, hot flashes, perivaginal itching, dyspareunia, and vaginal discharge.
- Menstrual periods stopped 1 year ago after several months of erratic cycles.
- She has had no vaginal bleeding in the past year.

Question 1 What would you like to ask this patient about her symptoms?

ADDITIONAL HISTORY

- Her fatigue has increased gradually over the past 2 years.
- She has hot flashes many times during the day and is frequently awakened at night.
- Her vaginal symptoms have occurred gradually and are not accompanied by abdominal pain or dysuria.
- She denies any history of vaginal infections.
- She has had one sexual partner for 20 years.

Question 2 What would you like to ask about her past medical history?

PAST MEDICAL HISTORY
- No history of migraines, gallbladder disease, deep venous thrombosis, or hepatic disease.
- Has a long history of hypercholesterolemia but has never had chest pain or been diagnosed with heart or cerebrovascular disease.
- No personal or family history of breast cancer.
- Normal mammogram last year.
- Is on no medications and has no allergies.

Question 3   What would you like to ask her about her lifestyle?

LIFESTYLE HISTORY
- She eats a low-fat diet and tries to watch her weight and cholesterol, but she admits her diet is low in calcium and high in phosphate.
- She used to walk regularly but got "out of the habit."
- She does not smoke or drink alcohol.

PHYSICAL EXAMINATION
- Alert thin female with no acute distress; mild kyphosis especially at the upper thoracic spine.
- T = 37 orally; P = 80 and regular; RR = 15 and unlabored; BP = 142/75 right arm.

HEENT, Skin
- Skin is thin and dry without rashes.
- PERRL, fundi without hemorrhages or exudates.
- Pharynx clear.

Lungs, Cardiac
- Good chest excursion; lungs clear to auscultation and percussion.
- Cardiac with RRR without murmurs or gallops.

Abdomen, Extremities
- Abdomen soft, nontender, without organomegaly or masses.
- Extremities with full pulses without edema.

Breasts, Pelvic

- Breasts symmetrical without masses, tenderness, or nipple discharge; axillae without adenopathy.
- Pelvic with dry perivaginal and vaginal tissues; decreased estrogen effect; pap pending; no uterine or adnexal masses.

Neurological

- Oriented x 4.
- Strength and sensation normal and symmetrical.
- DTR 2+ and symmetrical.
- Gait normal.

Question 4 What are the pertinent positives and negatives on exam?

Question 5 What laboratories would you order?

LABORATORY RESULTS

- FSH increased.
- Chemistries, including calcium and phosphate, normal.
- CBC including HCT normal.
- Liver function tests normal.
- Lipid profile shows increased LDL and decreased HDL.
- Mammogram consistent with postmenopause without masses or abnormal calcifications.
- Dual energy x-ray densitometry consistent with decreased bone mineral density.

Question 6   What recommendations for management should be made for this patient?

26

Allergic Rhinitis

DEFINITION

- A clinical condition of increased humoral immunity that is IgE-mediated (type I hypersensitivity) and occurs in response to environmental antigens resulting in inflammation of the upper respiratory tract.

EPIDEMIOLOGY

- Allergic (sometimes called atopic) rhinitis is the most common allergic condition. Its prevalence is estimated at 20% of the U.S. population.
- It is becoming more common, especially in industrialized countries.
- Peak symptoms occur in decades 2, 3, and 4, but children (average age 10) are also affected.
- There is a clear genetic predisposition for allergic disease.
    - There is a 13% prevalence if neither parent is atopic, 30% if one is atopic, and 50% if both parents are atopic.
    - Over 20 genes have been implicated in allergic disease, including interleukin-4 (IL-4,) IL-4 receptor, cytokine, interferon gamma (INFγ), β adrenergic receptor, 5 lipoxygenase, and leukotriene C4 synthetase genes.
- Intrauterine and childhood exposure to allergens increases the risk of allergic rhinitis and other allergic disorders, such as asthma.
- Common allergens include:
    - Seasonal aeroallergens (5 to 70μm in size): flowering plants trees, grasses, ragweed, fungus.
    - Perennial aeroallergens: dust mites, animal dander, roaches, latex, mice feces and urine.
    - Food allergens: eggs, milk, corn, nuts, shellfish.
- The bedroom is the location of allergen exposure that correlates with the greatest risk for allergic disease.
- Childhood infections with some intracellular pathogens (hepatitis A, *toxoplasmosis gondii*, *Helicobacter pylori*) are associated with less risk for developing allergies, whereas a history of vaccination to hepatitis B, pertussis, and polio increases the risk of allergy. Theoretically, the viral infections prime the immune system to respond to environmental antigens with cellular immunity, whereas the vaccinations prime for increased humoral immunity like that seen in allergic disease.
- Exposure to environmental pollutants, such as nitrogen dioxide and sulfur dioxide, can increase the allergic response to allergens.

PATHOPHYSIOLOGY

- Allergens are ingested by macrophages, dendritic cells, and B lymphocytes (antigen presenting cells or APCs). They are then processed and presented on the surface of these cells for interaction with T helper lymphocytes (CD4 cells) (Fig. 26-1).

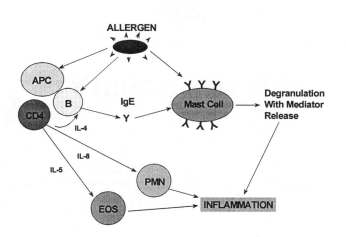

Fig. 26-1 Cellular Interactions in Allergy

- In allergic patients, the number of dendritic cells and B lymphocytes in the respiratory mucosa is increased, which favors the stimulation of humoral immunity.

- In allergy, interleukin-4 (IL-4) is preferentially released by the CD4 cell (TH$_2$ phase of cytokine production) resulting in B lymphocyte proliferation. B cells undergo an "isotype switch" such that they switch from producing IgM to producing large amounts of IgE.

- IgE binds to the mast cell via high affinity Fc receptors with resultant mast cell degranulation and release of vasoactive (ex. histamine), chemotactic, and inflammatory (ex. leukotrienes) mediators.

- Other interleukins (IL-8, IL-5) are also released and activate neutrophils (PMNs) and eosinophils (EOS). A high level of activity of IL-5 may be the crucial step in moving from allergic sensitization to actual symptomatic disease.

- IL-4 and IL-5 also promote adhesion molecule expression on endothelial and epithelial cells leading to more migration of inflammatory cells, especially neutrophils and eosinophils.

- The allergic response then is one of vascular and cellular responses that cause inflammation. This process occurs episodically in response to allergen exposures, but can lead to chronic changes in the respiratory mucosa with persistent symptoms.

- A variety of clinical effects occur depending on the allergen, the individual, and the tissue most targeted for allergic response. In allergic rhinitis.

    - The nasal mucosa becomes edematous with increased mucus production.

    - Inspiratory effort with negative nasal airway pressure results in nasal collapse and airway obstruction. Eustachian tube blockage can result in serous otitis and can lead to otitis media.

    - Upper respiratory inflammation is associated with lower airway inflammatory responses and can be associated with asthma.

    - There is often a late-phase response mediated by memory T cells and eosinophils in which symptoms recur 4 to 12 hours after the initial exposure.

PATIENT PRESENTATION

History

Family history of allergy, allergen exposure, perennial or seasonal symptoms, underlying respiratory disease, childhood infections and vaccinations.

Symptoms

Nasal congestion, rhinorrhea, postnasal drainage, sore throat, cough (especially when lying down), hoarseness, sneezing, itchy nose, watery eyes, headache, ear ache, loss of smell and taste, fatigue, daytime somnolence.

Examination

Shiners, Dennie Morgan infraorbital creases, allergic salute, swollen pale nasal mucus membranes, nasal and pharyngeal erythema, nasal polyps, serous otitis; children may develop high arched palate and dental overbite (facial remodeling due to persistent mouth breathing).

DIFFERENTIAL DIAGNOSIS

- Infectious rhinitis (rhinovirus, adenovirus)
- Rhinitis medicamentosa
- Gustatory, vasomotor, atrophic or drug-induced rhinitis
- Sinusitis
- Cerebrospinal fluid rhinorrhea
- Adenoidal hyperplasia
- Nasal polyps
- Septal deviation, adenocarcinoma of the nasal mucosa
- Foreign bodies
- Otitis media
- Ciliary dyskinesia syndrome

KEYS TO ASSESSMENT

- A nasal smear that reveals numerous eosinophils confirms allergy.
- Sinus films (plain x-ray or computed tomography) can evaluate for associated sinusitis.
- Allergy testing:
  - Skin testing: epidermal injection as a test dose followed by dermal injection.
    1) The size of the response correlates with degree of symptoms.
    2) Anaphylaxis is a small risk.
    3) False positives (sensitization to an allergen without actual symptoms from it) and false negatives can occur.
  - Serum antibody testing (radioallergosorbent testing [RAST]) is expensive and slow but has no risk for anaphylaxis (also can have false positives and negatives).

KEYS TO MANAGEMENT

- Allergen avoidance
  - Decontaminate surfaces with 1:10 dilution of bleach, encase pillows and mattresses.
  - Provide pet free areas (especially the bedrooms).
  - Use dehumidifiers and wear a mask when vacuuming.

- Antihistamines
  - In general, use antihistamines alone for seasonal rhinitis and in combination with decongestants (pseudoephedrine, naphazoline, oxymetazoline) for perennial rhinitis.
  - "First generation" antihistamines (ex. diphenhydramine) can cause irritability, insomnia, hypertension, arrhythmias, and seizures.
  - "Second generation" antihistamines (azelastine, cetirizine, fexofenadine, loratadine) are more effective with less side effects and may decrease associated asthma symptoms.
- Antiinflammatories
  - Nasal steroids cause symptomatic relief in up to 90% or patients and are superior to antihistamines in relieving nasal symptoms.
  - Nasal cromolyn should be considered for children.
  - Leukotriene antagonists (e.g., Montelukast) can also be effective in relieving symptoms.
  - Oral steroids should be used only for intolerable symptoms, such as total nasal obstruction and impaired sleep; "steroid bursts" (e.g., 30 mg X 3 days) or long-acting injections are an option during highly symptomatic periods.
- Immunotherapy
  - Decreases histamine and IgE, induces T cell anergy, produces antibodies that block IgE activity, and causes a shift away from antibody production.
  - Dosing schedules require several injections per week for several weeks, then weekly or biweekly injections for the duration of the season (or continuously for perennial rhinitis); continue for at least 2 years.
  - Provides excellent long-term allergy control for most patients and may prevent future asthma.
  - Generally safe; 3% will get some systemic reaction (50% of which are due to dosing errors); monitor patients for 20 minutes after injection.
  - New nasal immunotherapy can be done at home safely and effectively.
- Anticholinergics
  - Intranasal ipratropium can relieve rhinorrhea but does not treat inflammation.
- Future therapies
  - Humanized monoclonal antibody to IgE.
  - Humanized monoclonal antibody to IL-4 and IL-5.
  - Allergen-specific DNA vaccines.
  - Injection of proteins from tick saliva that can block histamine.
  - CCR3 receptor blockers: prevent eosinophil chemotaxis.

Pathophysiology → # Clinical Link

What is going on in the disease process that influences how the patient presents and how he or she should be managed?

What should you do now that you understand the underlying pathophysiology?

Pathophysiology	Clinical Link
Strong genetic component to the risk for allergic disease. In addition, an increased risk for allergic disease can begin with intrauterine allergen exposure.	A family history is important, and pregnant mothers with a family history of allergies should consider reducing their allergen exposure.
The amount of allergen exposure during childhood is correlated with the risk for allergic disease. The exposure of greatest risk occurs in the bedroom.	Children with a family history of allergies should have their allergen exposure limited as much as possible, especially in the bedroom.
Allergy is type I (IgE-mediated) hypersensitivity and is the result of a powerful humoral immune response.	Childhood infections with intracellular pathogens stimulate cellular immunity and reduce the risk of allergies. Certain vaccinations, which work through stimulating humoral immune responses, may increase the risk for allergic disease.
Antigen presentation to the immune system results in activation of the T helper (CD4) cells that produce large amounts of IL-4 which in turn stimulates the production of IgE by the B lymphocyte.	Future therapies for allergy may include monoclonal antibodies that block the activity of IL-4 and IgE.
IgE binding to the surface of mast cells causes the release of histamine and other cytokines. This, along with activation of PMNs and eosinophils, results in vascular and cellular responses that cause inflammation.	Antihistamines and antiinflammatories are the mainstays of pharmacologic management for allergic rhinitis. Intranasal steroids are the most effective form of treatment, along with second-generation antihistamines, such as loratadine. The leukotriene antagonists offer another antiinflammatory alternative.
Inflammation of the nasal mucosa results in the symptoms of allergic rhinitis including nasal congestion and serous otitis.	Decongestants such as pseudoephedrine can be used in combination with antihistamines and antiinflammatory drugs to relieve nasal congestion and open the eustachian tubes.

Suggested Reading

Anonymous. (2000). Best articles relevant to pediatric allergy and immunology. Selected by members of the section on allergy and immunology of the American Academy of Pediatrics from articles appearing in the medical literature between December 1, 1998 and November 30, 1999. *Pediatrics, 106*(2 Pt 3), 429-476.

Barnes, P. J. (2000). New directions in allergic diseases: Mechanism-based anti-inflammatory therapies. *Journal of Allergy & Clinical Immunology, 106*(1 Pt 1), 5-16.

Berger, A. (2000). Th1 and Th2 responses: What are they? *British Medical Journal, 321*(7258), 424.

Blaiss, M. S. (2000). Cognitive, social, and economic costs of allergic rhinitis. *Allergy & Asthma Proceedings, 21*(1), 7-13.

Christodoulopoulos, P., Cameron, L., Durham, S., & Hamid, Q. (2000). Molecular pathology of allergic disease. II: Upper airway disease. *Journal of Allergy & Clinical Immunology, 105*(2 Pt 1), 211-223.

Corren, J. (2000). Allergic rhinitis: Treating the adult. *Journal of Allergy & Clinical Immunology, 105*(6 Pt 2), S610-S615.

Fireman, P. (2000). Rhinitis and asthma connection: Management of coexisting upper airway allergic diseases and asthma. *Allergy & Asthma Proceedings, 21*(1), 45-54.

Fireman, P. (2000). Therapeutic approaches to allergic rhinitis: Treating the child. *Journal of Allergy & Clinical Immunology, 105*(6 Pt 2), S616-S621.

Haselden, B. M., Kay, A. B., & Larche, M. (2000). Peptide-mediated immune responses in specific immunotherapy. *International Archives of Allergy & Immunology, 122*(4), 229-237.

Holgate, S. T. (2000). Science, medicine, and the future. Allergic disorders. *British Medical Journal, 320*(7229), 231-234.

Howard, T. D., Meyers, D. A., & Bleecker, E. R. (2000). Mapping susceptibility genes for asthma and allergy. *Journal of Allergy & Clinical Immunology, 105*(2 Pt 2), S477-S481.

Howarth, P. H. (2000). Leukotrienes in rhinitis. *American Journal of Respiratory & Critical Care Medicine, 161*(2 Pt 2), S133-S136.

Huss, K., & Huss, R. W. (2000). Genetics of asthma and allergies. *Nursing Clinics of North America, 35*(3), 695-705.

James, J. M., & Burks, A. W., Jr. (2000). Food allergy: Current diagnostic methods and interpretation of results. *Clinical Allergy & Immunology, 15*, 199-215.

Kato, M., Kato, Y., Takeuchi, K., & Nakashima, I. (2000). Local levels of soluble tumor necrosis factor receptors in patients with allergic rhinitis are regulated by amount of antigen. *Archives of Otolaryngology—Head & Neck Surgery, 126*(8), 997-1000.

Kay, G. G. (2000). The effects of antihistamines on cognition and performance. *Journal of Allergy & Clinical Immunology, 105*(6 Pt 2), S622-S627.

Kramer, M. F., Ostertag, P., Pfrogner, E., & Rasp, G. (2000). Nasal interleukin-5, immunoglobulin E, eosinophilic cationic protein, and soluble intercellular adhesion molecule-1 in chronic sinusitis, allergic rhinitis, and nasal polyposis. *Laryngoscope, 110*(6), 1056-1062.

Larsen, J. N., & Lowenstein, H. (2000). Allergen vaccines for specific diagnosis. *Clinical Allergy & Immunology, 15*, 1-51.

Le Souef, P. N., Goldblatt, J., & Lynch, N. R. (2000). Evolutionary adaptation of inflammatory immune responses in human beings. *Lancet, 356*(9225), 242-244.

Meltzer, E. O. (2000). Role for cysteinyl leukotriene receptor antagonist therapy in asthma and their potential role in allergic rhinitis based on the concept of "one linked airway disease." *Annals of Allergy, Asthma, & Immunology, 84*(2), 176-185.

Metson, R. B., & Gliklich, R. E. (2000). Clinical outcomes in patients with chronic sinusitis. *Laryngoscope, 110*(3 Pt 3), 24-28.

Mygind, N., Dahl, R., & Bachert, C. (2000). Nasal polyposis, eosinophil dominated inflammation, and allergy. *Thorax, 55*(Suppl 2), S79-S83.

Mygind, N., Dahl, R., & Bisgaard, H. (2000). Leukotrienes, leukotriene receptor antagonists, and rhinitis. *Allergy, 55*(5), 421-424.

Mygind, N., Laursen, L. C., & Dahl, M. (2000). Systemic corticosteroid treatment for seasonal allergic rhinitis: A common but poorly documented therapy. *Allergy, 55*(1), 11-15.

Nakai, Y., Ohashi, Y., Kakinoki, Y., Tanaka, A., Washio, Y., Nasako, Y., Masamoto, T., Sakamoto, H., & Ohmoto, Y. (2000). Allergen-induced mRNA expression of IL-5, but not of IL-4 and IFN-gamma, in peripheral blood mononuclear cells is a key feature of clinical manifestation of seasonal allergic rhinitis. *Archives of Otolaryngology—Head & Neck Surgery, 126*(8), 992-996.

O'Hollaren, M. T. (2000). Update in allergy and immunology. *Annals of Internal Medicine, 132*(3), 219-226.

Parronchi, P., Brugnolo, F., Sampognaro, S., & Maggi, E. (2000). Genetic and environmental factors contributing to the onset of allergic disorders. *International Archives of Allergy & Immunology, 121*(1), 2-9.

Philpot, E. E. (2000). Safety of second generation antihistamines. *Allergy & Asthma Proceedings, 21*(1), 15-20.

Pien, L. C. (2000). Appropriate use of second-generation antihistamines. *Cleveland Clinic Journal of Medicine, 67*(5), 372-380.

Platts-Mills, T. A., Rakes, G., & Heymann, P. W. (2000). The relevance of allergen exposure to the development of asthma in childhood. *Journal of Allergy & Clinical Immunology, 105* (2 Pt 2), S503-S508.

Poley, G. E., Jr., & Slater, J. E. (2000). Latex allergy. *Journal of Allergy & Clinical Immunology, 105*(6 Pt 1), 1054-1062.

Rihoux, J. P. (2000). Perennial allergic rhinitis and keratoconjunctivitis. *Thorax, 55*(Suppl 2), S22-S23.

Robinson, D. S. (2000). Allergen immunotherapy: Does it work and, if so, how and for how long? *Thorax, 55*(Suppl 1), S11-S14.

Romagnani, S. (2000). The role of lymphocytes in allergic disease. *Journal of Allergy & Clinical Immunology, 105*(3), 399-408.

Schoenwetter, W. F. (2000). Allergic rhinitis: Epidemiology and natural history. *Allergy & Asthma Proceedings, 21*(1), 1-6.

Shiohara, T. (2000). Viral infections, allergy and autoimmunity: A complex, but fascinating link. *Journal of Dermatological Science, 22*(3), 149-151.

Skoner, D. P. (2000). Complications of allergic rhinitis. *Journal of Allergy & Clinical Immunology, 105*(6 Pt 2), S605-S609.

Strachan, D. P. (2000). Family size, infection and atopy: The first decade of the "hygiene hypothesis." *Thorax, 55*(Suppl 1), S2-10.

Szalai, C., Bojszko, A., Beko, G., & Falus, A. (2000). Prevalence of CCR5delta32 in allergic diseases. *Lancet, 355*(9197), 66.

Takafuji, S., & Nakagawa, T. (2000). Air pollution and allergy. *Journal of Investigational Allergology & Clinical Immunology, 10*(1), 5-10.

Togias, A. (2000). Unique mechanistic features of allergic rhinitis. *Journal of Allergy & Clinical Immunology, 105*(6 Pt 2), S599-S604.

Upton, M. N., McConnachie, A., McSharry, C., Hart, C. L., Smith, G. D., Gillis, C. R., & Watt, G. C. (2000). Intergenerational 20 year trends in the prevalence of asthma and hay fever in adults: The Midspan family study surveys of parents and offspring. *British Medical Journal, 321*(7253), 88-92.

von Mutius, E. (2000). The environmental predictors of allergic disease. *Journal of Allergy & Clinical Immunology, 105*(1 Pt 1), 9-19.

Warner, J. A., Jones, C. A., Jones, A. C., & Warner, J. O. (2000). Prenatal origins of allergic disease. *Journal of Allergy & Clinical Immunology, 105*(2 Pt 2), S493-S498.

Yunginger, J. W., Ahlstedt, S., Eggleston, P. A., Homburger, H. A., Nelson, H. S., Ownby, D. R., Platts-Mills, T. A., Sampson, H. A., Sicherer, S. H., Weinstein, A. M., Williams, P. B., Wood, R. A., & Zeiger, R. S. (2000). Quantitative IgE antibody assays in allergic diseases. *Journal of Allergy & Clinical Immunology, 105*(6 Pt 1), 1077-1084.

Case Study

Allergic Rhinitis

INITIAL HISTORY

- A 27-year-old female graduate nursing student presents in December with a 5-week history of itchy eyes and nasal congestion with watery nasal discharge.
- She also complains of a "tickling" cough, especially at night.
- Over the past few days, she has developed facial pain and headache, and her nasal discharge has become purulent.

Question 1   What is your differential diagnosis based on the information you now have?

Question 2   What other questions would like to ask this patient about her symptoms?

ADDITIONAL HISTORY

- The patient complains of repetitive sneezing and has recently developed earache, especially on the right.
- She seems to get these "colds" that last for weeks every winter; her symptoms seem to improve in the spring.
- She has a cat but is not aware of any allergies.
- Her cough is somewhat productive but she can tell that the phlegm comes down from the back of her throat.
- Her nasal congestion is worse on the right than the left but definitely involves both nares.
- She denies any trauma to her face.
- She has no significant medical history and is on no medications.

Question 3 What questions would you like to ask her about her family and her childhood?

FAMILY AND CHILDHOOD HISTORY

- Her mother had asthma as a child and her sister has multiple allergies.
- She was always sick during the winter months as a child.
- Her mother had cats in the house during her pregnancy and throughout the patient's childhood, they routinely slept at the foot of her bed.
- She grew up in Chicago.
- She has never had any serious childhood infections and received the usual vaccinations.

Question 4 How would you interpret her history at this point?

PHYSICAL EXAMINATION

- Well appearing 27-year-old white female in no acute distress, sniffling frequently.
- Afebrile, T = 37° F orally, RR = 18 and unlabored (breathing through her mouth at rest); BP 125/70 sitting.

Skin

- Without rashes.

HEENT

- PERRL; fundi benign.
- Sclera red and slightly swollen with frequent tearing.
- Face tender over right maxillary sinus; sinus transilluminates poorly.
- Outer nares with red irritated skin.
- Internal nares with red, boggy, moist mucosa; purulent discharge visible on the right; no evidence of polyps.
- Pharynx erythematous without exudate; purulent postnasal drainage visible.
- Right tympanic membrane with mild serous otitis; left normal; hearing slightly decreased on the right.

Neck

- No palpable cervical, supraclavicular, infraclavicular, or axillary adenopathy.
- Thyroid nonpalpable.

Chest
- Lungs clear to auscultation and percussion.
- No wheezing even on forced expiration.

Cardiac, Abdomen, Extremities, Neurological
- Exam unremarkable.

Question 5   What do you think of her exam findings?

Question 6   What diagnostic tests would you obtain?

LABORATORY RESULTS
- White blood count (WBC) and differential normal.
- Nasal smear positive for PMNs, eosinophils, and numerous bacteria.
- RAST
    - House dust mite = 4+
    - Cat = 2+
- Sinus x-ray reveals thickened mucosa with an air/fluid level in the right maxillary antrum.

Question 7   How would you interpret these laboratory results?

Question 8   How would you manage this patient now?

27

Human Immunodeficiency Virus Disease*

DEFINITION

- A clinical condition caused by infection with the hman imunodeficiency vrus (HIV). In most cases, HIV infection leads to the acquired immune deficiency syndrome (AIDS).

- AIDS is defined by the Center for Disease Control and Prevention as HIV infection with an associated indicator disease including (1) certain opportunistic infections; (2) certain cancers, such as Kaposi's sarcoma, lymphomas, and invasive cervical or anal carcinomas; (3) wasting syndrome; (4) associated neurologic diseases; and (5) recurrent pneumonias; or HIV infection and a CD4 <200 (or CD4% <14).

EPIDEMIOLOGY

- The two major types of lentiviruses that infect humans are HIV-1 and HIV-2. It is believed that zoonotic transfer of these simian immunodeficiency viruses may have occurred at several times, giving rise to genetically distinct HIV strains.

- Both HIV-1 and HIV-2 are spread principally by sexual transmission, perinatal transmission, or through infected blood or body fluids (intravenous drug abuse [IVDA], transfusion, etc.).

- The global epidemic (or pandemic) of HIV-1 infection continues to and is growing most rapidly in the nations of Central and South America, South-East Asia, and in the subcontinent of India, although the largest number of HIV-infected persons is still in sub-Saharan Africa. In most of the world, heterosexual and perinatal transmission are the most common forms.

- Recent data suggest that about 34 million adults and approximately 2 million children are infected by HIV-1, and estimates from the World Health Organization predict that between 40 and 100 million persons will be infected by the end of 2001.

- The overall incidence of AIDS peaked in 1993 and has since declined 37%. However, the proportion of those infected in minorities continues to grow such that now over half of people in the U.S. with AIDS are non-Hispanic blacks and Hispanics.

- In the United States, the proportion of all AIDS cases has decreased in men who have sex with men and IV drug abusers.

- There is no HIV-2 pandemic, it is still mostly restricted to West Africa (e.g., Cameroon, Ivory Coast, Senegal). Compared to HIV-1, persons can be infected with HIV-2 for much longer periods without developing disease. There is evidence that HIV-2 infected persons may be at a decreased risk for acquiring HIV-1 infection.

PATHOPHYSIOLOGY

Characteristics of the HIV Virus

- HIV is a retrovirus with single stranded RNA contained within a capsid and an envelope, as well as 3 important enzymes (reverse transcriptase, integrase, and protease).

---

*Richard P. Keeling and Valentina L. Brashers contributed this chapter.

- There are two major groups of HIV-1 viruses, those that infect T helper (CD4) lymphocytes (T-cell trophic) and those that infect macrophages (monocyte trophic).

- The viral capsid within the envelope is composed of several proteins including p24 and p18 which, along with viral RNA, can be used clinically to detect the presence of virus in the body.

- The viral envelope has on its surface a **g**lyco**p**rotein (**gp**120) in combination with gp41; this molecule binds to the CD4 receptor on T helper lymphocytes and on macrophages.

- Fusion of the virus to the host cell requires three steps.
  - Binding of gp120/gp41 to the CD4 molecule on macrophages and CD4 cells.
  - Interaction of the virus with chemokine receptors on the host cells.
    1) CXCR-4 (fusin) on CD4 cells (T cell trophic) and CCR5 on macrophages (monocyte trophic).
    2) 10% of Caucasians are heterozygous for a defective CCR5 and have a slower rate of infection and disease progression; 1% are homozygous and resistant to infection.
  - Conformational changes of the bound molecules (prehairpin to hairpin).

- The virus produces **reverse transcriptase**, such that when it enters the cell it can make DNA from its RNA which then integrates (using **integrase**) into the host DNA. There it reproduces more viral RNA and makes a large polypeptide which is then cleaved into its active parts (by **protease**). The virus is then reassembled and shed from the cell into the blood.

- The virus also produces regulatory proteins which feed back on the integrated viral DNA; 4 promote virus production and 1 (nef) downregulates replication. Other genes code for drug resistance.

- There is enormous genetic diversity of HIV-1 due to (1) the incredible rate of HIV replication and (2) HIV has a high mutation rate (1 out of every 3 replication cycles results in the production of a mutant form of the virus). This allows the virus to adapt rapidly to any selective pressures that it may encounter, including antiretroviral drugs and host immune responses.

- Drug resistant mutations have been identified for all currently available antiretroviral drugs. In any one individual, approximately 3300 viruses are produced each day with one of these mutations.

- This viral diversity limits the likelihood of finding an effective vaccine, which means that multiple drug combinations are vital to preventing the sequential acquisition of broad spectrum resistance.

Natural History and Immunology of HIV Infection

- Primary infection occurs most commonly through mucous membranes and significant viremia occurs within days with extensive seeding of the lymphoid system.

- Symptomatic primary infection (acute retroviral syndrome) occurs in 80% to 90% of HIV infected patients. The time from infection to the onset of symptoms is usually 2 to 4 weeks. Symptoms include fever, adenopathy, pharyngitis, rash, myalgias, and headache.

- Once infection has occurred, viral replication begins at an astonishing pace with billions of viruses produced daily.

- The half-life of HIV in plasma is 1 to 2 days; 30% of HIV in plasma is replaced daily by viral replication such that the entire HIV population turns over in 14 days.

- HIV replication is maintained from newly infected CD4 cells, such that 99% of the virus in the bloodstream at any moment is from newly infected cells. Billions of CD4 cells are produced, infected, and destroyed daily (lifespan = 1.2 days).

- The virus establishes long-term, latent, nonproductive infection in some inactive CD4 cells (memory cells). The virus also establishes latent infection in dendritic cells of the lymph nodes and the glial cells of the CNS. This infection of "sanctuary sites" has been found to occur very early during the course of the primary infection and makes eradication of the virus very difficult.

- Cellular immunity is the primary mode of viral (and CD4 cell) killing:
  - T cytotoxic lymphocytes (CD8 cells) recognize infected T helper cells (CD4 cells) and macrophages and directly destroy these cells and the viruses they contain.
  - Cellular immunity is facilitated by the secretion of cytokines from uninfected CD4 cells called the TH_1 cytokines. During the course of HIV infection, the virus induces many of the CD4 cells to shift from the TH_1 mode of cytokine production (favors cellular immunity) to the TH_2 cytokine profile (favors humoral immunity). Humoral immunity is less effective for HIV killing.
- Other ways that the virus decreases CD4 cell numbers and function include:
  - Certain HIV strains (syncytia-inducing) cause infected CD4 cells to coalesce with noninfected CD4 cells rendering them nonfunctional.
  - HIV reduces the amount of glutathione (O_2 radical scavenger) in CD4 cells inducing apoptosis.
  - HIV causes the production of "free" glycoprotein (gp120) and releases it into the bloodstream, which attaches to uninfected CD4 receptors and causes immune destruction of healthy CD4 cells.
- After several weeks, a steady state and clinical latency is achieved in which the immune system is able to decrease the amount of virus in the blood by killing infected CD4 cells, and the bone marrow is able to maintain production of adequate numbers of newly produced and functional CD4 cells.
- Viral replication continues at a very high rate in the blood, and at a slower rate in lymph nodes and other sanctuary sites. The level of decrease of virus in the blood (viral load or viral titer) that the immune system is able to achieve determines the rate of clinical deterioration.
- Over time, the ability of the marrow to produce CD4 cells falls below that necessary to replenish the killed CD4 cells and immunosuppression results. The clinically latent phase gives way to a 2 to 4 year phase of chronic symptoms and rising viral titers but not yet life-threatening illness.
- Late in the clinical latent period, the structure of lymph nodes begins to break down releasing more active virus into the circulation. Viral titers rise dramatically and CD4 levels fall below the level necessary to prevent life-threatening opportunistic infections (<200, AIDS).

AIDS

- Loss of normal CD4 cell activity disrupts virtually every aspect of immune function, especially cellular immunity.
- Common opportunistic infectious agents include fungi (candida, cryptococcus, histoplasmosis), parasites (*Pneumocystis carinii* [PCP], Toxoplasmosis gondii, cryptosporidiosis), mycobacteria (tuberculosis [TB], avium complex [MAC]), viruses (herpes simplex, HHV-8, varicella-zoster, cytomegalovirus [CMV], Epstein-Barr virus), and bacteria (listeria, nocardia, legionella, salmonella).
- Common AIDS-associated malignancies include Kaposi sarcoma, lymphoma, and anal and cervical cancer.
- **HIV-associated wasting syndrome**
  - Defined as the involuntary loss of 10% of body weight with chronic fever, weakness, or diarrhea in the absence of other related illnesses contributing to the weight loss. The newer expanded definition includes malnutrition as well as metabolic causes.
  - It is correlated with poor prognosis and may occur early in disease progression.
  - Causes include anorexia (depression, financial difficulties, oropharyngeal disease, side effects of medications), malabsorption (GI diseases), and metabolic abnormalities (low testosterone or growth hormone, cytokine abnormalities [especially tumor necrosis factor, TNF]).

PATIENT PRESENTATION

History

History of exposures (number of incidents of unprotected sex, sexual networks, IVDA, transfusions); other sexually transmitted diseases (STDs); pregnancy; menstrual history; addiction history; recurrent infections; coinfections, such as hepatitis B or C; opportunistic infections; neoplasms; depression; changes in sleep patterns; family, living, and work environment; vaccination history.

Symptoms

Fever; night sweats; weakness; adenopathy; pharyngitis; rash; myalgias; headache; weight loss; seborrhea; skin rashes and pain; mouth pain; anal pain; dysphagia; dyspnea; cough; chest pain; abdominal pain; vaginal bleeding, blurred vision; diarrhea; memory loss; confusion.

Examination

Fever, muscle wasting; rashes; skin lesions; oral lesions; perianal lesions; adenopathy; masses; pulmonary consolidation (crackles); pleural rub; cardiac dysfunction (cardiomegaly, S3, pericardial rub); abdominal tenderness; focal neurologic deficits; cognitive deficits.

DIFFERENTIAL DIAGNOSIS

- Other viral infections: mononucleosis, influenza, hepatitis
- Other immunocompromised states; congenital, drug-induced
- Opportunistic infections (listed above)
- Malignancies
- Depression

KEYS TO ASSESSMENT

Screening

- The CDC recommends that all patients in hospitals which have a high rate of newly diagnosed with AIDs patients (1/1000 discharges) should be tested, as well as all pregnant women.
- Other indications for testing include persons with STDs, high risk categories (IVDA, men who have sex with men with a history of high risk behavior), heterosexual with >1 partner in the past 12 months, persons with active TB, occupationally exposed persons, and blood or tissue donors.
- The average time from exposure to seroconversion is 70 days; >95% of infected individuals will seroconvert by 6 months.

Diagnosis of HIV infection

- The ELISA test followed by the Western blot confirms the diagnosis of HIV infection.
- Viral titers (polymerase chain reaction [HIV RNA PCR] or branched chain DNA [bDNA]), also called viral load, can be measured within hours to days of infection.
- AIDS is diagnosed when there is a positive antibody and viral titer plus CD4 <200 or opportunistic infection.

Laboratory testing once HIV infection is confirmed

- Viral load assay (HIV RNA PCR or bDNA)
- CD4 cell count
- Complete blood count (CBC) with differential and platelet count
- Chemistry panel including fasting lipid profile

- Urinalysis
- Chest x-ray
- PAP smear in women
- Serologies: syphilis, toxoplasmosis gondii, hepatitis A, B, and C, CMV, varicella-zoster
- PPD

Clinical Staging of HIV infection

- Category A: asymptomatic or acute retroviral syndrome.
- Category B: symptomatic disease but with conditions not listed in category C, such as thrush, vulvovaginal candidiasis, seborrheic dermatitis, eosinophilic folliculitis, cervical dysplasia, fever, diarrhea, oral hairy leukoplakia, herpes zoster, pelvic inflammatory disease, listeriosis, or peripheral neuropathy.
- Category C: AIDS indicator condition (candida of esophagus or lung; invasive cervical cancer; extrapulmonary histoplasmosis, coccidioidomycosis or cryptococcosis; cryptosporidiosis; CMV; extracutaneous, herpes simplex; HIV-associated dementia; HIV-associated wasting; Kaposi sarcoma; CNS lymphoma; non-Hodgkin's lymphoma; MAC, tuberculosis; nocardiosis; *Pneumocystis carinii* pneumonia; progressive multifocal leukoencephalopathy; salmonella septicemia; strongyloidiasis; toxoplasmosis).
- These categories can be further subdivided 1 through 3 depending on the associated CD4 count.

MANAGEMENT

- Treatment decisions should be made after careful consideration of the patient's wishes and preferences, and is generally based on HIV RNA levels and CD4+ cell counts.
- When to begin antivirals in adults and adolescents is still controversial. It is now recognized that eradication of HIV infection cannot be achieved with current antiretroviral therapy, that active antiretroviral therapy is associated with substantial toxicity, and that the difficulty of long-term adherence to current treatment regimes leads to the development of drug resistance.
- The goals of treatment are to reduce the amount of HIV in the plasma to undetectable (<50 copies/ml) and to achieve the recovery of immunity (increased CD4 count).
- Treatment requires careful monitoring for drug levels, CD4 and HIV levels, drug toxicities, and other complications of the infection.
- Antiretroviral treatment requires the simultaneous initiation of combinations of at least three drugs to prevent resistance (highly active antiretroviral therapy, HAART). Current antiretroviral drugs include:
  - Those that inhibit reverse transcriptase activity:
    1) Nucleoside reverse transcriptase inhibitors (NRTIs) such as AZT (zidovudine), 3TC (lamivudine), didanosine (ddI), zalcitabine (ddC), stavudine (d4T), abacavir (ABC), and emtricitabine (FTC).
    2) Non-nucleoside reverse transcriptase inhibitors (NNRTIs) such as nevirapine, delavirdine, efavirenz, and capravirine.
  - Those that inhibit protease activity (protease inhibitors, [PI]) such as indinavir, ritonavir, saquinavir, nelfinavir, amprenavir, and tripranavir.
- Currently, the most common initial regimens include two NRTIs plus a PI or an NNRTI. Combination antiretrovirals are now available that include more than one drug from more than one class.
- Drug toxicities are numerous including diarrhea, pancytopenia, dyslipidemias, lipodystrophy, lactic acidemia, hypertriglyceridemia, nephrolithiasis, and insulin resistance.

- Adherence is a crucial issue because even short viral bursts can result in increased seeding of lymphoid reservoirs and increased likelihood of drug resistance. However, even excellent adherence to these complicated drug regimes cannot prevent the eventual development of drug resistance.

- Management of patients who develop resistance includes sequencing of antivirals, newer agents, and multiple combinations of drugs.

- Many experimental drugs that attack other steps in viral replication (eg. attachment inhibitors, chemokine antagonists, integrase inhibitors, fusion inhibitors) or that bolster immune function (eg interleukin 2 (IL-2), interferons) are being evaluated.

- Prophylaxis to prevent opportunistic infections (TB, MAC, PCP, and CMV) is begun when the CD4 count falls to specified levels.

- Studies are looking at treatment simplification or withdrawal therapy after successful response.

- Vaccinations should include hepatitis A and B, Haemophilus influenza, Pneumovax, influenza, and tetanus-diphtheria.

- Postexposure prophylaxis consists of 2 or 3 drugs and should be given soon after exposure.

- Women should receive optimal therapy regardless of pregnancy status.

  - Perinatal transmission prevention is optimized by the use of combination therapy using 2-3 drugs (with possible delay of protease inhibitor until after first trimester) and can reduce transmission rates from 25% to 2%. In countries where HAART is not available, concentrated treatment with AZT during the intrapartum period reduces transmission significantly.

  - Cesarean section reduces risk further and infected mothers should not breastfeed.

- Persons with HIV infection, even when their viral loads are undetectable, should be considered infectious.

Pathophysiology

$\rightarrow$

Clinical Link

What is going on in the disease process that influences how the patient presents and how he or she should be managed?

What should you do now that you understand the underlying pathophysiology?

HIV is not one virus—it is many viruses including HIV-1, HIV-2, and several subgroups and clades with differing geographic distributions and virulence factors.	Worldwide transmission patterns of HIV differ and are constantly changing. New types of HIV infection are being described and it is unlikely that a true "global" vaccine will be developed.
HIV infection involves binding of the viral envelope to the target cells (macrophages and CD4 lymphocytes) via a complex series of steps that require the interaction of numerous viral and host cell receptors and chemokines.	Genetic alterations in viral and host cell surface characteristics may explain some of the differences observed in infectivity. Furthermore, purposeful alterations in these factors may provide future therapies to prevent HIV infection.
Three important enzymes are coded by the viral RNA and include reverse transcriptase, integrase, and protease. Activity of each of these enzymes is necessary for viral reproduction inside the host cell.	Current therapies for HIV include 2 classes of drugs that inhibit reverse transcriptase, and drugs that inhibit protease. Integrase inhibitors are in development.
HIV replication occurs at an incredible rate, and is associated with numerous mutations. These mutations can lead to increased virulence and to drug resistance.	In any individual, the virus that is present in his/her body is constantly changing. Careful drug adherence is necessary to prevent resistance. Unprotected sex is ill-advised even between two HIV positive adults. Furthermore, an individual's initial infection may be with a virus that is already drug resistant.
HIV killing by the immune system relies on CD8 cell-mediated cellular immunity which destroys infected CD4 cells. HIV tends to shift the immune system from the TH_1 cytokine pattern that promotes cellular immunity to the TH_2 pattern of humoral immunity. Humoral immunity is less effective for HIV killing.	Experimental therapies for HIV include immune modulating drugs (e.g., IL-2 and interferons) that shift the TH_2 cytokine pattern back to the TH_1 pattern, thus improving cellular immunity and viral killing.
Immunodeficiency occurs when infected CD4 cell killing exceeds bone marrow replenishment with healthy cells, and when lymph nodes break down and release virus. When CD4 levels fall below 200/ml and viral load rises, opportunistic infections develop that have a very high morbidity and mortality.	The monitoring of the CD4 count and viral load is crucial to initiating antiviral therapy, monitoring responses to therapy, and predicting the occurrence of the many infections of AIDS. Aggressive antiretroviral therapy and prophylaxis for opportunistic infections has improved quality of life and outcomes for many patients, but drug toxicities are often severe.

Suggested Reading

Agnoli, M. M. (2000). Immune reconstitution in the HAART era, part 1: Immune abnormalities in HIV/AIDS. *Journal of the Association of Nurses in AIDS Care, 11*(1), 78-81.

Altfeld, M., & Rosenberg, E. S. (2000). The role of CD4(+) T helper cells in the cytotoxic T lymphocyte response to HIV-1. *Current Opinion in Immunology, 12*(4), 375-380.

Anonymous. (2001). The cost-effectiveness of testing HIV for genetic signs of drug resistance as a guide to the choice of therapy. *Annals of Internal Medicine, 134*(6), S89.

Baggaley, R., & van Praag, E. (2000). Antiretroviral interventions to reduce mother-to-child transmission of human immunodeficiency virus: Challenges for health systems, communities, and society. *Bulletin of the World Health Organization, 78*(8), 1036-1044.

Bozzette, S. A., Joyce, G., McCaffrey, D. F., Leibowitz, A. A., Morton, S. C., Berry, S. H., Rastegar, A., Timberlake, D., Shapiro, M. F., & Goldman, D. P. (2001). Expenditures for the care of HIV-infected patients in the era of highly active antiretroviral therapy. *New England Journal of Medicine, 344*(11), 817-823.

Bulterys, M., & Fowler, M. G. (2000). Prevention of HIV infection in children. *Pediatric Clinics of North America, 47*(1), 241-260.

Cannon, M. J., Dollard, S. C., Smith, D. K., Klein, R. S., Schuman, P., Rich, J. D., Vlahov, D., & Pellett, P. E. (2001). Blood-borne and sexual transmission of human herpesvirus 8 in women with or at risk for human immunodeficiency virus infection. *New England Journal of Medicine, 344*(9), 637-643.

Carpenter, C. C., Cooper, D. A., Fischl, M. A., Gatell, J. M., Gazzard, B. G., Hammer, S. M., Hirsch, M. S., Jacobsen, D. M., Katzenstein, D. A., Montaner, J. S., Richman, D. D., Saag, M. S., Schechter, M., Schooley, R. T., Thompson, M. A., Vella, S., Yeni, P. G., & Volberding, P. A. (2000). Antiretroviral therapy in adults: Updated recommendations of the International AIDS Society-USA Panel. *Journal of the American Medical Association, 283*(3), 381-390.

Cefalo, R. C. (2001). Trial of shortened zidovudine regimens to prevent mother-to-child transmission of human immunodeficiency virus type 1. *Obstetrical & Gynecological Survey, 56*(3), 138-139.

Chen, Y. H., Xiao, Y., & Dierich, M. P. (2000). HIV-1 gp41: Role in HIV entry and prevention. *Immunobiology, 201*(3-4), 308-316.

Crowe, S. M., & Sonza, S. (2000). HIV-1 can be recovered from a variety of cells including peripheral blood monocytes of patients receiving highly active antiretroviral therapy: A further obstacle to eradication. *Journal of Leukocyte Biology, 68*(3), 345-350.

Cunningham, A. L., Li, S., Juarez, J., Lynch, G., Alali, M., & Naif, H. (2000). The level of HIV infection of macrophages is determined by interaction of viral and host cell genotypes. *Journal of Leukocyte Biology, 68*(3), 311-317.

De Clercq, E. (2000). Inhibition of HIV infection by bicyclams, highly potent and specific CXCR4 antagonists. *Molecular Pharmacology, 57*(5), 833-839.

De Clercq, E. (2000). Novel compounds in preclinical/early clinical development for the treatment of HIV infections. *Reviews in Medical Virology, 10*(4), 255-277.

Deeks, S. G. (2000). Determinants of virological response to antiretroviral therapy: Implications for long-term strategies. *Clinical Infectious Diseases, 30*(Suppl 2), S177-S184.

Deeks, S. G. (2001). Nonnucleoside reverse transcriptase inhibitor resistance. *JAIDS: Journal of Acquired Immune Deficiency Syndromes, 26*(Suppl 1), S33.

Deeks, S. G., Wrin, T., Liegler, T., Hoh, R., Hayden, M., Barbour, J. D., Hellmann, N. S., Petropoulos, C. J., McCune, J. M., Hellerstein, M. K., & Grant, R. M. (2001). Virologic and immunologic consequences of discontinuing combination antiretroviral-drug therapy in HIV-infected patients with detectable viremia. *New England Journal of Medicine, 344*(7), 472-480.

Dejucq, N. (2000). HIV-1 replication in CD4+ T cell lines: The effects of adaptation on co-receptor use, tropism, and accessory gene function. *Journal of Leukocyte Biology, 68*(3), 331-337.

DeSimone, J. A., Pomerantz, R. J., & Babinchak, T. J. (2000). Inflammatory reactions in HIV-1-infected persons after initiation of highly active antiretroviral therapy. *Annals of Internal Medicine, 133*(6), 447-454.

Detels, R., Tarwater, P., Phair, J. P., Margolick, J., Riddler, S. A., Munoz, A., & The Multicenter AIDS Cohort Study. (2001). Effectiveness of potent antiretroviral therapies on the incidence of opportunistic infections before and after AIDS diagnosis. *AIDS, 15*(3), 347-355.

Dezube, B. J. (2000). The role of human immunodeficiency virus-I in the pathogenesis of acquired immunodeficiency syndrome-related Kaposi's sarcoma: The importance of an inflammatory and angiogenic milieu. *Seminars in Oncology, 27*(4), 420-423.

Distler, O., Cooper, D. A., Deckelbaum, R. J., & Sturley, S. L. (2001). Hyperlipidemia and inhibitors of HIV protease. *Current Opinion in Clinical Nutrition & Metabolic Care, 4*(2), 99-103.

D'Souza, M. P., Cairns, J. S., & Plaeger, S. F. (2000). Current evidence and future directions for targeting HIV entry: Therapeutic and prophylactic strategies. *Journal of the American Medical Association, 284*(2), 215-222.

Dwyer, M. L. (2000). Advanced practice nursing for children with HIV infection. *Nursing Clinics of North America, 35*(1), 115-124.

Edgeworth, R. L., & Ugen, K. E. (2000). Immunopathological factors for vertical transmission of HIV-1. *Pathobiology, 68*(2), 53-67.

Eron, J. J., Jr. (2000). HIV-1 protease inhibitors. *Clinical Infectious Diseases, 30*(Suppl 2), S160-S170.

Esparza, J., & Bhamarapravati, N. (2000). Accelerating the development and future availability of HIV-1 vaccines: Why, when, where, and how? *Lancet, 355*(9220), 2061-2066.

Fantuzzi, L., Conti, L., Gauzzi, M. C., Eid, P., Del Corno, M., Varano, B., Canini, I., Belardelli, F., & Gessani, S. (2000). Regulation of chemokine/cytokine network during in vitro differentiation and HIV-1 infection of human monocytes: Possible importance in the pathogenesis of AIDS. *Journal of Leukocyte Biology, 68*(3), 391-399.

Fleming, P. L., & Jaffe, H. W. (2001). AIDS among heterosexuals in surveillance reports. *New England Journal of Medicine, 344*(8), 611-613.

Fowler, M. G., Simonds, R. J., & Roongpisuthipong, A. (2000). Update on perinatal HIV transmission. *Pediatric Clinics of North America, 47*(1), 21-38.

Freedberg, K. A., Losina, E., Weinstein, M. C., Paltiel, A. D., Cohen, C. J., Seage, G. R., Craven, D. E., Zhang, H., Kimmel, A. D., & Goldie, S. J. (2001). The cost effectiveness of combination antiretroviral therapy for HIV disease. *New England Journal of Medicine 344*(11), 824-831.

Fung, H. B., Kirschenbaum, H. L., & Hameed, R. (2000). Amprenavir: A new human immunodeficiency virus type 1 protease inhibitor. *Clinical Therapeutics, 22*(5), 549-572.

Furrer, H., Opravil, M., Rossi, M., Bernasconi, E., Telenti, A., Bucher, H., Schiffer, V., Boggian, K., Rickenbach, M., Flepp, M., Egger, M., & The Swiss HIV Cohort Study. (2001). Discontinuation of primary prophylaxis in HIV-infected patients at high risk of *Pneumocystis carinii* pneumonia: Prospective multicentre study. *AIDS, 15*(4), 501-507.

Goedert, J. J. (2000). The epidemiology of acquired immunodeficiency syndrome malignancies. *Seminars in Oncology, 27*(4), 390-401.

Goetz, M. B. A., Morreale, A. P., Rhew, D. C., Berman, S. C., Ing, M. D., Eldridge, D., Justis, J. C., & Lott, E. (2001). Effect of highly active antiretroviral therapy on outcomes in Veterans Affairs medical centers. *AIDS, 15*(4), 530-532.

Gotch, F., Rutebemberwa, A., Jones, G., Imami, N., Gilmour, J., Kaleebu, P., & Whitworth, J. (2000). Vaccines for the control of HIV/AIDS. *Tropical Medicine & International Health, 5* (7), A16-A21.

Hader, S. L. M., Smith, D. K. M., Moore, J. S. P., & Holmberg, S. D. M. (2001). HIV Infection in women in the United States: Status at the millennium. *Journal of the American Medical Association, 285*(9), 1186-1192.

Harrigan, P. R., & Cote, H. C. (2000). Clinical utility of testing human immunodeficiency virus for drug resistance. *Clinical Infectious Diseases, 30*(Suppl 2), S117-S122.

Jellinger, K. A. (2001). AIDS-related focal brain lesions in the era of highly active antiretroviral therapy. *Neurology, 56*(5), 696.

Jiang, S., & Debnath, A. K. (2000). Development of HIV entry inhibitors targeted to the coiled-coil regions of gp41. *Biochemical & Biophysical Research Communications, 269*(3), 641-646.

Johnson, S. C., & Gerber, J. G. (2000). Advances in HIV/AIDS therapy. *Advances in Internal Medicine, 45,* 1-40.

Kaplan, J. E., Hanson, D., Dworkin, M. S., Frederick, T., Bertolli, J., Lindegren, M. L., Holmberg, S., & Jones, J. L. (2000). Epidemiology of human immunodeficiency virus-associated opportunistic infections in the United States in the era of highly active antiretroviral therapy. *Clinical Infectious Diseases, 30*(Suppl 1), S5-14.

Kass, N. E., Taylor, H. A., & Anderson, J. (2000). Treatment of human immunodeficiency virus during pregnancy: The shift from an exclusive focus on fetal protection to a more balanced approach. *American Journal of Obstetrics & Gynecology, 182*(4), 856-859.

Kennedy, I., & Williams, S. (2000). Occupational exposure to HIV and post-exposure prophylaxis in healthcare workers. *Occupational Medicine (Oxford), 50*(6), 387-391.

Kilby, J. M., Goepfert, P. A., Miller, A. P., Gnann, J. W., Jr., Sillers, M., Saag, M. S., & Bucy, R. P. (2000). Recurrence of the acute HIV syndrome after interruption of antiretroviral therapy in a patient with chronic HIV infection: A case report. *Annals of Internal Medicine, 133*(6), 435-438.

Kourtis, A. P. M., Bulterys, M. M., Nesheim, S. R. M., & Lee, F. K. P. (2001). Understanding the timing of HIV transmission from mother to infant. *Journal of the American Medical Association, 285*(6), 709-712.

Kunches, L. M., Meehan, T. M., Boutwell, R. C., & McGuire, J. F. (2001). Survey of nonoccupational HIV postexposure prophylaxis in hospital emergency departments. *JAIDS: Journal of Acquired Immune Deficiency Syndromes, 26*(3), 263-265.

Lamothe, B., & Joshi, S. (2000). Current developments and future prospects for HIV gene therapy using interfering RNA-based strategies. *Frontiers in Bioscience, 5,* D527-D555.

Lewis, W. (2000). Cardiomyopathy in AIDS: A pathophysiological perspective. *Progress in Cardiovascular Diseases, 43*(2), 151-170.

Little, S. J. (2000). Transmission and prevalence of HIV resistance among treatment-naive subjects. *Antiviral Therapy, 5*(1), 33-40.

Loetscher, P., Moser, B., & Baggiolini, M. (2000). Chemokines and their receptors in lymphocyte traffic and HIV infection. *Advances in Immunology, 74,* 127-180.

Loveday, C. (2001). Nucleoside reverse transcriptase inhibitor resistance. *JAIDS: Journal of Acquired Immune Deficiency Syndromes, 26*(Suppl 1), S24.

Luzuriaga, K., & Sullivan, J. L. (2000). Viral and immunopathogenesis of vertical HIV-1 infection. *Pediatric Clinics of North America, 47*(1), 65-78.

Lyon, D. E., & Truban, E. (2000). HIV-related lipodystrophy: A clinical syndrome with implications for nursing practice. *Journal of the Association of Nurses in AIDS Care, 11*(2), 36-42.

Matsushita, S. (2000). Current status and future issues in the treatment of HIV-1 infection. *International Journal of Hematology, 72*(1), 20-27.

Miller, V. (2001). Resistance to protease inhibitors. *JAIDS: Journal of Acquired Immune Deficiency Syndromes, 26*(Suppl 1), S50.

Mofenson, L. M., & McIntyre, J. A. (2000). Advances and research directions in the prevention of mother-to-child HIV-1 transmission. *Lancet, 355*(9222), 2237-2244.

Moodley, P., Wilkinson, D., Connolly, C., & Sturm, A. W. (2001). Impact of HIV-1 infection on response to treatment of sexually transmitted infections. *AIDS, 15*(4), 542-543.

Mosier, D. E. (2000). Virus and target cell evolution in human immunodeficiency virus type 1 infection. *Immunologic Research, 21*(2-3), 253-258.

Moss, R. B., Jensen, F. C., & Carlo, D. J. (2000). Insights into HIV-specific immune function: Implications for therapy and prevention in the new millennium. *Clinical Immunology, 95* (2), 79-84.

Nathanson, N., & Mathieson, B. J. (2000). Biological considerations in the development of a human immunodeficiency virus vaccine. *Journal of Infectious Diseases, 182*(2), 579-589.

Nielsen, K., & Bryson, Y. J. (2000). Diagnosis of HIV infection in children. *Pediatric Clinics of North America, 47*(1), 39-63.

O'Brien, W. A. (2000). Resistance against reverse transcriptase inhibitors. *Clinical Infectious Diseases, 30*(Suppl 2), S185-S192.

Omrani, A. S., & Pillay, D. (2000). Multi-drug resistant HIV-1. *Journal of Infection, 41*(1), 5-11.

Panel on Clinical Practices for the Treatment of HIV Infection. (2000, February). *Guidelines for the use of antiretroviral agents in HIV-infected adults and adolescents*. Menlo Park, CA: Henry J. Kaiser Family Foundation.

Pani, A., & Marongiu, M. E. (2000). Anti-HIV-1 integrase drugs: How far from the shelf? *Current Pharmaceutical Design, 6*(5), 569-584.

Paterson, D. L. M., & Singh, N. M. (2001). Adherence to protease inhibitors. *Annals of Internal Medicine 134*(7), 625.

Picker, L. J., & Maino, V. C. (2000). The CD4(+) T cell response to HIV-1. *Current Opinion in Immunology, 12*(4), 381-386.

Pierson, T., McArthur, J., & Siliciano, R. F. (2000). Reservoirs for HIV-1: Mechanisms for viral persistence in the presence of antiviral immune responses and antiretroviral therapy. *Annual Review of Immunology, 18*, 665-708.

Piscitelli, S. C., Bhat, N., & Pau, A. (2000). A risk-benefit assessment of interleukin-2 as an adjunct to antiviral therapy in HIV infection. *Drug Safety, 22*(1), 19-31.

Qaqish, R. B., Fisher, E., Rublein, J., & Wohl, D. A. (2000). HIV-associated lipodystrophy syndrome. *Pharmacotherapy, 20*(1), 13-22.

Ruprecht, R. M., Hofmann-Lehmann, R., Rasmussen, R. A., Vlasak, J., & Xu, W. (2000). 1999: A time to re-evaluate AIDS vaccine strategies. *Journal of Human Virology, 3*(2), 88-93.

Sewell, A. K., Price, D. A., Oxenius, A., Kelleher, A. D., & Phillips, R. E. (2000). Cytotoxic T lymphocyte responses to human immunodeficiency virus: Control and escape. *Stem Cells, 18*(4), 230-244.

Sewell, W. A. C., Mazhude, C. S. R., Murdin-Geretti, A. L., Jones, S. S. P., & Easterbrook, P. J. (2001). Interrupting antiretroviral treatment needs particular care. *British Medical Journal, 322*(7286), 616.

Sterling, T. R., Vlahov, D., Astemborski, J., Hoover, D. R., Margolick, J. B., & Quinn, T. C. (2001). Initial plasma HIV-1 RNA levels and progression to AIDS in women and men. *New England Journal of Medicine, 344*(10), 720-725.

Tomasselli, A. G., & Heinrikson, R. L. (2000). Targeting the HIV-protease in AIDS therapy: A current clinical perspective. *Biochimica et Biophysica Acta, 1477*(1-2), 189-214.

Weinstein, M. C. P., Goldie, S. J. M., Losina, E. P., Cohen, C. J. M., Baxter, J. D. M., Zhang, H. B., Kimmel, A. D. A., & Freedberg, K. A. M. (2001). Use of genotypic resistance testing to guide HIV therapy: Clinical impact and cost-effectiveness. *Annals of Internal Medicine 134*(6), 440-450.

Wise, J. (2001). Breast feeding safer than mixed feeding for babies of HIV mothers. *British Medical Journal, 322*(7285), 511.

Case Study

Human Immunodeficiency Virus Disease

INITIAL HISTORY

- A 32-year-old white female is admitted to the hospital with a 5-day history of fever, dyspnea, productive cough, and right sided pleuritic chest pain.
- She states she has had pneumonia several times in the past 3 years.
- She is currently on oral contraceptives but is taking no other medications and has no allergies.

Question 1   What else would you like to ask this patient about her history of present illness and past medical history?

ADDITIONAL HISTORY

- The patient denies any chills, vomiting, headache or rashes.
- She was told that her previous pneumonias were "just the usual kind" and were effectively treated with antibiotics.
- She has not smoked since she left college 10 years ago.
- She denies any history of lung disease, heart disease, or other hospitalizations.
- She has had a long history of vaginal yeast infections and was recently told that her PAP smear was abnormal but "not cancer."
- She states her overall health has not been good lately, with fatigue and a 7 pound unintentional weight loss over the past 6 months.

Question 2   What about her history concerns you, and what else would you like to ask her now?

MORE HISTORY

- She has had occasional night sweats and has had mild anorexia for the past few months.
- She denies any recent travel and does not know anyone with tuberculosis or other unusual infections; her PPD was last checked while she was college and was negative.
- She has had 4 sexual partners in the past year and has had occasional unprotected sex with each.
- She has no children and works as an accountant in a large local firm. She denies any history of toxin exposure.

PHYSICAL EXAMINATION

- Thin, ill appearing female with occasional productive cough.
- T = 39° F degrees orally, RR = 25, BP 110/70 sitting.

Skin

- Seborrhea around the nose, cheeks, and scalp.

HEENT

- PERRL; fundi without lesions.
- Nares and tympanic membranes without lesions.
- Pharynx reveals a thick cheesy exudate on the soft palate and tongue.

Neck

- Palpable cervical adenopathy.
- Thyroid nonpalpable.

Chest

- Lungs with dullness to percussion, increased tactile fremitus, inspiratory crackles and egophony over the right lower lobe.
- Cardiac rhythm regular without murmurs or gallops.

Abdomen, Extremities, Neurological

- No abdominal masses or tenderness.
- No pedal edema; pulses full; palpable inguinal adenopathy.
- Alert and oriented; neurologic exam nonfocal.

Pelvic

- Erythema and mild excoriation of the perineum.
- Thick white vaginal discharge.
- No adnexal masses.
- PAP smear obtained.

Question 3   What do you think of her additional history and her exam findings?

Question 4 What diagnostic tests would you obtain?

LABORATORY RESULTS
- HIV ELISA positive.
- White blood count (WBC) 9,000 /mm^3 with 90% PMNs ; HCT 37%; PLTs = 190,000/mm^3.
- Serum chemistries normal.
- Chest x-ray reveals right lower lobe infiltrate consistent with lobar pneumonia.
- Sputum gram stain positive for numerous PMNs and gram-positive diplococci.
- Sputum culture positive for *Streptococcus pneumoniae*.
- Blood cultures negative.
- O$_2$ saturation 96%.
- PPD negative.
- Hepatitis serology negative.
- Oral and vaginal smear KOH positive for yeast.
- PAP smear reveals inflammation and mild dysplasia without carcinoma.

Question 5 How would you interpret these laboratory results and what would you do next?

HOSPITAL COURSE
- The patient responds to antibiotics, and hydration.
- Western blot is positive.

Question 6 What additional labs would you order now?

ADDITONAL LABORATORY RESULTS

- HIV RNA PCR = 25,000 copies/ml
- CD4 count = 400/mm^3
- Lipid profile normal
- Serologies all negative

Question 7 How should this patient be managed?